NUTRITION IN MEDICAL PRACTICE

ROBERT E. HODGES, M.D.

Professor of Internal Medicine
Chief, Section of Nutrition
School of Medicine
University of California
Davis, California

With contributions by

RAYMOND D. ADELMAN, M.D.

Associate Professor of Pediatrics
Director, Pediatric Nephrology
Department of Pediatrics
School of Medicine
University of California
Davis, California

W. B. SAUNDERS COMPANY • PHILADELPHIA • LONDON • TORONTO

W. B. Saunders Company: West Washington Square
Philadelphia, PA   19105

1 St. Anne's Road
Eastbourne, East Sussex BN21 3UN, England

1 Goldthorne Avenue
Toronto, Ontario M8Z 5T9, Canada

Library of Congress Cataloging in Publication Data

Hodges, Robert Edgar, 1922–

Nutrition in medical practice.

1. Nutrition.   2. Nutritionally induced diseases.   I. Title.
[DNLM: 1. Nutrition.   2. Nutrition disorders–
Complications.   3. Diet–Adverse effects. QU 145.3
H689n]

QP141.H52   613.2   77–11337
ISBN 0–7216–4706–5

Nutrition in Medical Practice   ISBN   0-7216-4706-5

Last digit is the print number: 9   8   7   6   5   4   3   2

This book is dedicated to my wife, NORMA, whose unfailing encouragement and understanding have made the task of writing a pleasure.

I am also grateful to my son, KARL, whose meticulous care in verifying references and in proofreading manuscripts has lightened the load immeasurably.

PREFACE

Despite the current wave of interest in nutrition among both lay and medical persons, one fact is obvious: most doctors have an inadequate fund of knowledge about nutrition. It is true that many physicians whose practices require that they have special knowledge of nutrition have taken steps to acquire the necessary information. This is especially evident among pediatricians, diabetologists, cardiologists, and recently, surgeons who are interested in parenteral nutrition. But the vast majority of the medical profession in the United States know very little about the science of nutrition as it may apply to their practice of medicine.

This state of affairs arises not from any fault of physicians themselves, but rather from the traditional design of the curriculum in American medical schools. Rightly or wrongly, the curriculum planners assumed that ours is a wealthy society, quite able to afford an abundance of good food: perhaps they equated quantity with quality. They also assumed that basic scientists and clinicians in the various specialties could teach whatever nutrition might be needed by future doctors. In this climate it became popular for medical students and house officers to memorize a few favorite diets for specific conditions or disorders and leave the rest to hospital dietitians. For a time there was little incentive to change this state of affairs.

During the past decade, however, a new and very important development, parenteral feeding of patients, has underscored the lack of adequate nutritional education of most physicians. Realization of the need for more knowledge has led to a flurry of interest in nutrition, but many who visit their medical libraries are disappointed to find that the information they seek is not readily available. This book represents an effort to provide useful information that is applicable to the patient, and to help the reader find more information when needed.

Undernutrition is not the most common form of malnutrition in the United States; overnutrition and improper nutrition are seen more frequently. Obesity is very easily diagnosed but seldom effectively treated. The hyperlipidemias and their atherosclerotic consequences may be minimized by an appropriate diet, and substantial evidence suggests that excessive use of salt may contribute to hypertension.

Even the apparently inevitable demineralization of the skeleton that occurs with advancing age, especially in women, may result in part from a diet that provides a surplus of phosphorus in relation to calcium.

In an effort to reverse the trend toward neglect of nutritional topics the author has endeavored to present the nutritional aspects of medical practice as they apply to each of the major organ systems. A deliberate effort was made to avoid encyclopedic description of each and every deficiency disease, because these have been published repeatedly in many other books. Instead, emphasis has been placed on the importance of assessing the nutritional status of patients, and provision of adequate nutrients to patients who are malnourished.

The author hopes that this book will serve as a stimulus to teach applied nutrition in medical schools. Some experts hold that nutrition as a separate subject need not be taught in medical schools; that it can be acquired in bits and pieces from biochemists, from physiologists, and from the clinical courses currently taught. In answer to this, the author suggests that this method has been employed during the past thirty years, yet our medical profession needs more knowledge. Now we have an opportunity to introduce nutrition into virtually every medical school curriculum and to give this subject sufficient emphasis to provide future physicians with a fund of nutritional knowledge that will enable them to give better care to their patients.

ROBERT E. HODGES, M.D.

CONTENTS

EVALUATION OF THE NUTRITIONAL STATUS OF PATIENTS

Robert E. Hodges, M.D.
and
Raymond D. Adelman, M.D.

INTRODUCTION

Although nutritional habits exert a profound influence upon the health of people of all ages, the medical profession has generally devoted surprisingly little time and effort to this subject. Nutritional evaluation is not taught to most medical students, so it is little wonder that they fail to learn how to take a nutritional history or to look for telltale signs of malnutrition when performing a physical examination. Pediatricians should be given credit for the best performance in this area, probably because growth and development of infants and children rapidly reflect the nutritional status of the patient. But adults "come in all sizes," and most physicians have learned to accept a wide range of nutritional conditions as within normal limits, or as they often note on their charts, "WNL". Indeed, one of the earliest abbreviations many medical students learn to use is *WD, WN, W♀*, meaning "well developed, well-nourished, white female". Regrettably, the second observation is likely to be wrong, for a substantial number of adult patients in this country are overweight. It would be much better to teach medical students in this country to use their eyes and to devote a few minutes to the use of such simple instruments as a measuring bar, a scale, skin-fold calipers, and a tape measure. The value of these measurements may well be much greater than that of expensive and time-consuming laboratory tests.

In the following pages, the topic of nutritional evaluation will be subdivided by age group because of profound differences in physiologic needs, dietary habits, and socio-economic status of individuals in different phases of life. These phases are arbitrarily designated as childhood (including infancy), adolescence, adulthood, and old age.

NUTRITIONAL EVALUATION OF CHILDREN

Nutritional evaluation of the child begins with the history, which should include the type and quantity of food ingested, the presence of food additives in the diet, and the presence or absence of chronic disease, eating difficulties, and ethnic food preferences. Exclusive intake of milk in a 12-month-old child will often be accompanied by iron deficiency anemia, since cow's milk contains little iron. Children raised on goat's milk will, in addition, suffer from folate deficiency. An exclusive diet of vegetables and fruits in the young infant may provide adequate calories but inadequate protein, leading to protein malnutrition. Most children receive some vitamin supplements, either in a pill or liquid form, or as additives to commonly ingested foods, such as the addition of vitamin A and vitamin D to commercial milk preparations. But some children may ingest foods lacking these additives, such as tortillas with neither iron nor thiamin. Occasionally, children may be given toxic amounts of vitamins, leading to hypervitaminosis, such as can occur with vitamins A and D. In addition, certain drugs affect nutritional status. Dilantin has long been recognized as a cause of folate and vitamin D deficiency. Children with chronic diseases, including cardiac, renal, pulmonary, and gastrointestinal diseases, may have marked nutritional deficiencies resulting from anorexia or from inadequate absorption of food. In addition, there may be feeding difficulties that interfere with the adequate ingestion of food. This may be especially troublesome in children with cerebral palsy, mental retardation, or in premature babies. One common scene of undernutrition is the hospital, where children with lingering illnesses are maintained for long periods of time on dextrose and electrolyte solutions lacking in both adequate calories and protein. They may receive vitamins in their intravenous infusions but these do not compensate for lack of protein or lack of adequate calories (Bistrian et al., 1976).

Information about the community has an important bearing on the problems of the individual. Knowledge of the common health problems, as well as the level of health care available in a community, aids the physician in anticipating problem areas for a given patient or for members of a given family. For example, although fluid milk sold in grocery stores and supermarkets throughout most of the United States is fortified with vitamin D, it is still possible to buy milk in certain rural areas that has not been pasteurized, homogenized, or fortified. Similarly, legal requirements for enrichment of commercially prepared farinaceous foods — including breads, flour, and breakfast cereals —insure the addition of iron, riboflavin, thiamine, and niacin. But in communities where hominy grits or rice are staple items of the diet, it is important to recognize that the intake of these essential nutrients may be lower than average.

The problem of endemic goiter which once was prevalent throughout the "Goiter Belt" of the North-Central states has been largely eliminated by a combination of events; iodization of table salt, feeding of trace minerals, including iodine, to both dairy cattle and meat-producing animals, and the use of organic iodine-containing compounds in the manufacture of bread. Iodine deficiency is no longer a likely cause of goiter in the United States.

The quality of drinking water is, however, a continuing problem. Excessive amounts of nitrates and nitrites in well-water may result in methemoglobinemia in infants. The fluoride content of water has been a topic of widespread concern on the part of many parents. Some are anxious to have municipal water supplies fluoridated in order to reduce dental caries in their children. Others oppose fluoridation, either because they object to the general principle of adding a "chemical" to their water supply or because they fear that fluorides may cause, in some obscure fashion, one or more of the diseases for which the etiology remains unknown. And the hardness or softness of the water is believed to have a bearing on the development of coronary heart disease in subsequent years; hard water communities tend to have a lower incidence than soft water communities. These and many other aspects of community health should be considered by the physician when talking with and examining patients (Stitt et al., 1973; Fomon, 1974).

Physical Findings

On physical examination, signs of nutritional deficiency may be apparent. Skin changes may include hyperkeratosis, dermatitis, edema, ecchymoses, and petechiae. Changes in the color and texture of the hair can signal protein malnutrition. Bossing of the skull, enlargement of the joints, and costochondral beading may reflect vitamin D deficiency or some other disorder of bone metabolism. The presence of xerosis or inflammation of the eyes should be noted as well as the condition of the teeth, all mucous membranes, the tongue, and the lips. One should also look for enlargement of the thyroid gland, the liver, and the spleen, but these findings are nonspecific. The physical examination is of value primarily in identifying interference with growth and development and usually gives a low percentage of positive signs. In addition, there is marked observer variability and a great deal of overlap in signs produced by specific deficiencies.

Anthropometric Measurements. A most important aspect of the physical examination is accurate measurement of the weight, the height or length, and the skin-fold thickness. Weight should be measured with the patient unclothed on a calibrated beam scale. In a child under two years of age, length measurement is performed with the subject in the supine position, and with the eyes gazing directly upward while the top of the head is held in contact with a fixed headboard and the heels held in contact with a moveable footboard. In a child over three years of age, height is measured, preferably using a block at right angles to a mounted rule or stadiometer. Bare heels, buttocks, shoulders, and head should touch the vertical measuring surface while the block is lowered to the crown of the head. Both height and weight should be plotted on standard growth charts for children (Tables 1–1 through 1–8). Children who have a low weight for age, height for age, or low weight for height may suffer from calorie, protein, or essential nutrient deficiency, and deserve further evaluation. For example, one should be concerned about nutritional deficiency in a child whose height for age is perhaps at the 25th percentile but whose weight for age is under the 3rd percentile; or in the child whose height and weight for age are both under the 3rd percentile; or in the child whose height and weight over time cross percentile lines — going, for example, from the 50th percentile at one age to the 5th percentile at a later age. These changes may also indicate an underlying chronic disease process. Children whose weight for height is greater than the 95th percentile may be presumed to be obese. This rule may generally be applied to children under age nine. In children older than nine years, a more accurate estimate of body fat content can be obtained through evaluation of skin-fold thickness. This can discriminate the individual whose excess weight is due to excess body fat from the individual whose excess weight is due to increased body musculature. The best sites for measuring skinfold thickness are the triceps area and the subscapular area. Skin-fold thicknesses exceeding the 90th or 95th percentile reflect obesity in the individual. Skin-folds can be measured using either the Lange or the Harpenden calipers, which apply a fixed pressure to the skin surface. This type of measurement, in children and infants, requires practice and patience. The triceps skin-fold should be measured with the arm flexed. The measurement is taken midway between the acromion and olecranon, 1 cm below a pinched skin-fold. Readings should be made approximately three seconds after application of the caliper.

Text continued on page 13

TABLE 1–1 LENGTH AND WEIGHT OF GIRLS AS A
FUNCTION OF AGE

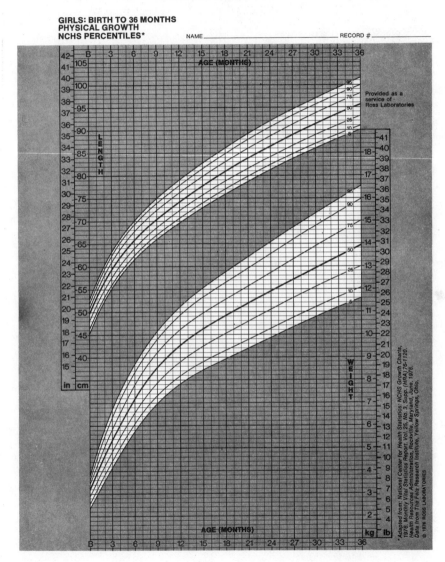

TABLE 1–2 HEAD CIRCUMFERENCE OF GIRLS BY AGE, LENGTH AND WEIGHT ARE PLOTTED BELOW

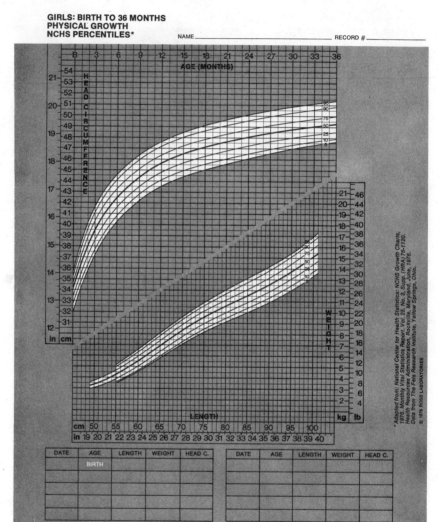

TABLE 1–3 STATURE AND WEIGHT OF GIRLS, AGE 2–18 YEARS, ARE PLOTTED BY AGE

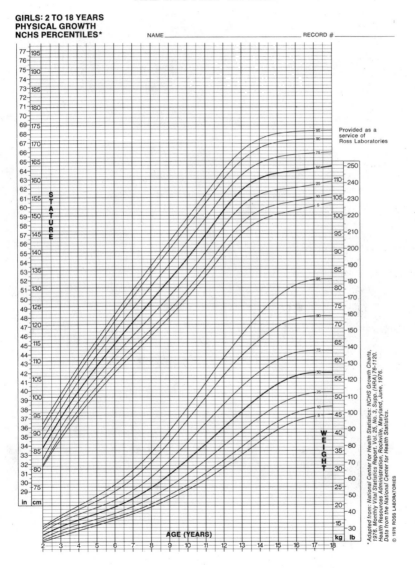

GIRLS: 2 TO 18 YEARS
PHYSICAL GROWTH
NCHS PERCENTILES*

NAME_____ RECORD #_____

Provided as a
service of
Ross Laboratories

* Adapted from: National Center for Health Statistics: NCHS Growth Charts, 1976. Monthly Vital Statistics Report, Vol. 25, No. 3, Supp. (HRA) 76-1120. Health Resources Administration, Rockville, Maryland, June, 1976. Data from the National Center for Health Statistics.

© 1976 ROSS LABORATORIES

TABLE 1–4 STATURE AND WEIGHT OF PRE-PUBESCENT GIRLS ARE PLOTTED AGAINST EACH OTHER

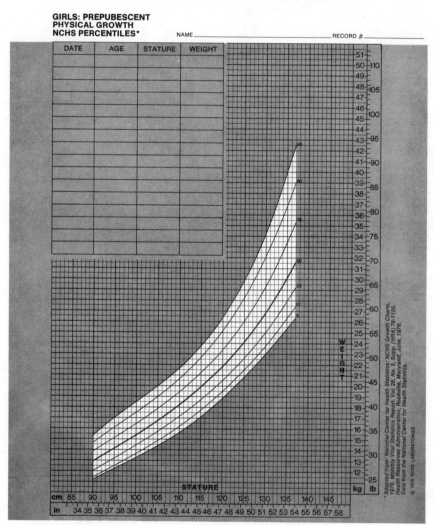

GIRLS: PREPUBESCENT
PHYSICAL GROWTH
NCHS PERCENTILES*

TABLE 1-5 LENGTH AND WEIGHT OF BOYS AS A FUNCTION OF AGE

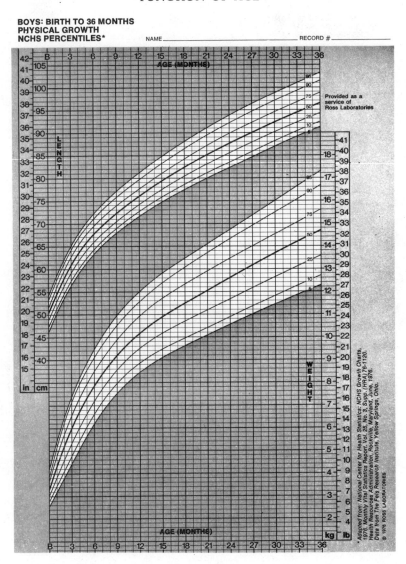

BOYS: BIRTH TO 36 MONTHS
PHYSICAL GROWTH
NCHS PERCENTILES*

NAME _____ RECORD # _____

Provided as a
service of
Ross Laboratories

* Adapted from: National Center for Health Statistics: NCHS Growth Charts, 1976. Monthly Vital Statistics Report, Vol. 25, No. 3, Supp. (HRA) 76-1120. Health Resources Administration, Rockville, Maryland, June, 1976. Data from The Fels Research Institute, Yellow Springs, Ohio.

© 1976 ROSS LABORATORIES

TABLE 1–6 HEAD CIRCUMFERENCE OF BOYS, PLOTTED BY AGE, LENGTH AND WEIGHT

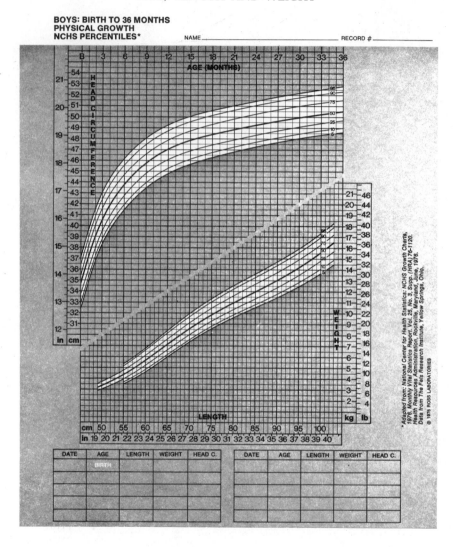

TABLE 1–7 STATURE AND WEIGHT OF BOYS, AGE 2–18 YEARS, PLOTTED BY AGE

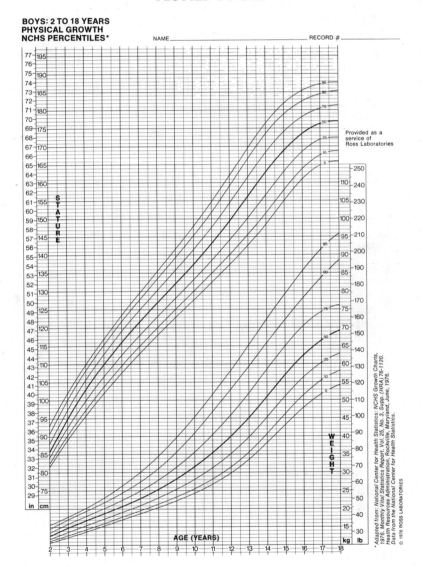

TABLE 1–8 STATURE AND WEIGHT OF PRE-PUBESCENT BOYS ARE PLOTTED AGAINST EACH OTHER

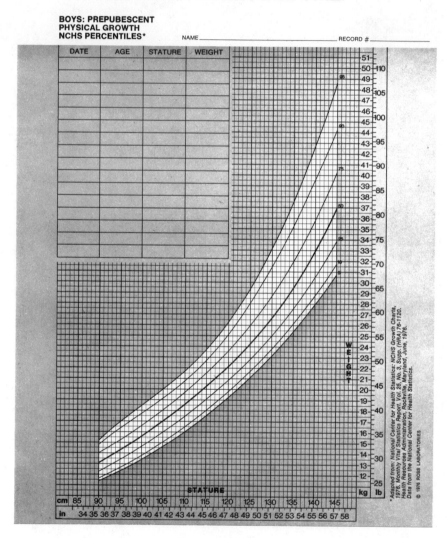

The subscapular skin-fold measurement is made at a point inferior and lateral to the inferior angle of the scapula. Although this skin-fold requires the individual to undress, it seems to be more accurate than the triceps skin-fold measurement.

Measurement of the circumference of the upper arm midway between the acromion and olecranon has been described by Martorell and others (1976) as a useful anthropometric indicator of nutritional status. In studies in Guatemalan children, it was possible to calculate the cross-sectional arm muscle area and compare this with skin-fold thickness. It was found that although Guatemalan children had reduced arm muscle and fat areas, the relative reduction in fat was greater than that of muscle. The conclusion was that energy, rather than protein, was the main nutritional problem in these children. The simple mathematical formulas used to estimate muscle area and fat area are given on pages 18 and 28.

Laboratory Tests

The laboratory can be used sparingly for nutritional assessment of the average child. Since iron deficiency anemia is the most common nutritional problem, with the exception of obesity, in children in the United States, it is appropriate to get at least a measurement of hemoglobin or hematocrit, and if this is abnormal other hematologic measurements should be made. The concentration of cholesterol in the serum should also be determined routinely, not only because cholesterol levels may reflect a familial hyperlipidemia, but also because malnutrition is often accompanied by abnormally low concentrations of cholesterol in the serum. Other laboratory tests depend upon the type of community assessed, the individual, the time of year, and other factors. For example, the child receiving Dilantin for a convulsive disorder should be assessed for folate deficiency. Children living in cloudy climates with no vitamin D supplementation of their food should have alkaline phosphatase activity determined and those with elevated alkaline phosphatase should also have wrist roentgenograms. Other blood and urine tests may be done when indicated.

ADOLESCENCE

Nutritionists have been perplexed for many years over how to estimate the nutrient requirements of children during the period of time commonly termed adolescence. Few people can even define the term adolescence, let alone understand its physiological and nutritional implications. It is well known, of course, that this is a transition from childhood to adulthood, that it is a period of rapid growth, of endocrine changes, of strong emotions, and of wide-ranging physical and intellectual demands. During adolescence, the velocity of growth increases for the only time during the 18 year growth period (Heald, 1969). The period of adolescence is much longer than many people realize — extending from age 12 through age 21 for females, and age 14 through 25 for males (Pearson, 1969). Although the same methods are employed in the evaluation of nutritional status of adolescents — namely, dietary history, anthropometric measurements of height, weight, arm circumference, and skin-fold thickness, and the same hematological and biochemical tests — the interpretation is much different (McGanity, 1976). The essence of the problem lies in the fact that individuals begin their "growth spurt" at different times and so one person of a given age may be physically preadolescent, another may be developing rapidly, and a third may have completed his or her development and achieved adult characteristics. Obviously, both the energy needs and the requirements for essential nutrients vary widely from one individual to another (Hodges and Krehl, 1965; Hodges, 1976).

A proposed solution to this dilemma is based on the sexual maturation of individuals and not on their chonological age or their height or their weight. Heald has devised a system for evaluating the state of sexual maturity of boys and girls ranging from infantile through adult characteristics. He has shown that individuals at similar levels of sexual maturation have similar nutrient requirements. For the physician who deals with substantial numbers of adolescent patients this classification could be highly valuable (Heald, 1976).

Laboratory tests for assessment of the nutritional status of adolescents are essentially the same as those for adults. Girls run a substantial risk of becoming anemic, so attention should be paid to their hematologic status. In both boys and girls, measurement of plasma levels of cholesterol and triglycerides is advised because familial hyperlipidemias can be readily detected at this age and appropriate measures can be taken to reduce lipid levels. Obviously, the efficacy of these preventive efforts cannot be ascertained until a number of years have passed, but the authors believe that they may prove to be effective.

NUTRITIONAL STATUS OF ADULTS

Most clinicians find it difficult to distinguish between well-nourished and malnourished persons, largely because there are no uniform criteria yet established. Severe malnutrition is obvious, yet many of the clinical findings associated with malnutrition can occur as a result of some other condition. Accordingly, the most accurate method for determining malnutrition of varying degrees of severity is to employ multiple indices, including dietary history, physical examination, anthropometric measurements (Figures 1–1 through 1–5) and laboratory studies. In the patient with few or no abnormalities, the assumption is that the nutritional status is good, whereas patients who have multiple abnormalities are almost certainly malnourished.

Nutritional Components of the Medical History

Most hospital charts have been found to contain little if any information about what the patient eats or doesn't eat, yet eating (and drinking) habits may play an all-important role in a patient's illness (Butterworth and Blackburn, 1975). Valuable information can be elicited by means of a few carefully directed questions interwoven in the medical history. These might include:

Height and weight at various stages of life, such as at graduation from high school, at time of marriage, on entry into military service, or upon application for insurance or employment.

Those *dietary and living habits* affected by occupation, level of physical activity, and time of arising:

Breakfast — no breakfast? juice? toast, eggs, bacon, and coffee? some other breakfast?

Lunch — no lunch? eaten at home, at the office? from a vending machine, "brown-bagged"? if a housewife, leftovers?

Dinner — an entree, salad, vegetables, fruits, bread, potatoes, dessert? some combination of these?

Snack items — candy, soft drinks, nuts, potato chips, corn curls, popcorn, and so on.

Alcohol — number of drinks per day.
          (12 oz. beer = 1 oz. whiskey = 3 oz. wine)

Use of salt —
Non salter: never adds salt;
Taster: tastes food, then salts to taste;
Salter: salts most foods before tasting.

Rate of eating —
Eats slowly: 30 minutes or more;
Average eater: about 20 minutes;
Fast eater: about 10 minutes.

Food preferences — favorite foods, least popular foods, food intolerances, and religious, social, or personal factors.

Meals Away from Home — number per week.

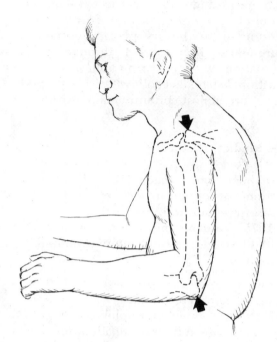

Figure 1–1 To find the midpoint of the arm, first identify the acromion and the olecranon (arrows).

Figure 1–2 Then place the tip of the middle finger of one hand on the acromion and the tip of the middle finger of the other hand on the olecranon. By extending the thumbs toward each other, it is easy to identify the midpoint, which should be marked with a pen.

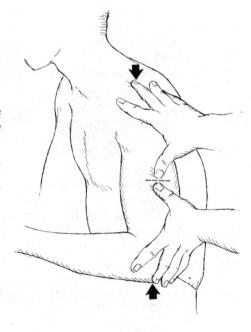

Figure 1-3 Arm circumference is measured with a steel rule calibrated in millimeters. Care must be taken to exert the same amount of tension on the tape each time a measurement is made.

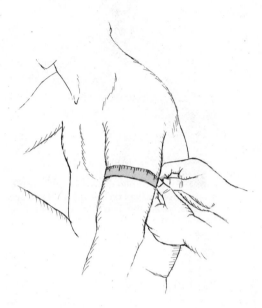

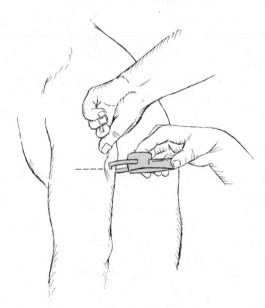

Figure 1-4 The skin-fold thickness is measured over the triceps muscle. A fold of the skin is gently grasped with thumb and forefinger of one hand while thickness is measured with a caliper (Lange). Three measurements should be made in succession allowing the calipers to exert pressure for 3 seconds before each reading. The average of the three readings is recorded.

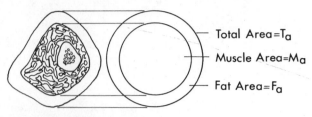

C=circumference, S=skinfold thickness

$$T_a = \frac{C^2}{4\pi}$$

$$M_a = \frac{(C-\pi s)^2}{4\pi}$$

$$F_a = T_a - M_a$$

Figure 1–5 From two measurements; arm circumference (c) and skin-fold thickness (s), it is possible to calculate the approximate area of the cross-section of the arm at mid-point. This is called the Total Area (Ta) and is equal to $C^2/4\pi$. Similarly, Muscle Area (Ma) is equal to $(C-\pi s)^2/4\pi$. And Fat Area (Fa) is the difference between Total Area and Muscle Area (Ta − Ma).

The following questions are deliberately repetitious and serve to verify or correct the information obtained in the preceding diet history.

Number of cups of coffee (tea) per day
Number of bottles (cans) of soft drinks per day
Number of snacks (of any kind) per day
Number of servings of meat per week
Number of quarts of milk consumed per week
Number of eggs eaten per week
Number of drinks per week (How much liquor, wine, or beer purchased weekly? How many helped drink it?)

The Physical Examination

General Appearance. (Sick or well, alert or obtunded, happy or sad). Apparent age compared with actual age.

Hair. Sheen, color, texture (note eyebrows, eyelashes, body hair, and lanugo hair). Depigmentation of hair occurs in children subjected to severe malnutrition or to prolonged illness, whereas alopecia is more common in adults (Figure 1–6).

Skin. Color, texture, turgor, and hair distribution may vary with age, race, sex, and exposure to sun and wind, as well as nutritional staus. The physician must use clinical experience as a guide, but *unusual* findings may indicate nutritional deficits. A debilitated surgical patient often has thin, inelastic skin with poor turgor (Plate 1)

Lanugo hair may be absent and pigmentation increased, especially at such pressure points as heels, sacrum, elbows, and scapulae. This reflects both caloric and protein lack. There is often a bleeding tendency, manifested by bruises, petechiae, and ecchymoses. Excessive bruising as a result of subcutaneous injections or venipuncture may indicate deficiency of vitamin K. Follicular hyperkeratosis may signify deficiency of vitamin A or of ascorbic acid. Perifollicular hemorrhages may signify scurvy.

Eyes. Palpebral fissures and extra-ocular motion may be affected by nutritional deficiency of thiamine. Strabismus with diplopia is common in alcoholic patients with a poor intake of food. The familiar Wernicke-Korsakoff's syndrome results in part from a lack of thiamin. Nystagmus may also be apparent.

Normally, the sclera is white, with a few superficial vessels coursing through the conjunctiva. With increasing age, the amount of vascularity may increase. In addition, yellowish plaques known as pingue-

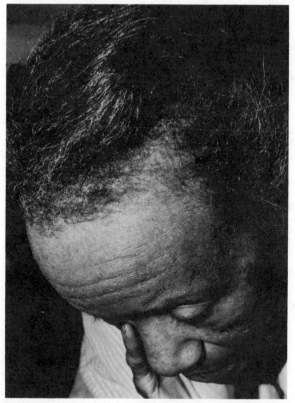

Figure 1–6 Alopecia in a malnourished woman. This occurs commonly in patients who are deficient in protein. It is one of many manifestations of arrested growth and repair of tissues in people who are malnourished.

culae develop on the nasal side of the iris. These are not of nutritional significance. Patients with deficiency of riboflavin may have increased vascularity of the bulbar conjunctivae (Plate 2). In tropical countries, a deficiency of vitamin A may be accompanied by the appearance of Bitot's spots. These may not be pathognomonic, but they certainly suggest vitamin A deficiency. The Bitot's spot is generally located along the equator of the eye, more often lateral to the iris and generally outside the limbus. It has the appearance of a white bubbly exudate, or of a small droplet of cottage cheese. If scraped away, a roughened, slightly erythematous base remains.

The normal luster of the eye and the transparency of the cornea depend in large part upon the secretion of tears and of oily sebaceous material. Lack of either vitamin A or vitamin C can lead to Sjögren's syndrome, which is characterized by diminished secretory activity of the lachrymal, salivary, and other mucus-secreting glands. In addition, there may be decreased secretion by the sebaceous glands.

The eyes may also give an indication of familial hyperlipidemias. In some patients with hypercholesterolemia, cholesterol deposits appear as soft yellow-white plaques in the tissues of the upper or lower lids. Many patients develop circumferential deposits of cholesterol around the iris. This is called "arcus senilis" or "arcus corneae" and may indicate abnormal cholesterol metabolism, though it is almost a universal finding in aged patients. It should be noted, however, that this finding is much more easily observed in persons with a deeply pigmented iris (brown eyes) than in persons with less pigmentation (blue or green eyes), because the cholesterol deposit appears gray or pale blue. Although the arcus becomes more prevalent with advancing age, there is evidence of a positive relationship between this finding and premature atherosclerosis (Schrott et al., 1972). It is a good rule to obtain lipoprotein studies in any young or middle-aged patient who is found to have a well-developed arcus senilis, xanthelasma, or other xanthomata.

Another indirect sign of nutritional problems relates to the eyelids. In any form of seborrheic dermatitis, the eyebrows may be involved in a scaling dermatitis (Figure 1–7). The resulting dandruff flakes often fall into the eyes where they cause irritation of the bulbar and palpebral conjunctivae. Any patient with blepharitis and scaling of the eyebrows may have one of the four deficiency syndromes characterized by seborrheic dermatitis. These are deficiencies of zinc, riboflavin, vitamin B_6, or essential fatty acids. Of course, the commonest form of seborrheic dermatitis is idiopathic, but a few well-directed questions will indicate whether the patient's diet is obviously adequate or questionably deficient.

During adolescence, a great many young people develop abundant secretions of their sebaceous glands, especially those of the face.

The tongue provides a great deal of valuable information about nutritional status. The normal red color may be replaced by a peculiar red-purple shade, sometimes described as "magenta" (Plate 3). This has often been attributed to deficiencies of riboflavin or pyridoxine or niacin, but in the experience of the author, administration of these vitamins either alone or with all of the other water-soluble vitamins has routinely failed to correct the abnormal color. Once these patients have been given adequate amounts of calories and protein and vitamins and essential minerals, however, the color of the tongue can revert to normal within a few days.

Another obvious color change results from severe anemia with its accompanying pallor, not only on the tongue, but also of mucous membranes, nail beds, and palms. Certain deficiencies — notably folate, vitamin B_{12} and iron — may be accompanied by smoothness of the tongue. This has been attributed to "atrophy of the filiform papillae" but in the case of vitamin B_{12}, at least, the smooth tongue may have been hereditary rather than acquired. No one seems to have recorded the ultimate condition of the tongue of patients who were once deficient in these nutrients, then treated with adequate supplements.

Recent studies in humans have confirmed animal studies that showed impairment of the special senses in vitamin A deficiency. Not only was night blindness a common feature, but loss of taste, loss of smell, and impairment of vestibular balance also occurred. In experimental animals, vitamin A deficiency results in a decreased intake of food, which in turn probably explains the failure of young animals to grow at a normal rate if they have inadequate vitamin A.

Examination of the neck will disclose the presence or absence of an enlarged thyroid gland, or goiter. As mentioned above, goiter was formerly a common expression of iodine deficiency in the North-Central portions of the United States, but the food supply now contains ample amounts of iodine. Goiter still occurs in a small number of people and it is still more common in women than in men, but most goiters probably arise from genetic or enzymatic defects, or as a result of ingestion of a goitrogenic compound. Although foods of the brassica family — such as mustard, turnip, and cabbage — contain goitrogens, the amount is small and does not likely cause human goiter in this country.

Examination of the thorax gives information about the patient's degree of fatness. The layer of subcutaneous tissue surrounding the thorax is proportional to the patient's eating habits. Measurement of the skin-fold thickness with calipers (see pages 4, 13, and 17) is often used as a guide to the degree of fatness of a patient. A point worth remembering is that most people, when standing unclothed with arms hanging naturally, have no visible gap between their arms and their thorax, regardless of their degree of leanness or fatness. But if a patient has recently lost a large amount of weight, perhaps 20 or 30 pounds in a short time, a gap may be seen between the upper arm and the thorax. Gynecomastia may occur in men as a result of alcoholism, especially when serious liver disease has developed as a consequence. In such instances, there often are other clues to the etiology: palmar erythema, tremor of the outstretched hands, and vascular nevi, or "spiders", on the face and shoulders and the upper anterior aspects of the chest.

The abdomen gives us information about the patient's energy balance, since most overweight patients have an increased abdominal girth. An old saying was that the presence or absence of obesity could be ascertained by employing the "ruler test". This consists of laying a long straight ruler (yardstick) along the midline of the abdomen of a supine, relaxed patient. If the ruler touches the xyphoid process of the sternum and the symphysis pubis at the same time, the patient is said not to be "fat". Most nutritionists, however, prefer to use more scientific measures of obesity, based upon height, weight, skin-fold thickness, and body composition.

Enlargement of the liver, with or without jaundice or ascites, provides presumptive evidence of hepatic disease. A large number of the malnourished patients seen in hospitals in this country have liver disease as a result of excessive use of alcohol. The familiar picture of a dejected patient with emaciated extremities, distended abdomen, magenta-colored tongue, red palms, and spider angiomata is all too common. This type of patient represents one of the most serious challenges to the ability of the physician, especially because such patients are literally nutritional derelicts. Examination of the male genitalia may disclose soft, atrophic testicles in cases of advanced malnutrition accompanying alcoholism.

The extremities provide much evidence of the patient's nutritional status. The general contour of arms and legs tells the examiner whether the patient is over- or undernourished and whether the patient has been in good or poor nitrogen balance. Strength, coordination, and range of motion give evidence for or against such a neurologic deficit as that seen in the thiamin-depleted alcoholic patient.

As mentioned below, the muscle mass can be estimated by a simple calculation based on the triceps skin-fold thickness and the circumference of the arm midway between the acromion and the olecranon.

In certain nutritional disorders, the skin gives valuable information. In scurvy, for example, the presence of both petechiae and hyperkeratotic hair follicles surrounded by a hemorrhagic halo may be detected first on the forearms and on the anterolateral aspects of the thighs. Vitamin A deficiency may produce similar hyperkeratosis of hair follicles on the extremities and trunk, but there is no hemorrhagic component. The "liver palms" of the alcoholic patient, mentioned above, involve hyperemia of the thenar and hypothenar eminences of the hands.

Just as the skeleton gives evidence of rickets or scurvy in children, so does it give valuable nutritional information in adults. Most people reach the peak of skeletal mineralization shortly after they achieve their maximum height. With each subsequent year thereafter, the skeleton loses a fraction of its mineral content and its structural shape changes gradually with the physical stresses that are applied. The result is exaggeration of the cervical and thoracic curves of the spine, shortening of the stature, and bowing of the legs. In many elderly people, this process results in considerable disability. It is difficult to make an arbitrary decision as to what is "normal" and what is frankly pathological. Perhaps the most objective test is a comparison of the patient's current height with his or her maximal height. A loss of two to four inches over a span of 50 years is not at all uncommon, but twice this amount is regarded as abnormal. Similarly, the patient with dorsal kyphosis so extreme as to prevent lying supine on the examining table represents an abnormal degree of change. Much evidence suggests that the average American diet provides an imbalance between calcium and phosphorus and that this may contribute to the loss of about 1 per cent of skeletal minerals each year of adult life. At present we do not have enough evidence to state that skeletal demineralization can be prevented in all persons, but studies under way (Lutwak, 1975) may provide these answers (see Chapter 6).

Laboratory Tests

Contrary to popular opinion, it is not usually necessary to obtain special tests in order to evaluate the nutritional adequacy of most patients. Recently there has been considerable notoriety generated by individuals who advertise their ability to make nutritional diagnoses. These include not only computerized evaluations of diet questionnaires, but detailed analyses of many nutrients in samples of urine, blood, hair, and even fingernails. The author believes that some of these methods can be useful in investigation of unusual forms of malnutrition but does not favor the routine application of expensive and often inexact procedures to the average patient.

Laboratory procedures that are commonly employed in most modern hospitals and clinics can be used effectively to obtain a wealth of information about the nutritional status of patients. These include a routine urine analysis, a complete blood count (erythrocyte count, hemoglobin, hematocrit, white blood cell count, and differential count), and performance of the routine biochemical tests referred to as SMA 6/60 — which detects chloride, sodium, CO_2, potassium, BUN, and glucose — and SMA 12/60 — which measures total protein, albumin, calcium, phosphorous, cholesterol, uric acid, bilirubin, creatinine, alkaline phosphatase, creatine phosphokinase (CPK), lactic dehydrogenase (LDH), and serum glutamic oxaloacetic transaminase (SGOT). These tests will tell the physician whether the patient is excreting blood, albumin, glucose, bilirubin, or acetone in his or her urine. It will tell the physician whether the patient is anemic, and if so, what the patient's hematologic indices are. Abnormalities of leukocytes or platelets will be apparent. The biochemical tests (SMA 6/60 and 12/60) will provide information about electrolyte balance, glucose level, nitrogenous substances, plasma proteins, calcium and phosphorous metabolism, bilirubin levels, and four enzymes that become elevated in a variety of disorders, including hepatic, pancreatic, and coronary heart disease.

Specific nutritional information can be quickly gleaned from these data. Most malnourished patients have two or more of these abnormalities:

1. Anemia, often normocytic and normochromic
2. Hypoalbuminemia
3. Hypocholesterolemia
4. A low ratio of BUN/Cr (normal = 10 to 20) in plasma

In addition, many malnourished patients, especially those with a history of alcohol abuse, will have elevation of their plasma levels of bilirubin and one or more of the enzymes.

Special tests are also available in many hospitals. If anemia is present, measurement of serum iron and total binding capacity may be indicated. Serum levels of folate and vitamin B_{12} should be measured in the event a patient's anemia is macrocytic in character or in the event of alcoholism or medication with such anticonvulsants as phenobarbital or dilantin. Alcohol often lowers folate levels, but if liver disease exists, the vitamin B_{12} level may be elevated.

Another special test is the time-honored prothrombin time supplemented by the activated partial thromboplastin time (PTT), both of which reflect the adequacy of vitamin K in the diet and the ability of the liver to synthesize specific coagulation factors.

Absorption studies may also be helpful in evaluating malnourished patients. The simplest of these include:

1. *Serum carotene level.* This provides some index of the patient's ability to digest and absorb fatty substances (assuming that the patient had recently been eating foods containing carotenes).
2. *Fecal fats.* The patient is fed a diet containing 100 gm of fat per day for three days, then a fecal sample is collected for 24 hours. This

sample should contain less than 30 per cent fat by dry weight, or less than 6 gm per 24 hour specimen.

3. *Lactose tolerance test* (to detect lactase deficiency). A test dose of lactose is given orally (usually either 100 gm or 1 gm/kg) and plasma levels of glucose are measured at 0, 30, 60, 90, 120 and 180 minutes. Failure to elevate glucose levels greater than 20 mg/dl is a positive test.

4. *D-xylose test.* The fasting patient is given 25 gm d-xylose orally and urine is collected for 5 hours. Normally 5 to 8 gm are excreted in that period of time.

5. *Schilling test.* Patients with defective secretion of intrinsic factor (IF) cannot absorb vitamin B_{12} adequately. The patient is given, orally, a dose of vitamin B_{12} tagged with ^{58}Co. After a suitable interval, the patient is given a "flushing dose" of non-radioactive vitamin B_{12}. The amount of radioactivity excreted in the urine during the next 24 hours reflects the amount of the original radioactive dose absorbed. If absorption is impaired, another dose of ^{58}Co-labeled vitamin B_{12} is given along with IF to determine absorption.

Judicious use of these tests can give the physician an excellent appraisal of a patient's nutritional status. Under unusual circumstances, it may be desirable to measure specific essential nutrients in plasma or urine. These tests may not be available, even in modern hospitals. They can be obtained from special laboratories known to the Director of Laboratories in your hospital. A partial list of such tests includes tests for retinol, riboflavin, nicotinic acid, ascorbic acid, copper, zinc, vitamin E — all found in serum — and for thiamine, riboflavin, xanthurenic acid (after tryptophan load test), vitamin B_6, and pantothenic acid — from urine samples (Sauberlich, 1974).

As nutrition becomes more a part of routine medical practice, there will undoubtedly be a wider selection of laboratory procedures available to the practicing physician. Meanwhile a great deal of information is available from routine sources. It is important to keep in mind that there is no single test to distinguish between well-nourished and malnourished individuals. Of the common laboratory tests, the serum albumin and the ratio of BUN/Cr correlate quite well with general nutritional status. In addition, the concentration of hemoglobin, the level of cholesterol, and the total number of lymphocytes reflect the overall nutritional status.

We have found that nutritional status can be effectively estimated from the data collected by performing a history, a physical examination, and laboratory tests as described above.

We classify each patient as being in Classes I to IV for energy status and for protein status. In addition, evidence of any specific essential nutrient deficiency is noted:

Class I is within normal limits.
Class II is moderate malnutrition.
Class III is marked malnutrition.
Class IV is very severe malnutrition.

In deciding upon the severity of the malnutrition in a given patient, we consider all available data and choose an approximate average (Table 1–9).

Anthropometric Measurements

For some unexplained reason, most physicians have been reluctant to use anthropometric measurements in their routine evaluation of adult patients. Pediatricians, however, routinely utilize height and weight as an index of the rate of growth and, consequently, of the nutritional status of infants and children. But even pediatricians may be reluctant to utilize other helpful and simple measurements, such as circumference of the head, circumference of the upper arm, and skin-fold thickness. Circumferential measurement of the arm has been used for many years in surveys where estimates of the overall nutritional status of a population group were needed. Under such circumstances, it has been possible to identify groups of individuals who are most severely in need of limited food resources (Anderson, 1975). A refinement of this technique allows investigators to calculate the upper arm cross-sectional area of muscle and of fat (Martorell et al., 1976). Upper arm circumference is measured to the nearest millimeter, using a steel tape to avoid the errors introduced by the stretching of a cloth or paper tape. Measurements are made midway between the tip of the acromion and the olecranon process with the left arm hanging relaxed. Triceps skin-fold thickness is also measured in this location to the nearest tenth of a millimeter, using a Harpenden skin-fold caliper (the Lange caliper is equally acceptable) (Tables 1–10 to 1–12). Calculation of cross-sectional muscle mass and fat mass can be readily made by using the following formulas. The formula for estimation of muscle cross-sectional area is:

$$M_a = \frac{(C - \pi S)^2}{4\pi}$$

Similarly, calculation of the cross-sectional area of fat can be easily done by this method:

$$T_a = \frac{C^2}{4\pi}$$

$$F_a = T_a - M_a$$

In these calculations, M_a equals the muscle area, F_a equals the fat area, T_a equals total area, C equals the circumference of the arm in millimeters, and S equals the triceps skin-fold thickness in millimeters. These calculations allow the examiner to differentiate between fat and muscle when evaluating an individual patient. Previous use of the arm circumference as an index of protein-calorie malnutrition in early childhood has documented its value (Jelliffe and Jelliffe, 1969).

Morphology of hair roots provides another anthropometric index. Under a dissecting microscope, the hair bulb can be accurately classified as in the anagen (growth) phase or in a resting phase. Children who are well fed have a major proportion of anagen hair bulbs but children with protein-calorie malnutrition may have less than 50 per cent in the anagen phase. Furthermore, the diameter of the hair root correlates closely with standard weight-for-age in children.

THE ELDERLY

In the United States, care of the elderly is sadly neglected. Unlike Oriental cultures, in which elderly persons are respected and revered, old people in our country are all too often regarded as a burden. Many are placed in old people's homes, retirement centers, or "convalescent" hospitals. In such surroundings, they are served meals that are more or less nutritious, but there is little effort made to recognize either their preferences or their physiologic needs.

In attempting to evaluate the requirements of elderly people, a number of factors should be considered. These include the obvious need for information about the individual's mental condition, visual acuity, ability to move about, and economic status. An old person living alone in a city may find it a real chore to utilize public transportation in order to get to a shopping center where he or she can purchase groceries and other supplies. As a result, old people tend more and more to buy foods with a long shelf life and to neglect fresh fruits and vegetables, as well as other nutritious but perishable foods.

The physician can render a great service to elderly patients by taking time to discuss with them their usual eating habits, their access to grocery stores and supermarkets, their ability or inability to go shopping by themselves, and the availability of relatives and friends who can help them.

But malnutrition is not confined to the upstairs room or the lonely apartment of an elderly person. It can be found all too frequently in modern hospitals, especially with elderly hospitalized patients (Jordan, 1976). Physicians must learn to assess the nutritional status of

Text continued on page 37

TABLE 1-9 CONSULTATION SHEET ON WHICH ALL NUTRITIONAL DATA ARE SUMMARIZED AND NUTRITIONAL STATUS IS NOTED

LETTERHEAD

PATIENT STAMP

Nutritional/Metabolic Consultation

History and Current Diagnoses:

Physical Examination: Age_____ yrs   Sex_____   Height_____ cm   Weight_____ kg _____ % Normal

Laboratory and Anthropometric Measurements:

Protein Status		*Metabolic/Energy Status*		*Minerals and Vitamins*	
Serum Levels:		Fasting Blood Glucose _____ mg/dl		Serum Levels:	
Total Protein _____ gm/dl		Plasma Cholesterol _____ mg/dl		Na⁺ _____ mEq/l	Vit. B₁₂ _____ pg/dl
Albumin _____ gm/dl		Arm Fat Area _____ % NL		K⁺ _____ mEq/l	Folate _____ mg/dl
TIBC _____ mg/dl		Uric Acid _____ mg/dl		CO₂ _____ mEq/l	Carotene _____ μg/dl
BUN/Cr _____		Total Bilirubin _____ mg/dl		Cl⁻ _____ mEq/l	Protime _____ sec
Blood:		SGOT _____ mU/ml		Mg⁺⁺ _____ mEq/l	Control _____ sec
Hemoglobin _____ gm		Others:		Zn⁺⁺ _____ μg/dl	Others:
Lymphocytes % _____ total				Cu⁺⁺ _____ μg/dl	

Urine, 24 hr:
Cr/Height _____ mg/kg/cm
Nitrogen _____ mg/kg
Urea _____ mg/kg
Arm Muscle Area _____ % NL

Fe^{++} _____ µg/dl
Ca^{++} _____ mg/dl
Pi _____ mg/dl
Others:

Assessment of Nutritional and Metabolic Status:

Balances*: Protein _____ Energy _____ Minerals _____ Vitamins _____ Fluids _____ ml/day _____

Suggested Management:

Target Levels: kcal/d _____ Protein _____ gm
Starting Levels: kcal/d _____ Protein _____ gm
Type of Nutritional Support: Oral, Tube Feedings, IV, TPN
Diet Prescription:

Suggested Additional Studies:

Fellow/Resident/Student Signature   Faculty Attending Signature   Date

*I = Normal Range; II = Moderate Defect; III = Marked Defect; IV = Severe Defect

TABLE 1-10 MEDIAN (50th PERCENTILE) VALUES FOR TRICEPS SKIN-FOLD THICKNESS ARE 10–12 mm FOR ADULT MEN AND 17–22 mm FOR ADULT WOMEN*

Age Group	Age Midpoint, Years	No.	Arm Circumference Percentile, mm					Triceps Skin-Fold Percentiles, mm				
			5th	15th	50th	85th	95th	5th	15th	50th	85th	95th
					Males							
0.0–0.4	0.3	41	113	120	134	147	153	4	5	8	12	15
0.5–1.4	1	140	128	137	152	168	175	5	7	9	13	15
1.5–2.4	2	177	141	147	157	170	180	5	7	10	13	14
2.5–3.4	3	210	144	150	161	175	182	6	7	9	12	14
3.5–4.4	4	208	143	150	165	180	190	5	6	9	12	14
4.5–5.4	5	262	146	155	169	185	199	5	6	8	12	16
5.5–6.4	6	264	151	159	172	188	198	5	6	8	11	15
6.5–7.4	7	309	154	162	176	194	212	4	6	8	11	14
7.5–8.4	8	301	161	168	185	205	233	5	6	8	12	17
8.5–9.4	9	287	165	174	190	217	262	5	6	9	14	19
9.5–10.4	10	315	170	180	200	228	255	5	6	10	16	22
10.5–11.4	11	294	177	186	208	240	276	6	7	10	17	25
11.5–12.4	12	294	184	194	216	253	291	5	7	11	19	26
12.5–13.4	13	266	186	198	230	270	297	5	6	10	18	25
13.5–14.4	14	207	198	211	243	279	321	5	6	10	17	22
14.5–15.4	15	179	202	220	253	302	320	4	6	9	19	26
15.5–16.4	16	166	217	232	262	300	335	4	5	9	20	27
16.5–17.4	17	142	230	238	275	306	326	4	5	8	14	20
17.5–24.4	21	545	250	264	292	330	354	4	5	10	18	25
24.5–34.4	30	679	260	280	310	344	366	4	6	11	21	28
34.5–44.4	40	616	259	280	312	345	371	4	6	12	22	28

Females

Age group		n										
0.0–0.4	0.3	46	107	118	127	145	150	4	5	8	12	13
0.5–1.4	1	172	125	134	146	162	170	6	7	9	12	15
1.5–2.4	2	172	136	143	155	171	180	6	7	10	13	15
2.5–3.4	3	163	137	145	157	169	176	5	7	10	12	14
3.5–4.4	4	215	145	150	162	176	184	6	7	10	12	14
4.5–5.4	5	233	149	155	169	185	195	6	7	10	13	16
5.5–6.4	6	259	148	158	170	187	202	6	7	10	12	15
6.5–7.4	7	273	153	162	178	199	216	6	7	10	13	17
7.5–8.4	8	270	158	166	183	207	231	6	7	11	15	19
8.5–9.4	9	284	166	175	192	222	255	7	8	12	17	24
9.5–10.4	10	276	170	181	203	236	263	6	8	12	19	24
10.5–11.4	11	268	173	186	210	251	280	7	9	13	20	29
11.5–12.4	12	267	185	196	220	256	275	8	9	14	20	25
12.5–13.4	13	229	186	204	230	270	294	8	10	15	23	30
13.5–14.4	14	184	201	214	240	284	306	8	11	16	22	28
14.5–15.4	15	197	205	216	245	281	310	9	10	15	24	30
15.5–16.4	16	187	211	224	249	286	322	9	12	16	23	27
16.5–17.4	17	142	207	224	250	291	328	9	12	17	26	31
17.5–24.4	21	836	215	233	260	297	329	10	12	19	25	31
24.5–34.4	30	1153	230	243	275	324	361		14	22	29	36
34.5–44.4	40	933	232	250	286	340	374				32	39

*Frisancho, A. R., Amer. J. Clin. Nutr. 27:1052, 1974.

TABLE 1–11 COMPARISON OF DIAMETER AND CIRCUMFERENCE VALUES OF UPPER ARMS OF MALES AND FEMALES*

Percentiles for upper arm diameter and upper arm circumference for whites of the Ten-State Nutrition Survey of 1968–1970

Age Midpoint, Years**	Diameter Percentiles, mm					Arm Muscle Circumference Percentiles, mm				
	5th	15th	50th	85th	95th	5th	15th	50th	85th	95th
	Males									
0.3	26	30	34	40	42	81	94	106	125	133
1	32	34	39	44	46	100	108	123	137	146
2	35	37	40	44	46	111	117	127	138	146
3	36	38	42	46	48	114	121	132	145	152
4	38	39	43	48	50	118	124	135	151	157
5	39	41	45	50	53	121	130	141	156	166
6	40	43	47	51	53	127	134	146	159	167
7	41	43	48	52	55	130	137	151	164	173
8	44	46	50	55	59	138	144	158	174	185
9	44	46	51	58	64	138	143	161	182	200
10	45	48	53	59	64	142	152	168	186	202
11	48	50	55	62	67	150	158	174	194	211
12	49	52	58	66	70	153	163	181	207	221
13	51	54	62	71	77	159	169	195	224	242
14	53	58	67	74	84	167	182	211	234	265
15	55	59	70	80	86	173	185	220	252	271
16	59	65	73	83	89	186	205	229	260	281
17	66	69	78	86	92	206	217	245	271	290
21	69	74	82	91	97	217	232	258	286	305
30	70	77	86	94	100	220	241	270	295	315
40	71	76	86	96	101	222	239	270	300	318

Females

Age										
0.3	27	29	33	37	40	86	92	104	115	126
1	31	32	37	41	43	97	102	117	128	135
2	34	36	40	44	46	105	112	125	140	146
3	34	37	41	44	46	108	116	128	138	143
4	36	38	42	46	48	114	120	132	146	152
5	38	40	44	48	51	119	124	138	151	160
6	38	41	45	49	53	121	129	140	155	165
7	39	42	47	52	56	123	132	146	162	175
8	41	44	48	53	59	129	138	151	168	186
9	43	45	50	56	62	136	143	157	176	193
10	44	47	52	58	62	139	147	163	182	196
11	44	48	55	62	67	140	152	171	195	209
12	48	51	57	64	68	150	161	179	200	212
13	49	53	59	66	71	155	165	185	206	225
14	53	56	61	70	74	166	175	193	221	234
15	52	55	62	70	74	163	173	195	220	232
16	54	57	64	72	83	171	178	200	227	260
17	54	56	62	71	77	171	177	196	223	241
21	54	58	65	73	80	170	183	205	229	253
30	56	60	68	78	87	177	189	213	245	272
40	57	61	69	80	89	180	192	216	250	279

*The age group and n are the same as in Table 1-10.
**Frisancho, A. R., *Amer. J. Clin. Nutr.* 27:1052, 1974.

TABLE 1–12 THE MUSCLE AREA (M_a) OF THE FOREARM CAN BE CALCULATED FROM THE ARM CIRCUMFERENCE AND THE SKIN-FOLD THICKNESS. IT PROVIDES AN OBJECTIVE INDIRECT ESTIMATE OF PROTEIN STATUS*

Age Midpoint, Years	Male Arm — Muscle Area Percentiles, mm					Female Arm — Muscle Area Percentile, mm				
	5th	15th	50th	85th	95th	5th	15th	50th	85th	95th
0.3	522	703	892	1,244	1,414	591	670	866	1,058	1,272
1	791	928	1,201	1,500	1,690	756	821	1,084	1,304	1,460
2	978	1,082	1,284	1,525	1,686	885	991	1,241	1,551	1,693
3	1,027	1,163	1,384	1,670	1,842	928	1,068	1,298	1,516	1,628
4	1,106	1,224	1,451	1,805	1,973	1,040	1,143	1,390	1,693	1,828
5	1,171	1,342	1,579	1,930	2,193	1,119	1,227	1,516	1,825	2,045
6	1,275	1,435	1,700	2,019	2,220	1,163	1,333	1,563	1,902	2,174
7	1,342	1,485	1,815	2,152	2,386	1,213	1,384	1,700	2,096	2,433
8	1,506	1,647	1,987	2,398	2,729	1,322	1,513	1,818	2,239	2,758
9	1,522	1,637	2,074	2,645	3,188	1,473	1,625	1,955	2,477	2,978
10	1,608	1,832	2,239	2,753	3,239	1,528	1,727	2,115	2,637	3,066
11	1,801	1,987	2,406	3,000	3,544	1,551	1,842	2,335	3,018	3,486
12	1,874	2,126	2,603	3,401	3,902	1,781	2,052	2,558	3,183	3,582
13	2,012	2,273	3,013	3,998	4,661	1,905	2,178	2,711	3,382	4,014
14	2,231	2,645	3,544	4,358	5,601	2,186	2,430	2,952	3,883	4,358
15	2,375	2,729	3,867	5,060	5,826	2,126	2,387	3,031	3,838	4,279
16	2,741	3,331	4,184	5,363	6,266	2,316	2,510	3,198	4,096	5,386
17	3,373	3,743	4,771	5,826	6,713	2,289	2,502	3,058	3,968	4,612
21	3,748	4,273	5,315	6,529	7,411	2,466	2,679	3,341	4,164	5,089
30	3,837	4,634	5,802	6,912	7,918	2,486	2,856	3,606	4,772	5,889
40	3,938	4,563	5,820	7,183	8,041	2,566	2,926	3,724	4,991	6,195

*Frisancho, A. R., *Amer. J. Clin. Nutr.* 27:1052, 1974.

their patients, utilizing all of the facilities available to them. For example, several studies have indicated that malnutrition in the elderly also affects the rate of synthesis of protein and, consequently, the rate of growth of hair. Many elderly people, both men and women, lose much of their scalp hair. Malnutrition probably contributes to this loss. In addition, there is growing evidence that even moderate degrees of malnutrition impair the immunologic mechanisms of the body (Law et al., 1973). Indeed, the nutritional status of the elderly patient represents an area that has not been adequately explored. But attention to the principles cited above will provide an awareness of the common problems and a beginning of efforts to solve them.

SUMMARY

The nutritional status of patients, both ambulatory and hospitalized, can be estimated with a growing degree of confidence. The tools and techniques available for performing such estimates have been described in the foregoing paragraphs. It is not difficult to apply these techniques, nor do they consume a great deal of time. Furthermore, aside from the special laboratory procedures, the means for evaluating nutritional status are not expensive. Nutritional evaluations should become an integral part of the assessment of every patient, whether in the physician's office, in a hospital clinic, or in a hospital bed. The precision and accuracy of such assessment will depend in large measure upon the number of tests and procedures employed. Dependence upon one or two measurements carries a high probability of error, whereas evaluation of six or eight parameters greatly increases the likelihood of an accurate assessment of nutritional status. As additional experience with these techniques is gained, their true place in the practice of medicine will become obvious.

REFERENCES

Anderson, M. A.: Use of height-arm circumference measurement for nutritional selectivity in Sri Lanka school feeding. *Amer. J. Clin. Nutr. 28*:775, 1975.
Bistrian, B. R., Blackburn, G. L., Vitale, J., Cochran, D., and Naylor, J.: Prevalence of malnutrition in general medicine patients. *J.A.M.A. 235*:1567, 1976.
Butterworth, C. E., and Blackburn, G. L.: Hospital malnutrition. *Nutr. Today 10*:8, 1975.
Fomon, S. J. (Ed.): *Infant Nutrition.* Second edition. Philadelphia, W. B. Saunders Company, 1974.
Heald, F. P. (Ed.): *Adolescent Nutrition and Growth.* New York, Appleton-Century-Crofts, 1969.
Heald, F. P.: New reference points for defining adolescent nutrient requirements (loc. cit.). Chapter 16 in *Nutrient Requirements in Adolescence*, McKigney, J. I. and Munro, H. N. (eds.). Cambridge, MA, The MIT Press, 1976.

Hodges, R. E., and Krehl, W. A.: Nutritional status of teenagers in Iowa. *Amer. J. Clin. Nutr. 17*:200, 1965.

Hodges, R. E.: Vitamin and mineral requirements in adolescence (loc. cit.). Chapter 7 in *Nutrient Requirements in Adolescence*, McKigney, J. I. and Munro, H. N. (eds.). Cambridge, MA, The MIT Press, 1976.

Jelliffe, E. R. P., and Jelliffe, D. B.: The arm circumference as a public health index of protein-calorie malnutriton of early childhood. *J. Trop. Pediat. 15*:176, 1969.

Jordan, V. E.: Protein status of the elderly as measured by dietary intake, hair tissue, and serum albumin. *Amer. J. Clin. Nutr. 29*:522, 1976.

Law, D. L., Dudrick, S. J., and Abdou, N. I.: Immunocompetence of patients with protein-calorie malnutrition — the effects of nutritional repletion. *Ann. Intern. Med. 79*:545, 1973.

Lutwak, L.: Metabolic and biochemical considerations of bone. *Ann. Clin. Lab. Sci. 5*:185, 1975.

Martorell, R., Yarbrough, C., Lechtig, A., Delgado, H., and Klein, R. E.: Upper arm anthropometric indicators of nutritional status. *Amer. J. Clin. Nutr. 29*:46, 1976.

McGanity, W. J.: Problems of nutritional evaluation of the adolescent. Chapter 9 in *Nutrient Requirements in Adolescence*, McKigney, J. I. and Munro, H. N. (eds.). Cambridge, MA, The MIT Press, 1976.

Pearson, W. N.: The biochemical appraisal of nutritional status (loc. cit.). Chapter 6 in *Adolescent Nutrition and Growth*, Heald, F. P. (ed.). New York, Appleton-Century-Crofts, 1969.

Sauberlich, H. E., Dowdy, R. P., and Skala, J. H. (editors): *Laboratory Tests for the Assessment of Nutritional Status*. Cleveland, CRC Press, 1974.

Schrott, H. G., Goldstein, J. L., Hazzard, W. R., McGoodwin, M. M., and Motulsky, A. G.: Familial hypercholesterolemia in a large kindred: Evidence for a monogenic mechanism. *Ann. Intern. Med. 76*:711, 1972.

Stitt, F. W., Clayton, D. G., Crawford, M. D., and Morris, J. N.: Clinical and biochemical indicators of cardiovascular disease among men living in hard and soft water areas. *Lancet 1*:122, 1973.

2

NUTRITION IN PREGNANCY AND LACTATION

Robert E. Hodges, M.D.

Until quite recently, nutrition in pregnancy was confined to the domain of dietitians, a handful of nutritionists, and a smaller number of obstetricians who recognized the full potential of this topic. Since 1970, a number of things have happened to bring nutrition into closer focus, and to emphasize its role in the reproductive processes.

Much of the impetus came from the Committee on Maternal Nutrition of the Food and Nutrition Board (1970), which published a realistic evaluation of the situation at that time and made strong recommendations, a number of which were contrary to common obstetrical practice. Shortly thereafter, Pitkin, who had been striving to emphasize the importance of nutrition for pregnant women, stated, "The physician responsible for the care of pregnant women often finds himself in a difficult position. His knowledge of nutrition in general is deficient and formal instruction in the nutritional principles is notably absent from medical school curricula and graduate programs." This continues to be true today, although nutritional management of pregnancy has changed substantially in the past decade. Nonetheless, many older physicians still cling to their previous concepts and, as a result, many of their patients are understandably confused by conflicting advice. Recently, the lay press has given a surprising amount of emphasis to nutritional factors in the health and welfare of humankind. This has stimulated many young women to seek specific nutritional advice about the best diet for pregnancy. The following information will provide not only a brief review of the origin of some of the deeply ingrained ideas about nutrition in pregnancy, but also physiological facts based upon both animal experimentation and epidemiologic studies of human populations.

Many of today's practicing obstetricians learned in medical school that women should not be allowed to gain too much weight during pregnancy because excessive weight gain not only increased obstetrical problems, such as uterine inertia and prolonged labor, but also predisposed such women to preeclampsia and eclampsia. Furthermore, it was commonly believed that an excessive intake of salt favored the development of hypertension and preeclampsia. These ideas apparently arose as a result of studies done in Germany during and shortly after World War I (Warnekros, 1916; and Gessner, 1921). These two clinicians, among others, observed that during the period of wartime shortages, the incidence of eclampsia decreased very significantly, only to return to the previous levels after the close of the war (Table 2–1). Warnekros and others noted that the reduction in the incidence of eclampsia was greatest in the city hospitals but was minimal or lacking in rural areas. They assumed that the difference lay in the relative availability of food throughout the countryside, and the relative scarcity of food in the cities. This was especially true of meats and fats, and so Warnekros recommended that pregnant women restrict these items in their diets, and emphasize foods of plant origin. Gessner, on the other hand, was less impressed by the effects of diet, and surmised that, during wartime, women had to perform more physical activity, and so reduced their body fat. In all likelihood, neither of these explanations was correct. Wartime Germany was a country without public transportation, because railroads were fully committed to the war effort; and there were no buses and very few private automobiles. Furthermore, roadways were largely unpaved and became virtually impassable for all except horses. Few pregnant women, especially those experiencing the symptoms of preeclampsia, would be willing to ride many miles on horseback in order to be delivered at a hospital. It seems probable that the pregnant women who were having difficulties elected to stay at home rather than undertake such a journey.

Nonetheless, the statistics reported by these German obstetricians had a profound impact upon the feeding of pregnant women for half a century, not only in Germany but throughout the world.

Pregnancy is a normal physiologic event which should be given every opportunity to be successful. Recent animal studies indicate that diet can have a profound effect, either good or bad, on both the fetus and the mother, but the extent of this effect depends, in part, on the relative weights of the offspring and the mother (Table 2–2).

TABLE 2–1 TOXEMIA OF PREGNANCY IN GERMAN HOSPITALS

YEAR	UNIVERSITY FRAUENKLINIK			CHARITY, BERLIN			RUDOLPH-VIRCHOW HOSPITAL			BADEN AREA		
	Births	Eclampsia	%	Births	Eclampsia	%	Births	Eclampsia	%	Births	Eclampsia	%
1910	1,476	62	4.2	—	—	—	—	—	—	65,583	98	0.15
1911	1,775	56	3.1	—	—	—	—	—	—	63,031	104	0.16
1912	1,868	59	3.2	3,320	78	2.4	2,942	57	2.0	63,308	103	0.16
1913	2,004	52	2.6	3,570	84	2.4	3,464	42	1.2	60,901	119	0.20
1914	1,994	51	2.6	3,350	66	2.0	3,496	40	1.2	60,621	103	0.17
1915	1,794	32	1.8	2,518	36	1.4	3,511	42	1.2	45,643	58	0.13
1916	1,430	12	0.8	1,400	8	0.57	2,462	25	1.0	32,358	42	0.13
1917	—	—	—	—	—	—	—	—	—	29,779	24	0.08
1918	—	—	—	—	—	—	—	—	—	30,546	20	0.06
1919	—	—	—	—	—	—	—	—	—	47,240	70	0.15

Leading obstetrical authorities attributed these results to diminished food intake, particularly less protein and fat. This was the origin of the concept that pregnant women should limit their intake of animal proteins and restrict calories to avoid excessive weight gain. Actually the data above demonstrate the effect of poor transportation on the type of patients entering obstetrical hospitals during the war years. The sickest patients remained home.

TABLE 2–2   WEIGHT OF MOTHER AND OFFSPRING
OF VARIOUS SPECIES

SPECIES	MATERNAL WEIGHT kg	BIRTH WEIGHT SINGLE FETUS kg	USUAL NUMBER OF YOUNG	TOTAL BIRTH WEIGHT AS % MATERNAL WEIGHT
Human	56	3.2	1	5.7
Monkey (Rhesus)	8	0.5	1	6.3
Pig	130	1.2	8	6.8
Sheep (Hampshire)	70	4.0	2	11.4
Cat	3	0.1	4	13.2
Rabbit	2.5	0.05	7	14.0
Dog (Beagle)	8.4	0.27	5	16.1
Rat	0.15	0.005	7	23.4
Guinea Pig	0.7	0.085	3	36.3
Mouse	0.03	0.014	8	37.3

Partly as a result of the usual single offspring, humans have a relatively low fetal-to-maternal weight ratio. Consequently, the effects of maternal malnutrition during pregnancy would be expected to be more severe in lesser animals whose fetal-to-maternal ratio may rise as high as 37 per cent. This helps to explain the ease with which evidence of the adverse effects of maternal malnutrition can be demonstrated in rats and other small animals. (Modified from Dawes, G. W.: *Fetal and Neonatal Physiology: A Comparative Study of the Changes at Birth.* Year Book Medical Publishers, Inc., Chicago, 1969.)

MATERNAL NUTRITION

Recent studies of the nutritional status of pregnant animals have clearly demonstrated certain principles. Contrary to the previous belief that protein was all-important in pregnancy, it now appears that total energy is equally important. Studies done in rats (Widdowson and Cowen, 1972) showed that restriction of protein or limitation of calories delayed puberty, reduced fertility, and resulted in smaller numbers of animals in the litters. It also interfered with lactation. When malnutrion was very severe, puberty was greatly delayed but if young animals were fed an excellent diet and fully rehabilitated, their reproductive performance was essentially normal. In other experiments, undernutrition of pregnant rats or mice decreased the ultimate body weight of the offspring and caused various abnormalities, including deficient renal tubular function and retarded neuromotor development. Furthermore, it was observed that these offspring had impaired learning capacities (Roeder and Chow, 1972).

The effects of undernutrition during pregnancy have triggered a series of investigations and epidemiologic studies, chiefly because of the possibility that permanent impairment of intelligence or performance may result. Nutritionists, epidemiologists, and not a few politicians were quick to realize the potential significance of these findings. If women were subjected to poverty and malnutrition during pregnancy, would they give birth to inferior children? This question remains at least partially unanswered, but the available evidence will be presented and discussed.

Nutritional deficits other than those involving the total amount of food or the amount of protein can have equally devastating effects upon the progeny. Studies in rats have demonstrated that although a complete deficit of almost any essential nutrient may disrupt pregnancy, there are several essential nutrients which are especially important to the developing embryo. Even mild maternal deficiencies which do not produce serious illness or gross manifestations of deficiency are still enough to cause marked defects in the developing offspring. Deficiency of vitamin A can cause abnormalities in the development of the eyes, deficiency of folic acid may result in abnormalities of the mouth and throat, and deficiency of pantothenic acid may result in embryonic death or deformity such as exencephalia. Lack of riboflavin in the maternal diet can cause such malformations as cleft palate, hypoplasia of the mandible, and shortening of the limbs (Giroud, 1970). But deficiency of zinc is perhaps one of the most teratogenic situations discovered experimentally. Pregnant rats that are deficient in zinc have babies with severe developmental defects, especially of the extremities (Hurley et al., 1968). These are only a few of the examples of the potential damage that can result from even a brief and relatively mild deficiency of an essential nutrient. This list is by no means all-inclusive but it does include some of the worst offenders.

But nutritional problems that impair the outcome of pregnancy are by no means limited to deficiency syndromes. On the other side of the coin, there are numerous animal experiments that demonstrate potential damage to the embryo or fetus after the mother has been given excessive doses of certain nutrients. Overdosing a pregnant animal with vitamin A will have teratogenic effects (Kalter and Warkany, 1961). Similarly, an overdose of vitamin D can result in supravalvular aortic stenosis in guinea pigs, and presumably also in humans (Friedman and Roberts, 1966). Toxicity from overdosage with these two fat-soluble vitamins has been recognized for many years. But a surprising development is evidence that overdosing a pregnant animal with vitamin C may have disastrous effects upon the developing offspring. A rather poorly documented article described the induction of elective abortion by giving large doses of vitamin C orally to women who were presumed to be pregnant (Samborskaya and Ferdman, 1966). This becomes more believable when one considers studies performed in animals suggesting that hypervitaminosis C may cause embryonic deformity or fetal death (Mouriquand and Edel, 1953; Neuweiler, 1951); and in the area of human reproduction, a Canadian observed that ingestion of excessive amounts of vitamin C by the mother can result in a vitamin-dependent situation wherein the offspring have an abnormally high requirement for the vitamin (Cochrane, 1965).

Among the more important developments in the area of nutrition and reproduction is the recognition of a relationship between the timing of malnutrition and its impact upon developing organ systems, especially the brain. Although every student of embryology learns that a developing organism does so by proliferating cells rapidly (hyperplasia), and later by enlargement of those cells (hypertrophy), it did not become obvious for some time why various studies of malnutrition in pregnant animals produced disparate results.

A series of investigations in experimental animals led to clarification of the mechanisms involved (Winick and Noble, 1966; Winick, 1971; Levitsky et al., 1975). The impact of these observations was well summarized in a recent editorial which said, "Work with laboratory animals of various species has related malnutrition early in life to impaired brain growth and altered behavior later. . . . The social and political implications of such a situation are enormous." (Editorial: "Nutrition and the developing brain," 1972).

In 1973, the Swedish Nutrition Foundation held a symposium entitled "Early Malnutrition and Mental Development". The impact of this symposium was summarized in part: " . . . in spite of widely publicized opinion that malnutrition in early life jeopardizes mental development, the evidence to support this opinion . . . is scanty." "What seems probable is that there is an interaction between malnutrition and other environmental factors, especially social stimulation. . . . " (Barnes, 1976).

HUMAN STUDIES

For obvious reasons, human studies are very difficult to design and conduct. It becomes necessary to rely upon retrospective analysis of growth development and performance of populations that have suffered from some natural disaster such as drought, famine, or pestilence, or in a few instances, from the ravages of war. Some studies have compared the effects of maternal dietary practices with the outcome of pregnancy (Burke et al., 1943). In a group of 216 pregnant women whose diets were evaluated, only 14 per cent were judged to be excellent or good, whereas 17 per cent were considered poor or very poor. The state of health of the newborn infants was judged by examining pediatricians. Twenty-three of the 216 infants were judged to be in superior condition, whereas 33 were considered to be in the poorest group. This included infants with congenital malformations or with obvious prematurity. The mothers of children judged to be superior were found to be the same ones who generally consumed a good or excellent diet (56 per cent), compared with only 3 per cent of the mothers who gave birth to the poorest children. Conversely, only 9 per cent of the mothers whose offspring were judged to be superior consumed a poor or very poor diet, whereas 79 per cent of the mothers who produced the poorest children consumed a poor or very poor diet. This study certainly paved the way for a change in the prevailing attitude about the importance of maternal diet with regard to the welfare of the offspring.

Other studies of population groups added weight to the idea that maternal nutrition has a direct impact upon the welfare of the off-spring and is not concerned merely with the health of the mother. Throughout the world, obstetricians pondered their statistics and found that the results did not agree with the old dictum that the developing fetus is a "perfect parasite." Indeed, it became obvious that there is a relationship between maternal weight gain during pregnancy and the birth weight and growth and development of the infant (Singer et al., 1968). Furthermore, there is a positive relationship not only between the weight gain of the mother during pregnancy, but also her pre-pregnancy weight and the birth weight of the child (Niswander, 1969). And most importantly, it was shown conclusively that the birth weight of the child and its fetal age are related to perinatal mortality; the smaller the child, the greater the risk (Susser et al., 1972).

Some of the most convincing reports arose from wartime starvation. Probably the most severe degree of starvation occurred during the siege of Leningrad when the Germans protracted an attack over a period of 18 months. The city was encircled between August, 1941, and January of 1943. A careful analysis of the obstetrical records collected during the calendar year 1942 yields much valuable information (Antonov, 1947). The people suffered from severe and sustained hunger, relying during much of the period of time upon insufficient amounts of bread, which was itself of very poor quality. Even if one assumes that this bread had about 250 Kcal/100 gm (and it probably was considerably less), manual workers were receiving only 750 to 1250 Kcal/day and "mental" workers received about 50 to 60 per cent of that amount. The impact of this prolonged starvation was very obvious in women and their offspring. There was a sharp fall in the birthrate and amenorrhea was widely prevalent. In a major obstetrical clinic only 79 women were delivered during the second half of 1942, and there was reason to believe that their nutritional intake had been substantially better than that of most women in Leningrad. Fourteen of these women were employed in food industries, six were receiving military rations, and 17 were physicians, nurses, teachers, or other professionals. Nonetheless, the effect of malnutrition was quite apparent in these women and their offspring. During the first half of 1942, the stillbirth rate rose to 5.6 per cent, and the rate of premature births reached 41 per cent. Even children born at term had a considerable decrease in average birth weight, amounting to 500 to 600 gm less than normal. The physiologic loss of weight of newborn children continued for a longer period than usual and newborn infants were generally considered to be of low vitality. The morbidity of newborns was 32.3 per cent and the mortality was high: nine per cent of those born at term and 30.8 per cent of those born prematurely. Surprisingly, the capacity for breast feeding persisted even in severe degrees of starvation, but less milk was produced and breast feeding was considerably shorter than normal. The author contradicted the old idea that the fetus is a perfect parasite and recognized the need for adequate nutrition of pregnant women.

Another example of wartime famine was studied in Holland, where the Nazis inflicted starvation upon the Dutch people for a period of about six months during the "hunger winter" of 1944 to 1945. Early assessment of the effects of this period of starvation upon reproduction yielded some surprising results (Smith, 1947). Severe undernutrition resulted in amenorrhea in about 50 per cent of women and some menstrual abnormalities in an additional 20 per cent. Those women who did conceive were judged to be not essentially different from those who did not. In instances where the mother was deprived of adequate food during the third trimester of pregnancy, the birth weight and birth length were significantly reduced. Toxemia of pregnancy was not increased and may have been slightly decreased, and congenital malformations were slightly but not significantly increased. There was no significant effect upon the incidence of stillbirths or of neonatal deaths. Lactation was not significantly altered.

A quarter of a century after the first evaluation of the Dutch hunger winter another group of investigators (Stein et al., 1975) undertook a reassessment of the effects of famine upon the children born during that period of time. They were particularly interested in obtaining information relating to the possible effects of intra-uterine malnutrition upon the intelligence and performance of the offspring. Their studies were limited to male offspring because the Dutch had detailed records on individuals who had participated in universal military training, thus providing data on height, weight, and other health characteristics, as well as background information about the educational level, the civilian occupation and the approximate income of each individual. Presumably, these parameters would provide considerable information regarding the intelligence and level of performance of individuals. The results of this study were quite unanticipated. They found that the prevalence of anomalies of the central nervous system such as spina bifida, hydrocephalus, and cerebral palsy *was* increased in those individuals whose intra-uterine exposure to malnutrition occurred early in gestation. Fetal growth was also altered, in that birth weight and placental weight were reduced significantly, whereas birth length and head circumference were affected only slightly. These effects of prenatal nutrition on fetal growth were confined to deprivation during the third trimester of gestation. Prenatal deprivation in the third trimester also increased early mortality of infants. In fact, infant mortality after three months was extremely high among cohorts born during the famine period. Despite these findings, the authors failed to detect any effects of prenatal exposure to famine on the mental competence or state of health of adult survivors. They postulated that one of several factors might have produced this outcome: first, that brain impairment and potential mental impairment were removed by coincident excess mortality; second, that learning might compensate for depressed mental function; and third, that the normal brain possesses a sufficiently large reserve of brain cells that it is protected from functional impairment even in the face of substantial depletion. The authors favored this last explanation.

Although the hardships suffered by the Dutch were extremely difficult to bear, it seems obvious that their period of deprivation was of much shorter duration and probably of lesser intensity than that experienced by the residents of Leningrad. Furthermore, like the women of Leningrad, there undoubtedly were people in the Dutch community who managed to get additional supplies of food. If one considers the fact that the vast majority of young and middle-aged men in the Dutch community either had left Holland voluntarily to join the Allied forces or had been sent by the Germans to work in factories in Germany, it then becomes obvious that at least some of the pregnancies resulted from liaisons with German military personnel, and it is not too difficult to imagine that in some instances, the Germans provided items of food to their paramours.

A totally unexpected development was the observation by this same group of investigators (Ravelli et al., 1976) that the fatness or leanness of young men exposed to famine in utero and in early infancy was significantly affected. Exposure to famine during the last trimester of pregnancy and the first few months of life significantly lowered obesity rates, presumably because nutritional deprivation during the period of adipose tissue hyperplasia resulted in fewer adipose tissue cells. By contrast, exposure of the mother to famine during the first half of pregnancy resulted in significantly higher rates of subsequent obesity in her offspring. The authors postulated that this might have resulted from nutritional deprivation that affected the developing hypothalamic centers that regulate food intake and growth. Whatever the explanation, the data are very convincing.

ENERGY REQUIREMENTS DURING PREGNANCY

Old ideas die slowly, so it is not surprising that many pregnant women and not a few physicians still regard pregnancy as some form of illness. We cannot overemphasize the fact that normal *pregnancy is a healthful, physiologic event*, but it does require additional food; yet this does not endorse the old adage that a woman "is eating for two"; a concept that may have contributed more than its share to another old adage that a woman puts on ten pounds with each pregnancy. Actually, careful attention to diet will not only ensure that the developing fetus will have an excellent chance for normal development, birth, and survival, but it will also protect the mother from becoming depleted of essential nutrients or from depositing unwanted and unnecessary fat. The question is: how much is enough? The following information will provide guidelines and specific facts that permit accurate calculation of the needs of individual patients, whether they are adult or adolescent, tall or short, lean or obese.

With the onset of pregnancy many women, perhaps most, develop peculiar sensations and altered appetites. The "craving" for unusual foods is no myth. Primigravidas were found to have cravings for fruit or highly flavored foods. Aversions are also common early in pregnancy. These may be directed against fried foods, tea, coffee, and other commonly accepted foods (Taggart, 1961). But at the same time, most pregnant women experience an increase in appetite that may become manifest moments after a wave of nausea. This increase in appetite, unfortunately, cannot be relied upon to determine how much additional food a pregnant woman should eat. Instead, the physician must have certain guidelines to aid in making dietary recommendations. The first of these is to measure the patient's height and weight. The weight can be compared with standard height/weight charts, or it can be approximated by using the rule of thumb that allows 105 pounds for the first 5 feet of height and an additional 5 pounds for each additional inch. This method overestimates the weight of short women by approximately 5 to 10 pounds.

Some estimate of the woman's level of physical activity can be obtained by asking a few simple questions regarding the number of children in the household and their ages, the amount of walking, household chores, and other forms of physical activity she performs, and whether she is employed outside the home. Most women reduce their level of physical activity as they become heavier during the third trimester. A young adult woman who is reasonably active will need about 35 Kcal/kg of normal body weight when she is in the nonpregnant state. During pregnancy her energy requirement will increase to about 40 Kcal/kg of her nonpregnant body weight. For younger women, and especially for adolescent girls, the energy requirement, like other nutrient needs, is substantially greater. Reference to the 1974 Tables of Recommended Daily Dietary Allowances (Food and Nutrition Board, National Academy of Sciences, National Research Council) (Table 2–3) allows the physician or dietitian to approximate the energy needs, the protein requirements, and the amounts of essential vitamins and minerals needed by virtually any pregnant woman, assuming that allowance is made for differences in height and weight. For example, a young woman aged 20 who is 5'5" tall, would be expected by rule of thumb to weigh about 130 pounds. According to the RDA tables, her normal weight would be 128 pounds, or 58 kg. Her energy requirement would be 2100 Kcal in the nonpregnant state, and 2400 Kcal when she is pregnant.

The additional energy required during pregnancy is needed, of course, for the growth and development of the fetus, but it also must supply the mother with the nutrients necessary to permit a number of physiological adaptations to the pregnant state. By the end of 40 weeks of pregnancy she will have gained an average of 12.5 kg. The fetus will weigh about 3.3 kg, the placenta about 0.6 kg, and the amniotic fluid about 0.8 kg. Maternal weight gain consists of enlargment of the uterus, 0.9 kg; enlargement of the breasts, 0.4 kg; and expansion of the maternal blood, 1.25 kg. This leaves a balance of about 5 kg that is not otherwise accounted for. This additional weight can be explained by the deposition of adipose tissue during pregnancy, and by slight retention of fluid throughout the tissues.

A common recommendation for the energy requirements during pregnancy is an additional 300 Kcal/day. This probably represents a modest surplus during the first three months of pregnancy and a modest deficit during the last three months of pregnancy. An easier and more physiologic approach is for the physician to plot the patient's actual weight at the time of each office visit on a graph similar to the accompanying graph (Figure 2–1). This shows the normal prenatal gain in weight of healthy, pregnant women. Of course, many individual patients will fall above or below this line, but their weight curve *should parallel* this line very closely. If a patient was initially instructed to eat a diet that met her non-pregnant requirements and added approximately 300 additional Kcal of energy she might gain a bit too rapidly at first and be advised to reduce her food intake by about 200 Kcal/day (roughly equivalent to 3 slices of bread per day). If, on the other hand, during the second trimester of pregnancy she was found to be gaining a bit too slowly she might be advised to add approximately 200 Kcal of food per day to her regular diet. The physician faces one of his or her most difficult tasks when confronted by a pregnant woman who is grossly overweight and who asks for a reducing diet during pregnancy. The best advice is for this patient to

TABLE 2–3 RECOMMENDED DIETARY ALLOWANCES*

	"NONPREGNANT FEMALES"				Pregnancy	Lactation
	11–14 yr†	15–18 yr†	19–22 yr§	23–50 yr§		
Energy (Kcal)	2400	2100	2100	2000	+300	+500
Protein (gm)	44	48	46	46	+30	+20
Vitamin A (I.U.)	4000	4000	4000	4000	5000	6000
Vitamin D (I.U.)	400	400	400	–	400	400
Vitamin E (I.U.)	12	12	12	12	15	15
Ascorbic acid (mg)	45	45	45	45	60	80
Folacin (μg)	400	400	400	400	800	600
Niacin (mg)	16	14	14	13	+2	+4
Riboflavin (mg)	1.3	1.4	1.4	1.2	+0.3	+0.5
Thiamin (mg)	1.2	1.1	1.1	1.0	+0.3	+0.3
Vitamin B_6 (mg)	1.6	2.0	2.0	2.0	2.5	2.5
Vitamin B_{12} (μg)	3	3	3	3	4	4
Calcium (mg)	1200	1200	800	800	1200	1200
Phosphorus (mg)	1200	1200	800	800	1200	1200
Iodine (μg)	115	115	100	100	125	150
Iron (mg)	18	18	18	18	¶	18
Magnesium (mg)	300	300	300	300	450	450
Zinc (mg)	15	15	15	15	20	25

* Food and Nutrition Board, National Academy of Sciences – National Research Council, Eighth Edition 1974.
† Weight 44 kg (97 lb), Height 155 cm (62 in).
‡ Weight 54 kg (119 lb), Height 162 cm (65 in).
§ Weight 58 kg (128 lb), Height 162 cm (65 in).
¶ The increased requirements of pregnancy cannot usually be met by ordinary diets; therefore, the use of supplement iron is recommended.

WEIGHT GAIN IN NORMAL PREGNANCY

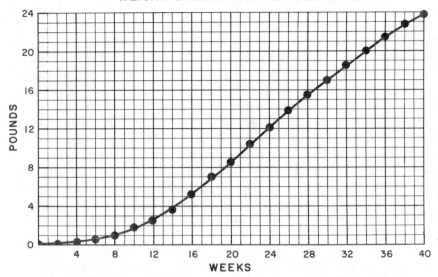

Figure 2–1 Weight gain in normal pregnancy. A normal pregnant woman of average height can be expected to gain only a few pounds during the first 3 months of pregnancy. But her weight gain will be almost linear between the 12th and the 40th weeks. Any major departure from this pattern of weight gain is cause for alarm. A dietary evaluation and a complete medical reexamination should be done promptly.

Even women who weigh much more or much less than average when nonpregnant can be expected to have a weight gain curve that has the same configuration as that shown above. This includes obese woman: pregnancy is not a good time to lose weight. Modified from figure published by U.S. Department of Health, Education, and Welfare, Social and Rehabilitation Service, Children's Bureau.

eat a well-balanced, healthful diet that permits her to *gain* weight at the same rate as any other pregnant woman until she delivers. Following pregnancy, appropriate dietary changes can assist her to lose weight. Pregnancy should *never* be considered a time for weight reduction.

The average pregnant woman did not plan on becoming pregnant on a specified date, and so did not see her obstetrician for an antenatal examination, nor did she attempt to follow an optimal diet for reproduction. Most women consult their physician after missing two or more menstrual periods. When told she is pregnant, a primipara usually asks for dietary advice. This is a unique opportunity for the physician to provide not only the patient, but also her family, with lasting nutritional principles because if the woman herself selects and prepares nutritious, well-balanced meals, her family will eat the same food. If, on the other hand, she subsists on "fast foods", snacks, and hastily prepared meals, both she and other members of her family are apt to have less than optimal nutrition. It therefore behooves the obstetrician to devote enough time to each new obstetrical patient to be sure that she understands a few basic principles. Many physicians find it helpful to have a dietitian talk with each patient, take a dietary history, and make adjustments in the food patterns when appropriate. One of the most important principles, however, is to avoid trying to inflict an unpalatable diet upon the pregnant woman. Unless her diet is completely unacceptable, she should be encouraged to persist in her customary food practices whenever possible, and changes should be made in a constructive fashion. For example, a woman of Latin-American origin who is particularly fond of Mexican food might find the typical American diet of meat, potatoes, vegetable, salad, and dessert to be unappetizing and unduly expensive. Similarly, an Oriental woman might prefer Chinese or Japanese cooking to the classic American cuisine. Nonetheless, the basic principles of the four major food groups can be applied to virtually every patient. These groups, of course, are (1) meats, fish, and poultry, or meat substitutes (cheese, eggs, nuts, peas and beans), (2) fresh fruits and vegetables (including one each of citrus fruits, green leafy vegetables, and deep yellow vegetables), (3) breads and cereals, and (4) milk (unless the individual is lactose intolerant) and milk products. The additional calories needed by a pregnant woman are best supplied in the form of larger servings of some of the food groups mentioned above, rather than in the form of concentrated carbohydrates.

PROTEIN ALLOWANCES

No one would deny that the pregnant woman needs additional protein during pregnancy in order to provide the amino acids necessary for the developing fetus, for the placenta and amniotic fluid, and for maternal changes, including enlargement of breasts and uterus and expansion of the blood volume. The amount of additional protein is still debated by experts. For example, studies performed in Guatemala showed that food supplements of either protein-containing foods or foods that provided additional energy were equally effective when given to pregnant women whose diets were obviously inadequate. Both types of supplements increased the weight of newborn children (Lechtig et al., 1974). The Recommended Dietary Allowances published by the National Academy of Sciences in 1968 suggested that a pregnant woman should be given an additional 10 gm of protein (in addition to the nonpregnant level of 65 gm). But the 1974 Recommended Dietary Allowances have decreased the nonpregnant protein allowance to 46 gm and increased the pregnant allowance to 30 gm, thus increasing the overall protein allowance from 65 gm to 76 gm/day. It is difficult to establish actual needs in humans and, in all probability, future committees of experts will change this recommendation. For the time being, however, an allowance of 76 gm seems to be ample. The average, well-balanced American diet contains slightly more than 30 gm of protein per 1000 Kcal, and so the woman who is consuming the recommended 2400 Kcal daily will receive an adequate amount. Once again, the increased amount of protein should be provided by a variety of foods of good quality. The old adage that a pregnant woman should "drink an extra quart of milk a day" is not very good advice, even though this would provide her with slightly more than the additional 30 gm of protein recommended per day. Whole milk contains more than twice the additional calories she needs, but even nonfat milk, which supplies fewer calories, is not ideal because some women are lactose intolerant (especially Blacks, Chicanos, American Indians, and Orientals), and will not drink large amounts of milk because of abdominal cramping, flatulence, and sometimes diarrhea. Furthermore, milk, although it is an excellent source of calcium, contains very little iron. Every pregnant woman who can tolerate milk should be encouraged to drink at least two 8 oz. glasses per day, but she should increase her use of other protein-containing foods at the same time.

CALCIUM ALLOWANCES

Calcium allowances represent another controversial topic. The recommended intake of calcium for nonpregnant women in the United States has been 800 mg for a number of years, whereas the majority of the world's populations consume about half this amount or even less. Yet pregnant women in such countries produce babies that seem to be as well developed as American babies, and the skeleton and teeth of the mothers are equally well calcified. We recommend that the pregnant American woman receive an additional 50 per cent increase for a total of 1200 mg of calcium, but at the same time we recommend an intake of 1200 mg of phosphorus. This one-to-one ratio of calcium to phosphorus may be more important than we have realized previously. The typical American diet contains two to four times as much phosphorus as calcium, and so the Ca to P ratio is from 0.5 to 0.25. Although the mineral content of a newborn infant's body shows a ratio of Ca to P $\cong$ 0.5, there is substantial reason to believe that a ratio of 1 to 1 is much better (Lutwak, 1969).

Calcium and phosphorus may be involved in the etiology of a harmless though annoying symptom of pregnancy: leg cramps, especially during the third trimester. It has been shown that reduction of milk intake or supplementation of the diet with calcium lactate or regular ingestion of aluminum hydroxide to promote fecal excretion of phosphates can prevent or relieve many cases of leg cramps in pregnancy (Page and Page, 1953). Usually, administration of aluminum hydroxide preparations is effective and there is seldom a need to remove milk from the diet.

For women who are lactose intolerant because of genetic loss of intestinal lactase, the problem of providing ample amounts of calcium in the diet becomes more difficult. Milk and milk products are the major sources of calcium in the American diet. In primitive days, corn and other grains were hand-ground using limestone grinding implements that added small but significant amounts of calcium salts to the flour. Modern milling techniques, of course, avoid this form of "contamination." Other sources of calcium are not always readily available. For example, the calcium contained in green, leafy vegetables is essentially unavailable because these same foods contain varying amounts of oxalates which, when combined with calcium, produce insoluble salts that cannot be absorbed. Similarly, at least some of the calcium present in whole grains is lost because of phytates and other compounds that can inhibit calcium absorption. A diet containing a variety of fresh fruits and vegetables will supply moderate amounts of calcium but nowhere near the recommended intake of 1200 mg daily. The use of small fish such as sardines or mackerel should be encouraged because of the high calcium content, but few women will eat these foods regularly. Cheeses that have been produced by fermentation processes can be tolerated by most people who are lactase deficient because the lactose has been largely hydrolyzed. A recent development which has yet to be fully evaluated is the marketing of fresh milk that has been incubated with lactase in order to hydrolyze part of the lactose prior to pasteurization. (For non-dairy foods rich in calcium, see Table 2–4.)

The amount of salt that should be recommended for the diet of a pregnant woman is yet another matter for controversy. As mentioned before, obstetricians of a few decades ago strongly recommended prophylactic restriction of sodium in the diet of pregnant women, and some even advocated the routine administration of diuretics in the hope of preventing edema of pregnancy, which they assumed was a precursor of preeclampsia and eclampsia. This ignores the physiologic changes that occur in pregnancy, including an increase in the glomerular filtration rate of the kidney and a tendency toward increased reabsorption of sodium by the renal tubules. The concept that sodium restriction is helpful has recently been challenged and there is some reason to believe that it may even be harmful (Pike and Smiciklas, 1972). Probably the best advice is for the pregnant woman to use the amount of salt she is accustomed to using, unless her clinical condition dictates otherwise (Pitkin et al., 1972).

TABLE 2–4 A FEW EXAMPLES OF NON-DAIRY
FOODS RICH IN CALCIUM

	CALCIUM: mg PER AVERAGE SERVING
Cereals	
Barley cereal, Gerbers, 1 cup	231
Oatmeal, 3/4 cup	153
Barley cereal, 1 oz., dry	264
Cereal, mixed, 1 oz., dry	277
Cereal Flours	
Cornmeal, whole grain, 1 cup	354
Soy flour, low fat, 1 cup	263
Wheat flour, self-rising, enriched, 1 cup	303
Fish	
Herring, canned, solids and liquids, 3-1/2 oz.	147
Mackerel, canned, 3-1/2 oz.	260
Sardines, Atlantic, canned in oil, 3-1/2 oz.	354
Smelt, Atlantic, canned, 3-1/2 oz.	358
Fruits	
Figs, dried, 3-1/2 oz.	126
Oranges, 1 large	96
Nuts	
Almonds, unblanched, 3-1/2 oz.	254
Brazil nuts, 3-1/2 oz.	186
Legumes and Seeds	
Soybean curd (Tofu) 4 oz.	154
Beans, common, dried, 1/2 cup	144
Garbanzo beans, dried, 1/2 cup	150
Sunflower seed kernels, 3-1/2 oz.	120
Syrups and Sugars	
Molasses, cane, third extraction, blackstrap, 3-1/2 oz.	579
Maple sugar, 3-1/2 oz.	180
Vegetables	
Broccoli, cooked, 1 cup	132
Spoon cabbage, raw, 3-1/2 oz.	165
Collards, cooked, 1/2 cup	152
Dandelion greens, cooked, 1/2 cup	140
Lambsquarter, cooked, 1/2 cup	258

SPECIAL PROBLEMS IN PREGNANCY

The Toxemias of Pregnancy

The term *toxemia* is used here to denote any syndrome occurring in a pregnant woman after the 20th week of gestation and characterized by the triad of hypertension, proteinuria, and edema. Although this is not a specific diagnosis it serves to characterize a condition or group of conditions that can be life-threatening to both mother and child. As noted earlier in this chapter, old-time obstetricians believed that there was a strong relationship between diet, salt retention and toxemia of pregnancy. At one time it was believed that deficiencies of specific vitamins or deficiency of protein might be related. Indeed, this idea was strengthened by the finding that mortality rates for toxemias of pregnancy were three times as great in low-income groups as they were in high-income groups according to data supplied by the U.S. Department of Health, Education, and Welfare (cited in Maternal Nutrition and the Course of Pregnancy, 1970). One of the mysteries of toxemia of pregnancy is the dramatic decrease in mortality during the past quarter century. In 1940, the mortality rate in the United States was 52.2 per 100,000 live births, but it dropped to 6.2 deaths per 100,000 births in the years between 1961 and 1965. The role played by nutrition remains obscure. In addition to the idea that total calories and total intake of protein might be related, there have been suggestions that the quality of protein consumed could have a bearing. Several investigators have suggested that vitamin B_6 may be related, since deficiency of this vitamin can cause nausea, vomiting, and disturbed metabolism of tryptophan (Wachstein and Graffeo, 1956). Members of the working group of the Committee on Maternal Nutrition (1970) concluded that even though there was no definite explanation for either the cause of toxemia or the dramatic decline in deaths from this condition since 1940, "Much greater emphasis should be placed on the value of a good diet during pregnancy, particularly for women entering pregnancy with poor nutritional status and poor dietary habits."

Vitamin and Mineral Supplements

Many nutrients are abundantly available in the well-balanced diet recommended for pregnant women. Nonetheless, it is recognized that not everyone eats as she should and this has been used as an excuse for recommending multiple vitamin and mineral supplements for all pregnant women. Of course, the decision should be made on an individual basis. A woman who is too busy or too unconcerned to eat a well-balanced diet may benefit from these supplements. On the other hand, some have suggested that if a woman does take supplements she may assume that all of her nutritional requirements are met and make no effort to consume a well-balanced diet. Regardless of one's philosophy, there are several nutrients that are apt to be in short supply in the diet of a pregnant woman.

The first of these is iron, which is notably deficient in the diet of most American women throughout their reproductive years. The Recommended Dietary Allowance for such women is 18 mg/day and the average diet contains about 6 to 7 mg of iron per 1000 Kcal. Since the recommendation for such women is only about 2100 Kcal/day, it is obvious that these women probably get an average of about 12 to 14 mg of iron rather than the recommended 18. It should be noted that the Food and Nutrition Board recognizes this problem and in a footnote to the RDA Tables they state, "This increased requirement cannot be met by ordinary diets; therefore, the use of supplemental iron is recommended."

The details of iron metabolism are presented in the chapter on hematology, but briefly it is important to recall here that the pregnant woman needs additional iron not only to meet the needs of her developing fetus but also to permit her to increase her red blood cell mass and its hemoglobin content. A healthy woman will increase her total blood volume by about 50 per cent during pregnancy, but the volume of erythrocytes is increased by only 20 to 30 per cent. This relative hydremia is reflected in lower hematologic values which may be misinterpreted as indicating a more severe degree of anemia than is actually present. Administration of medicinal iron is highly recommended for all pregnant women, and should be given in such a form as to minimize unpleasant gastrointestinal side reactions. Ferrous sulfate, which is the least expensive and most commonly used, is quite well absorbed, but it also carries a relatively high incidence of unpleasant reactions. Other forms of iron cause less distress, perhaps because they are less well absorbed. The usual dose of ferrous sulfate is 150 to 300 mg/day orally. If side reactions do occur, smaller doses given at more frequent intervals can be given a trial, or another preparation of iron can be used.

Folates

The second most common nutritional cause of anemia in pregnancy is a deficiency of folic acid. Theoretically, it should be a simple matter to provide most pregnant women with a diet that contains an abundance of folates, but in actual practice this cannot always be achieved. Part of the reason is that the microbiological methods formerly used for estimating the folate content of foods measure the polyglutamate forms of pteroic acid, whereas humans are not able to absorb and utilize 100 per cent of these compounds. Pteroylmonoglutamate is very well absorbed from the digestive tract but the polyglutamate forms must be enzymatically hydrolyzed before absorption can be completed. Accordingly, it has become customary to assume that only about 25 per cent of mixed glutamates represent the active folic acid content of a given food. This has resulted in a good deal of contradiction and confusion in food tables listing the folate content of various items. Megaloblastic anemia is not common in pregnancy but it does occur often enough to suggest that folate supplementation is justifiable in all pregnant women. Some authorities challenge this conclusion on a basis of a cost/benefit ratio, but folic acid is neither expensive nor harmful in modest doses and the extra folate may be of particular benefit to women who have multiple pregnancies. Many commercial preparations of folates are available, usually in combinations with other vitamins. The recommended level of intake of mixed folates is 800 μg per day (equivalent to 200 μg of folic acid) but it is customary to give tablets containing 0.25 mg as a daily dose.

Calcium

As mentioned above, the calcium requirements of a pregnant woman who consumes an additional 2 glasses of milk per day can easily be met. On the other hand, women who are lactose intolerant may have considerable difficulty getting an adequate amount of calcium. It is for this reason that calcium supplements may be desirable for some patients. Obviously, one will not wish to give calcium lactate to a woman who is lactose intolerant, but calcium carbonate or some other suitable salt of calcium can be given in doses of approximately 600 to 1200 mg daily as elemental calcium. Most pharmaceutical preparations containing calcium for prenatal purposes also contain iron and a number of vitamins. This necessitates care in avoiding an overdose of the fat-soluble vitamins, and it also may be wasteful.

Vitamin D

Until recently, it was assumed that there is no adult requirement for vitamin D since most individuals are exposed to sunlight, at least for a few minutes every day. It has been reported (Loomis, 1967) that people with heavily pigmented skin are not able to synthesize vitamin D in sufficient amounts by ultraviolet irradiation. Although this idea has been challenged, it seems wise to ensure that there is an adequate oral intake of vitamin D in all patients, either as part of their diet or as medicinal supplements. In pregnancy, however, the oral intake should not ordinarily exceed 400 I.U. (10 μg) per day.

Food Fads

Food fads are discussed in more detail elsewhere in this volume, but it is important to identify three common food fads and their potential influence on the outcome of pregnancy.

Vegetarian Diets. Many young people today have adopted the philosophy that vegetarian diets are desirable for religious, social, ecological, or other reasons. Physicians and nutritionists may, at first, be alarmed when a pregnant woman announces that she is a vegetarian. It is important to take a careful dietary history to determine what her actual food intake is, and whether she has been taking or needs to take dietary supplements. A carefully selected vegetarian diet can be fully nutritious, but many are not. Diets commonly known as "Zen macrobiotic diets" are apt to be grossly inadequate to meet the needs of a pregnant woman. On the other hand, lacto-ovo diets, which contain both milk products and eggs, are usually highly nutritious. People who are strict vegetarians (vegans) are likely to develop a deficiency of vitamin B_{12}, but with the exception of this nutrient, it is possible to meet all of the dietary requirements by feeding foods of plant origin. It is, however, difficult to obtain adequate amounts of calcium and of iron on such a diet.

Fasting. A particularly pernicious custom for a pregnant woman is that of fasting. Recent work indicates that even a brief period of starvation ketosis may have a disastrous effect upon the fetus (Churchill, 1968). Accordingly, physicians should strongly condemn this practice for any pregnant woman. Presumably, this also would apply to weight reduction diets that depend upon curtailment of carbohydrates to induce ketosis.

Megavitamin Therapy. A popular form of self-medication is megavitamin ingestion. This term, while not specifically accurate, does convey the meaning that very large doses of vitamins are consumed. In general, the amount given ranges between 100 and 1000 times the recommended level of intake. For many nutrients this might be harmless, but as mentioned previously, overdosage with vitamin A, vitamin D, and perhaps also with ascorbic acid during the first trimester of pregnancy may result in deformities of the developing child. A good general rule is to avoid, if possible, giving any medication or any unusual diet to any pregnant woman.

Teen-age Pregnancy

A girl who has not yet achieved her linear growth is usually nutritionally immature. Her muscles are not fully developed, her skeleton may not be fully mineralized, and her stores of several essential nutrients—notably iron, folic acid, vitamin A, and vitamin B_{12}—are much smaller than those of a well-fed adult woman. The nutrient requirements of an adolescent vary a great deal from one individual to another. Some girls achieve physical maturity early in their teens, whereas others are still developing in their late teens or early twenties. In general, however, a girl achieves reproductive maturity by about age 17. Whenever called upon to supervise pregnancy in a teen-age girl, the physician should take a careful developmental history as well as a diet history. If it is obvious that the girl is still in the period of rapid adolescent growth, her diet must supply sufficient energy, protein, and other essential nutrients to meet her growth requirements and, in addition, she will need extra amounts to meet the needs of pregnancy. Examination of the Food and Nutrition Board's Table of Recommended Daily Dietary Allowances (1974) will give a good estimate of the energy requirements, the protein needs, and other nutrient needs of an adolescent, and it is a simple matter to add to these the recommended increments of nutrients for pregnancy. In this situation, however, reliance upon the weight curve of pregnancy is no longer valid. It is not unusual for an adolescent girl to grow several inches and add many pounds within less than a year if she is undergoing her "growth spurt." If pregnancy is superimposed upon this period of rapid growth, her nutrient requirements may be truly remarkable. It is only by careful supervision and personal attention that the physician can ensure optimal nutritional support of such a patient.

Pica

Many people engage in a peculiar practice known as pica, or the ingestion of non-nutritious substances. The most common forms of pica are the ingestion of clay, the eating of cornstarch, or the eating of ice. From time to time efforts have been made to identify some innate craving or physiologic hunger with this practice, but to no avail. Pica is more common amongst women, especially in the Southeastern states of the United States and in certain parts of Europe. It is not something the patient will voluntarily relate, and sometimes it requires skillful questioning to elicit a history of pica. Pica during pregnancy can have several adverse effects, the most important of which are substitution of non-nutritious substances for a proper diet and the ingestion of useless minerals in clay, which may interfere with the absorption of essential nutrients. When pica is recognized in a pregnant woman, every possible effort should be made to discourage continuation of this habit. It may be necessary to provide the patient with dietary supplements if there is evidence of nutritional deficiencies.

Alcohol and Drugs

Pregnant women should avoid taking medications of any kind unless absolutely necessary. This applies not only to over-the-counter drugs and to megavitamin self-medication, but most especially to alcohol and the "hard drugs" used by some of today's young people, for these may have a devastating effect on the developing child. Infants whose mother used habituating or addicting drugs may be born with a drug-dependence that requires intensive care for the first few days of extrauterine life.

But alcoholism in a pregnant woman is a very serious threat to the fetus, either as a result of its own toxicity or because of its metabolic antagonism of folate, or perhaps as a result of a poor diet that so often accompanies alcohol abuse. Hanson and colleagues (1976) reported that 30 to 50 per cent of infants born to mothers who are severe alcoholics display the "fetal alcohol syndrome". In 41 cases, growth and performance were found to be abnormal in 80 to 97 per cent, craniofacial defects occurred in 49 to 92 per cent, and abnormalities of limbs were found in 41 to 49 per cent. Other defects were demonstrable in 22 to 49 per cent, including cardiac defects (mostly septal defects), genital abnormalities, hemangiomas, and deformities of the external ear. Children so afflicted may have short palpebral fissures, epicanthal folds, low nasal bridges with short or upturned noses, and long upper lips with narrow vermillion borders (Figure 2–2).

Characteristics of the fetal alcohol syndrome may also include hirsutism of the forehead and other parts of the body, asymmetrical maxillary hypoplasia, abnormal crease patterns of the palms, and congenital dislocation of the hips. In addition, the neonatal death rate has

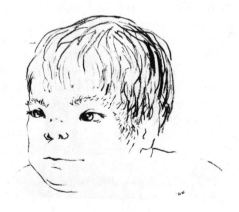

Figure 2–2 Composite drawing of a child showing the commonest features of the fetal alcohol syndrome. Although it is unusual for all of these to occur in the same child, they are depicted together for illustration. Note the narrow bitemporal diameter, wide-set eyes, narrow palpebral fissures, prominent epicanthal folds, and strabismus. There is excessive hair on the forehead and foreshortening of the mid-portion of the face, resulting in a saddle-nose. The upper lip is long, the mouth wide, the vermilion border thin, and the chin receding. Not shown are the diminished height and weight and the transverse palmar crease. Some reports describe psychomotor retardation and low IQs.

been observed to be as high as 17 per cent in the offspring of alcoholic mothers compared to only 2 per cent for nonalcoholic mothers. But even more devastating is the fact that of the survivors, 44 per cent of children whose mothers were alcoholic had an IQ of 79 or less by age 7 years, in contrast to only 9 per cent who had such a low IQ if their mothers did not use alcohol.

The question of whether social drinking can cause difficulties cannot be answered with finality, but the ancient Carthaginians used to admonish bridal couples not to drink wine on their wedding night lest they conceive a defective child.

NUTRITIONAL NEEDS OF THE LACTATING MOTHER

Breast feeding of infants is still the most desirable and physiological form of infant nutrition. Maternal benefits are also substantial: they include more rapid involution of the uterus, more rapid elimination of the adipose tissue often accumulated during pregnancy, some measure of birth control, and perhaps most importantly, emotional gratification of both mother and child. The nutritional requirements of lactation are not greatly different from those of pregnancy, with a few notable exceptions. The recommended increase in food intake should approximate 500 additional Kcal above the non-pregnant level but this, of course, varies with the age and size of the nursing infant. Similarly, the suggested additional 20 gm of protein may be adequate for the newborn child but quite insufficient for a child at age 10 to 12 months. Vitamin A intake should be 50 per cent greater than before pregnancy (1200 retinol equivalents). Most of these nutrients will be supplied automatically if the nursing mother selects her additional calories from a variety of foods representing each of the four major food groups. If she was taking supplements of iron, folate, calcium, and multiple vitamins during pregnancy, it probably would be advisable for her to continue to do so until she stops nursing her child. She should be cautioned about the potential for any drugs or medications which she might take appearing in breast milk and being absorbed by her offspring.

For a woman who is obese, the period of lactation may represent an opportunity for her to consume a well-balanced diet that supplies all of the essential nutrients necessary for both the mother and child but that has a modestly reduced caloric content. If the average pregnant woman would need 2600 Kcal daily, it would be permissible to reduce this by 500 Kcal, thus providing her with the potential for a weight loss of approximately 1 pound per week. This would permit her to lose at a rate of 4 pounds per month, or nearly 50 pounds in a year if she continues nursing for that length of time. It must be stressed, however, that more rigid restriction of energy intake should not be attempted because of the potentially adverse effects on her intake of other essential nutrients.

SUMMARY

In the past two decades, obstetricians and nutritionists have reexamined old ideas about the best diet for the pregnant woman and have concluded that many of them were in error.

The fetus is *not* a perfect parasite and the maternal diet *does* have an important impact on the outcome of pregnancy. The optimal rate of maternal weight gain has been depicted in graphic form: this has also been correlated with birth weight of the child. Neonatal death rate has been shown to have a negative correlation with birth weight.

There is no single diet for the pregnant woman. Her eating habits and preferences must be considered. On average she will need an additional 300 Kcal of energy along with increased amounts of calcium, protein, and many other essential nutrients. And it is safe to assume that most women of reproductive age consume inadequate amounts of iron both before and during pregnancy. Therefore, iron supplements are necessary. Similarly, folate intake may be inadequate, so many obstetricians give folate supplements.

Major hazards to the developing embryo are posed by starvation ketosis, deficiency of certain essential nutrients, or overdosage with vitamin A or vitamin D. And many common medications can have an adverse effect on the developing child. This is especially true of alcohol.

Therefore it is a good rule to advocate regular meals of balanced composition. Nutritional supplements must not be given in excess but modest supplements of iron and of folate may be needed. A pregnant woman should never take any medication that is not essential, and then only under the guidance of her physician.

Nutritional needs during lactation are similar to those during pregnancy but the energy demands increase progressively as the child grows. Here again, all unnecessary medications must be avoided.

REFERENCES

Antonov, A. N.: Children born during the siege of Leningrad in 1942. *J. Pediat.* 30:250, 1947.

Barnes, R. H.: Dual role of environmental deprivation and malnutrition in retarding intellectual development. *Amer. J. Clin. Nutr.* 29:912, 1976.

Burke, B. S., Beal, V. A., Kirkwood, S. B., and Stuart, H. C.: The influence of nutrition during pregnancy upon the condition of the infant at birth. *J. Nutrition* 26:569, 1943.

Churchill, J. A., Berendes, H. W., and Willerman, L.: Gestational acetonuria and some developmental measures in the offspring. Presented at the meeting of the American Public Health Association, Detroit, MI, 1968.

Cochrane, W. A.: Overnutrition in prenatal and neonatal life: a problem? *Canadian Med. Assoc. J.* 93:893, 1965.

Committee on Maternal Nutrition, Food and Nutrition Board, National Research Council, National Academy of Sciences: Maternal nutrition and the course of pregnancy. Washington, D.C., Superintendent of Documents, U.S. Government Printing Office, 1970.

Editorial: Nutrition and the developing brain. *Lancet* 2:1349, 1972.

Food and Nutrition Board, Natinal Research Council; Natinal Academy of Sciences. *Recommended Dietary Allowances,* eighth revised edition. Washington, D. C., 1974.

Friedman, W. R., and Roberts, W. C.: Vitamin D and the supravalvular aortic stenosis syndrome. *Circulation* 34:77, 1966.

Gessner, A.: Die badische Eklampsiestatistik für das Jahr 1919 im Lichte der Diatetik. *Zentrablatt für Gynäkologie* 45:1814, 1921.

Giroud, A.: *The Nutrition of the Embryo.* Springfield, IL, Charles C. Thomas, 1970.

Hanson, J. W., Smith, D. W., and Jones, K. S.: Fetal alcohol syndrome. *J.A.M.A.* 235:1458, 1976.

Hurley, L. S., Dreosti, I. E., Swenerton, H., and Gowan, J.: The movement of zinc in maternal and fetal rat tissues in teratogenic zinc deficiency. *Teratology* 1:216, 1968.

Kalter, H., and Warkany, J.: Experimental production of congenital malformations in strains of inbred mice by maternal treatment with hypervitaminosis A. *Amer. J. Pathol.* 38:1, 1961.

Lechtig, A., Habicht, J. P., Yarbrough, C., Delgado, H., Guzman, G., and Klein, R. E.: Influence of food supplementation during pregnancy on birth weight in rural populations of Guatemala. *Proceedings of the IX International Congress of Nutrition.* Basel, S. Karger, 1974.

Levitsky, D. A., Massaro, T. F., and Barnes, R. H.: Maternal nutrition and the neonatal environment. *Fed. Proc.* 34:1583, 1975.

Loomis, W. F.: Skin-pigment regulation of vitamin D biosynthesis in man. *Science* 157:501, 1967.

Lutwak, L.: Tracer studies of intestinal calcium absorption in man. *Amer. J. Clin. Nutr.* 22:771, 1969.

Mouriquand G., and Edel, V.: Sur l'hypervitaminose C. *Compt. Rend. Soc. Biol.* 147:1432, 1953.

Neuweiler, W.: Die Hypervitaminose und ihre Beziehung zur Schwangerschaft. *Internat. Z. für Vitaminforsch.* 22:392, 1951.

Niswander, K. R., Singer, J., Westphal, H., and Weiss, W.: Weight gain during pregnancy and prepregnancy weight: association with birth weight of term gestation. *Obstet. Gynecol.* 33:482, 1969.

Page, E. W., and Page, E. M.: Leg cramps in pregnancy. Etiology and treatment. *Obstet. Gynecol.* 1:94, 1953.

Pike, R. L., and Smiciklas, H. A.: A reappraisal of sodium restriction during pregnancy. *Internat. J. Gynecol. Obstet.* 10:1, 1972.

Pitkin, R. M., Kaminetzky, H. A., Newton, M., and Pritchard, J. A.: Maternal nutrition. A selective review of clinical topics. *Obstet. Gynecol.* 40:773, 1972.

Ravelli, G.-P, Stein, Z. A., and Susser, M. W.: Obesity in young men after famine exposure in utero and early infancy. *New England J. Med.* 2:349, 1976.

Roeder, L. M., and Chow, B. F.: Maternal undernutrition and its long-term effects on the offspring. *Amer. J. Clin. Nutr.* 25:812, 1972.

Samborskaya, E. P., and Ferdman, T. D.: Mechanism of termination of pregnancy by ascorbic acid. *Byulleten Eksperimental noi Biologii i Medicin* 62:96, 1966.

Singer, J., Westphal, M., and Niswander, K. R.: The relationship of weight gain during pregnancy to birthweight and infant growth and development in the first year of life: a report from the Collaborative Study of Cerebral Palsy. *Obstet. Gynecol.* 51:417, 1968.

Smith, C. A.: The effect of wartime starvation in Holland upon pregnancy and its product. *Amer. J. Obstet. Gynecol.* 53:599, 1947.

Stein, Z., Susser, M., Saenger, G., and Marolla, F.: *Famine and Human Development: The Dutch Hunger Winter of 1944–1945.* New York, Oxford University Press, 1975.

Susser, M. W., Marolla, F. A., and Fleiss, J.: Birthweight, fetal age and perinatal mortality. *Amer. J. Epidemiol.* 96:197, 1972.

Taggart, N.: Food habits in pregnancy. *Proc. Nutrition Soc.* 20:35, 1961.

Wachestein, M., and Graffeo, L. W.: Influence of vitamin B_6 on the incidence of preeclampsia. *Obstet. Gynecol.* 8:177, 1956.

Warnekros, K.: Kriegkost und Eklampsie. *Zentrablatt für Gynäkologie* 40:897, 1916.

Widdowson, E. M., and Cowen, J.: The effect of protein deficiency on the reproduction of rats. *Brit. J. Nutr.* 27:85, 1972.

Winick, M.: Cellular growth during early malnutrition. *Pediatrics* 47:969, 1971.

Winick, M., and Noble, A.: Cellular response in rats during malnutrition at various ages. *J. Nutrition* 89:300, 1966.

3

NUTRITION AND THE DIGESTIVE SYSTEM

Robert E. Hodges, M.D.

Because of the intimate association between nutrition and the digestive tract, it is easy to understand why physicians interested in diseases of this organ system should also have an interest in diets and their therapeutic potential, and for many years this was true. The past century might be characterized as the heyday of diet therapy. There were uncounted varieties of diets; some disease-oriented such as the "ulcer diet", the "colitis diet", the "gallbladder diet", and many others. Some diets were named after famous clinicians (Sippy, Meulengracht, and so on). But today, most gastroenterologists as well as a majority of other physicians regard diet therapy with suspicion, if not scorn, for many of the firmly held views of the past about "digestibility", "neutralization of gastric acid", and "avoidance of irritation" have been disproven. Furthermore, with a better understanding of the pathophysiology of the common diseases of the digestive tract, there has been a parallel development of pharmaceutical products that accomplish many of the things once attributed to diet therapy. But it would be a serious mistake to abandon all forms of diet therapy as useless. Instead, diets, like pharmaceutical agents, should be carefully prescribed with regard for the individual patient's needs, customs, and preferences. A fundamental understanding of the advantages and limitations of diet therapy will provide the physician with new and effective ways to treat patients.

OBJECTIVES OF MODERN DIETARY MANAGEMENT

General Principles of Diet Prescription

Unlike the physician of old, today's clinician does not rely upon a list of "old favorites" in treating each and every disease or symptom complex. Instead, the modern physician recognizes that the diet prescription should, for a patient of a given height and weight and level of physical activity, include the proper number of calories, an appropriate protein allowance, and a desirable balance between protein, carbohydrates, and fats. In addition, the diet must of course provide sufficient quantities of each of the essential vitamins and minerals, and it must be translated into meals that are pleasant and appealing to the patient. Basically, there are four ways in which a diet is modified for therapeutic purposes: (1) alterations in texture; (2) variations in frequency of feeding; (3) quantitative modifications (more or less of any given constituent such as sodium, fat, or protein); or (4) qualitative changes which consist of total elimination of an offending substance such as gluten, lactose, copper, or ethanol.

Specific Goals

A therapeutic diet seldom, if ever, provides a cure for a given disease or disorder, except starvation. Instead, the therapeutic goals of diet therapy are (1) to relieve symptoms; (2) to hasten recovery; (3) to provide optimal nourishment; and (4) to remove offending substances. Oftentimes, patients who have gastrointestinal disorders experience considerable relief of symptoms after the ingestion of a specific food item. This type of information is useful in managing the patient's problems, assuming of course, that there is no specific contraindication. The classical example is the relief a patient with a duodenal ulcer feels after drinking a glass of milk. In some instances, dietary therapy can hasten recovery. This is particularly true of the patient who is malnourished, either as a result of a restricted intake of foods or because of the effects of underlying disease. Correction of malnutrition may aid indirectly in recovery. With today's nutritional armamentarium, the physician can provide optimal nutrition for virtually any patient. Most of the time this can be done in the form of regular food with appropriate modifications. Sometimes it is necessary to resort to tube feeding of either a liquified diet or an elemental diet. And the last resort, of course, is total parenteral nutrition wherein the patient receives all nutrients intravenously. Recent experience has demonstrated that patients who are restored to a positive caloric and nitrogen balance often withstand specific forms of treatment such as surgical operation, chemotherapy, irradiation treatment, and so forth far better as a result of their improved nutritional status. And, of course, removal of an offending substance from the diet of a patient may result in substantial improvement. The most obvious example is abstinence from the use of alcohol by a patient who is suffering from the effects of alcohol abuse.

CLINICAL APPLICATIONS

A majority of patients admitted to a modern hospital are so busy undergoing diagnostic examinations or therapeutic procedures that they scarcely have time to consume the diet that has been ordered for them. This undoubtedly has contributed to the impression shared by so many physicians that diet therapy is of little importance in the clinical management of their hospitalized patients. On the contrary, appropriate application of the basic principles of nutrition will enable physicians to achieve greater levels of therapeutic success in shorter periods of time. Sometimes success consists merely of relieving symptoms, but more often it means correction of existing nutritional defects such as loss of body weight, low serum proteins, anemia, and the malaise that accompanies nutritional failure. In the following paragraphs, some of the more common disorders of the digestive tract are considered under their respective anatomical headings and appropriate dietary management is discussed. Admittedly, there are areas of controversy, but in most instances a conservative, "middle-of-the-road" course is recommended.

The Esophagus

Motor abnormalities of the esophagus are rather common in patients who are middle-aged or older. Any patient with symptoms of obstruction or dysphagia must undergo diagnostic procedures to rule out serious disorders. When the symptoms obviously result from spasm with or without a constriction ring, an appropriate change in the diet may be more effective than medications. In this instance, a change in the texture of the diet and in the frequency of feedings may solve the problem. It is wise to start with a liquid diet and with small, frequent feedings; then add soft or puréed foods, and finally, restore as many favorite foods as possible, so long as they do not cause dysphagia, pain, or regurgitation. Similarly, in patients who have reflux esophagitis with or without a hiatal hernia, diet may play a vital role. A great many patients with this syndrome are obviously overweight. An obese abdomen can result in increased intra-abdominal pressure that favors the reflux of gastric contents into the lower segment of the esophagus. This is exaggerated by ingestion of a large meal. The obvious form of diet therapy consists of smaller, more frequent meals and a substantial reduction in total caloric intake over a prolonged period of time in order to correct obesity and maintain normal body weight. It also is wise to prohibit the use of beverages, such as coffee and alcoholic drinks, that may stimulate gastric secretions.

A rather uncommon cause of dysphagia is the Plummer-Vinson syndrome that has been attributed to iron deficiency. Many of these patients do have iron deficiency anemia in addition to dysphagia. Some, but not all, have an anatomical "web" demonstrable either by X-ray or esophagoscopy. Treatment of the iron deficiency may be accompanied by subsidence of dysphagia but the true etiology of the syndrome is obscure. Provision of a nutritious diet that meets all nutrient requirements certainly contributes to recovery from the iron deficiency and often results in improvement of general well-being.

The Stomach — Physiology and Pathophysiology

Citizens of the United States are so accustomed to seeing television commercials showing stylized bottles shaped like the stomach that they tend to think of their own symptoms in terms of the announcer's vocabulary. Indeed the words "indigestion", "heartburn", and "acid stomach" are so ingrained in many patients that they can scarcely give an accurate description of their own symptoms. Nonetheless, a good many patients do complain of distress and some describe substantial relief after ingestion of certain foods, especially milk or other foods with temporary buffering capacity. Sometimes these patients carry with them one or another of the popular antacids advertised on television. Some, but by no means all, of these patients may actually have peptic ulcer disease. It is important to note whether the use of such antacids does or does not relieve their symptoms. Hendrix (1971) described the characteristics of "heartburn" and suggested that the pathophysiology involved three prerequisites: (1) material in the stomach that will irritate the esophagus if reflux occurs; (2) an incompetent sphincter that allows reflux into the cardia; and (3) sensitivity of the esophagus to the refluxed material. Such patients may have distress, particularly after a large meal and after bending over. The discomfort may be relieved by standing up, by drinking something, or by taking antacids. Hendrix suggested that a large volume of highly acid gastric juice, a certain amount of delay in gastric emptying, and incompetence of the lower esophageal sphincter all contribute to the syndrome.

The ambulatory patient can be managed by giving six small feedings a day, with the ingestion of no food for 2 hours before retiring. An ounce of non-absorbable antacid such as liquid aluminum hydroxide gel should be given an hour after each meal and at bedtime. Sometimes elevation of the head of the bed 6 or 8 inches and avoidance of tightly fitting garments around the abdomen will reduce the amount of acid reflux into the lower segment of the esophagus. Attention should be paid to the patient's description of those foods that cause "dyspepsia"; these should be avoided. It is also desirable for the patient to avoid coffee, decaffeinated coffee, and alcoholic beverages (Nutrition Reviews, 1976).

Peptic Ulcer Disease. The distress of a peptic ulcer may be closely similar to that of "heartburn" described above or it may manifest itself as a form of hunger or as merely an unpleasant sensation in the general region of the epigastrium. There are many different types of response to eating and to the taking of antacids. Many, but by no means all, patients with peptic ulcer will describe a painful sensation associated with hunger and a pleasant relief of distress after the ingestion of foods. Sometimes patients report that consuming milk and other protein-containing foods gives prompt relief. They may also volunteer that certain foods, especially citrus fruit juices, carbonated beverages, coffee, tea, and alcoholic beverages, aggravate their distress. But there are so many exceptions to these generalizations that it is not safe to assume that a patient either does or does not have a peptic ulcer on the basis of history alone. Nor can the patient's description of symptoms be used as a successful guide to appropriate therapy.

The best dietary approach to peptic ulcer is yet to be determined. There are many different ideas about the potential benefits or the harm of prescribing diets for these patients, and each proponent or adversary can quote one or several reports to document any given position. The facts are that the traditional concepts have been challenged, as well they should be. Nonetheless, physicians must guard against reckless abandon in their haste to "throw out the old and bring in the new". The time-honored tradition of feeding patients small quantities of bland, neutral foods at frequent intervals is based upon the ability of many foods to buffer the hydrochloric acid secreted by the stomach and the subjective relief reported by many patients who have been given this type of diet. Fordtran (1973) believes that the gastric pH throughout a 24 hour period is actually *lower* in those patients who receive frequent feedings than it is in those who eat a regular diet. Isenberg (1975) recognizes that the wisdom or folly of frequent milk feedings is still disputed and would rather rely more heavily upon use of antacids, particularly those containing aluminum hydroxide. Certainly the original Sippy diet and most modifications thereof should be avoided. Hartroft (1964) described an increased incidence of coronary artery disease in patients with peptic ulcer who had been treated with the Sippy diet as compared with similar patients who had received some other form of treatment. This work was repeated and fully confirmed a few years later in Great Britain. McMillan and Freeman (1965) described the milk-alkali syndrome occurring in patients who had been treated with calcium carbonate as an antacid. This induced hypercalcemia which, in turn, impaired renal function. Even the aluminum hydroxide antacids may induce metabolic problems, as evidenced by the report of Lotz and others (1968) of a phosphorus depletion syndrome resulting from vigorous administration of antacids. It is apparent that either diet or antacids may neutralize excess gastric acid and either form of therapy may cause undesirable side effects. Perhaps some combination of the two is worthwhile. Until there is further evidence on the subject, the author prefers to prescribe a diet supplying a proper number of calories and composed of attractive foods that are familiar to the patient. Any food that causes distress is omitted. Because hunger may be accompanied by abundant secretion of gastric juices it seems wise to give interval feedings between meals. And administration of an antacid preparation 1 hour after a meal should aid in neutralization of excess acid. In addition, a generous dose of antacid should be given at bedtime and additional amounts taken throughout the night as indicated by the clinical situation. There is one point of general agreement in the controversy over diet and peptic ulcer: virtually everyone agrees that alcoholic beverages and coffee, and even decaffeinated coffee should be totally forbidden (Nutrition Reviews, 1976). The evidence for prohibiting the use of tea and carbonated soft drinks is less convincing.

Stress Ulcers and Steroid Ulcers. Surgeons have recognized for many years that any patient undergoing a major surgical procedure may develop peptic ulceration of the stomach during the postoperative period. Similarly, ulceration of the gastric mucosa develops with some regularity in patients who have sustained severe cutaneous burns or in patients with cerebral trauma. A similar type of phenomenon is seen in some patients who receive large doses of adrenocortical steroids for prolonged periods of time. A number of methods have been employed in an effort to prevent or control this phenomenon, including administration of aluminum hydroxide antacids, nasogastric gavage feedings of milk-based formulas or blended diets, and the administration of various medications including vitamin A. There does not seem to be any convincing evidence that any of these forms of treatment are effective. It is true that once the patient can tolerate gastric feedings, the risk of ulceration is substantially diminished but this may merely reflect improvement in the patient's general condition with a lessening of the degree of "stress". The most hopeful development is the availability of the new H-2-receptor blocker agents that appear to inhibit secretion of hydrochloric acid by gastric mucosa (Mainardi et al., 1974). Studies currently under way should clarify the value and limitations of this type of medication.

The author believes that appropriate dietary therapy combined with the use of nonabsorbable antacids and perhaps with the adminis- tration of the H-2-blocking agents represents the most effective way of dealing with clinical problems resulting from or associated with ex- cessive secretion of gastric digestive juices. Physicians must not ig- nore the strong impact of emotions on peptic ulcer disease nor the emotional value of eating. A patient deprived of food or forced to consume an unattractive formula in lieu of meals may suffer more from frustration and annoyance which, in turn, can have an impact on the secretory activity of the gastric mucosa. A strong case can be made for permitting the patient to eat familiar foods, even if these constitute foods with considerable bulk or even foods that are rather highly seasoned. If the patient likes them, and suffers no distress from eating them, they should be permitted. And, above all, patients should be taught to make mealtimes pleasant and relaxing.

The Small Bowel

Nutrition and diet are perhaps more closely related to the small bowel than to any other portion of the digestive tract because it is here that most of the processes of digestion and absorption occur. Disease or malfunctioning of the small bowel can lead to rapid and severe nutritional consequences. And, conversely, certain nutritional defi- ciencies can and do affect one or more of the multiple functions of the small bowel.

Anatomical and Motor Abnormalities of the Small Bowel. Mal- functioning or obstruction of the small bowel results in immediate interruption of the patient's nutritional input and this quickly leads to depletion of fluids and electrolytes unless appropriate measures are taken. Within a day or two the patient's carbohydrate reserves are exhausted and fatty acids then become the major source of energy. This, of course, results in varying degrees of ketosis and is accompa- nied by substantial losses of salt and water. For reasons not entirely understood, ingestion of carbohydrates permits the body to retain salt and water, whereas deficiency of carbohydrate has the opposite effect (Sigler, 1975). Indeed, this is the underlying principle that has led so many to believe that a carbohydrate-free diet is an effective way to lose weight. It is an effective way to lose water.

With prolonged malfunctioning of the small bowel, all the events leading to starvation and emaciation begin to take place. Protein, every molecule of which serves a useful purpose, is used as a source of energy and those proteins with the shortest half-life become depleted first. The concentration of albumin in the serum falls rapidly, hemoglobin declines at a somewhat slower rate, and both skeletal muscle and subcutaneous tissue become wasted and shrunken. At the same time, there is progressive loss of essential vitamins and minerals. Until recent years, physicians had to be content with peripheral infusions of isotonic solutions of glucose and saline. These prevented dehydration, electrolyte depletion, and ketosis but did nothing for the protein losses. Water-soluble vitamins often were added to the isotonic solutions and, for several decades, efforts were made to reverse the protein losses by infusing solutions of protein hydrolysates. These all represented important steps in the right direction, but they seldom achieved "total" nutrition so that those patients with a nonfunctioning small bowel could be maintained in good nutritional health. It was not until the advent of total parenteral nutrition about a decade ago that this picture changed dramatically.

Patients whose small bowel function has been only partly curtailed or those who have had complete interruption of bowel function but are beginning to recover should be fed enterally, but reintroduction of food must be accomplished gradually. Too often an impatient physician attempts to hasten the recovery of a patient's digestive tract by giving too much too soon. The result may be a serious setback in the form of abdominal distention, nausea, vomiting, and further impairment of the nutritional condition. The best advice is "make haste slowly". The patient who has been fed parenterally for days or weeks should not be given food abruptly. It is important to remember that digestive enzymes undergo temporary atrophy, so reintroduction of undigested foods must be undertaken slowly. The suppressed enzyme secretion that accompanies starvation requires only a few days for reasonable recovery, but attempts to feed a patient too rapidly will almost certainly lead to disappointment. The old regimen was "sips of water" followed by "clear liquids", then "full liquids". This was followed by administration of soft or puréed diet and, finally, regular foods were given. Today, we have few improvements on this regimen. The use of elemental diets which are composed of individual amino acids, simple carbohydrates, a very small amount of essential fatty acids, and vitamins and minerals in a convenient "packet" supplying 300 kilocalories represents a useful therapeutic adjunct. The regular dilution with 300 ml of water results in a formula that is quite hypertonic. Therefore it is wise to start with a more dilute solution such as 300 kcal in 600 ml of water. This can be used instead of a clear-liquid diet, which supplied chiefly water, sugar, and salt. Both the volume and the concentration of the elemental diet can be increased as rapidly as tolerated, and soon the patient is ready to begin eating foods again. The best evidence of recovery is a return of appetite, absence of nausea and vomiting, and restoration of normal bowel motility (Rosensweig, 1975).

Patients with inflammatory bowel disease (Crohn's disease) may have serious and long-lasting nutritional problems. Not only does their disease lead to caution in eating, but recurrent episodes of diarrhea are accompanied by losses of protein and blood in the stool. And in those patients with involvement of the terminal ileum, absorption of vitamin B_{12} and reabsorption of intrinsic factor are impaired. The resulting vitamin B_{12} deficiency can contribute to the anemia so often present in these patients.

Dietary management of regional enteritis, or of any inflammatory disorder of the small bowel should be undertaken on a rational basis. The sooner a physician accepts the fact that there is no curative diet, the sooner that physician will be able to achieve maximum benefit for the patient. Crohn's disease usually produces severe and prolonged malnutrition accompanied by all of its manifestations: protein wasting, anemia, impairment of immune mechanisms, impairment of wound healing, progressive weakness, and malaise. The modern physician can and should restore such a patient to nutritional adequacy and maintain the patient in that state. This is possible in almost every instance through the judicious use of one or more of the three major resources available: regular feedings, tube feedings, and parenteral feeding. Contrary to the opinion of a few, the author does not believe that Crohn's disease or any other inflammatory process of the digestive tract is specifically cured by nutritional methods. On the other hand, restoration of optimal nutritional conditions may permit the patient to undergo a spontaneous remission or may enable the surgeon to perform necessary procedures with a minimum of catabolic effect, and with the best possible opportunity for adequate wound healing. To repeat, total parenteral nutrition is a most valuable adjunct to the treatment of inflammatory bowel disease but it is not a specific cure.

Although many clinicians choose to argue about the virtues and evils of fiber in the diet, few seem to be aware of the more important issue: how the average patient's nutritional status can best be maintained. There is no single answer, but close attention to a great many details will achieve the desired result in most instances. For the hospitalized patient this may involve a stern prohibition against the all too frequent use of the "NPO" order as a method of being certain some diagnostic test has not been forgotten and will not be interfered with by a meal. Another worthwhile device is to make a point of visiting patients (preferably accompanied by a dietitian) at mealtimes to determine whether the patient is receiving the prescribed meals, and whether the meals are attractive and of proper temperature. Is the coffee lukewarm and the ice cream melted? Did anyone make it possible for the patient to gain access to his or her tray? How much can or will the patient eat at a single meal? Would the patient prefer other foods or in-between snacks or a different method of cooking? These and many other details can be elicited by a few friendly words. Contrast this with a disgruntled patient whose breakfast was held because an upper gastrointestinal series had been ordered, then canceled at the last minute because radiology has been swamped by some emergency, and so the patient's tray is ordered from the diet kitchen. It arrives late in the morning, often with soggy toast, cold eggs, and tepid coffee. While the patient is poking at the tray, another diet aide enters with an early lunch. By this time, the patient is so frustrated as to refuse to eat either one. Multiply this chain of events by several days each week, and it is easy to see why so many patients develop "hospital malnutrition". Sometimes the patient who complains of anorexia, abdominal cramping, and even nausea and vomiting is merely expressing resentment toward an unattentive nurse who failed to respond promptly to the call button. These, and a host of other factors, enter into patient acceptance of food, for food represents far more than merely a source of nutrients. It represents security, affection, and affluence and, of course, unavailability of food or unacceptable food has the opposite connotations. It is sometimes helpful to give patients small, attractive meals of their own choosing and augment these with oral or gavage feedings of an elemental formula. This type of formula can be administered through a catheter of very small caliber, which is generally well tolerated. And, of course, for the patient who is febrile, catabolic, and obviously malnourished, it may be necessary to resort to total parenteral nutrition.

Enzymatic Defects.   Enzymatic defects of the small bowel are of three general types: hereditary, such as lactase deficiency; acquired, such as tropical sprue; and secondary, such as the defects accompanying infantile diarrhea or adult enterocolitis. The most common "defect" is lack of lactase. In actual fact, there is much logic to the argument that persistence of lactase in the small bowel mucosa long after weaning may itself be an abnormality. More than half the people of the world have lactase deficiency by the time they reach adulthood. This is true of a majority of people of African origin, most Orientals, most Eskimos and American Indians, and many races whose ancestors lived along the shores of the Mediterranean Sea — substantial percentages of Spanish, Portuguese, French, Italian, Greek, and Jewish people.

Lactase deficiency (for lack of a better term) is defined as an abnormal response to an oral dose of lactose. Different techniques have been employed, but generally, either 1 gm/kg of body weight is given or 100 gm are given as a single dose. Blood is collected before, and at 30 minutes after administration of the test dose and measured for the concentration of glucose in serum. A rise of 20 mg per deciliter or more is interpreted as a normal finding. A smaller rise is indicative of inefficient hydrolysis of lactose into its glucose and galactose components.

About half of those individuals with an abnormal response will experience symptoms from drinking as little as 240 ml of milk (about 12.5 mg of lactose). Although lactose has been credited with having a favorable effect on calcium absorption, there are many people who refuse to drink milk because of the unpleasant symptoms it causes (Rosensweig, 1975; Woteki et al., 1976). Page and colleagues (1975a and 1975b) have studied the relationship between milk consumption and the results of lactose tolerance tests in individuals. They have also shown that lactose-hydrolyzed milk is well tolerated by people who are proved to be lactase-deficient. The symptoms of lactose intolerance may consist of cramping, bloating, flatulence, and in some instances, diarrhea. Few patients will volunteer the information that they cannot drink milk, and even when asked, they may say they can. But ask them, "*Do* you drink milk?" and they will say no. Then ask if they have ever used milk as a laxative; if they give an affirmative answer, the diagnosis is quite certain. Lebenthal has shown that there is a relationship between lactase activity and milk consumption in older children (1975). Those who do not drink milk are deprived of important sources of calcium, vitamin A, vitamin D, and riboflavin, as well as an inexpensive high quality protein. The American diet is top-heavy with phosphates, and the calcium supplied by milk helps to restore the Ca/P ratio towards the desirable level of one-to-one. Persons who can't or won't drink milk can be given fermented (hard) cheeses, fermented buttermilk, specially modified milk with the lactose hydrolyzed, or soy milk which has been fortified with calcium and other nutrients. In addition, a diet containing such small fish as sardines and herring provides important sources of calcium because of the presence of small edible bones, but few persons wish to eat sardines or herring on a daily basis. The green leafy vegetables, such as spinach and collards, contain substantial amounts of calcium but their high oxalate content interferes with calcium absorption. Similarly, the abundance of calcium in most whole grains is disappointingly ineffective because the phytates present in bran combine with calcium to make it unavailable.

Other enzymatic defects of the digestive tract are less common and less severe. A few instances of sucrase deficiency have been reported but this is usually not of great severity or long duration. Persons who have been starved or who have had a serious illness may have temporary suppression of most of the enzymes of the small bowel mucosa. Administration of food or of generous amounts of folic acid or of both may restore normal enzymatic activity within a few days.

The "steatorrheas" represent a group of disorders characterized by weight loss, abdominal cramping, flatulence, and the passage of voluminous foamy or foul-smelling stools. The old idea that a stool that floated in the toilet water was necessarily high in fat has been dispelled. Most stools float because they contain a large amount of gas. It is true, however, that intestinal malabsorption may involve both fat and carbohydrates, and that residual carbohydrates in the stool will support bacterial growth which, in turn, generates gas bubbles that result in a floating stool. On the other hand, there are many cases of malabsorption with steatorrhea in which the appearance of the stools is not particularly remarkable. One of the most fascinating forms of steatorrhea and malabsorption is commonly known as "gluten enteropathy" or celiac sprue (Nutrition Reviews, 1975). In this disorder, there may be a combination of nutritional defects, including inadequate absorption of sufficient energy to maintain normal body weight. In addition, absorption of protein, vitamins B_{12}, D, K, and folic acid, trace minerals, and even water, are delayed. One of the early symptoms of malabsorption is nocturia. This results from delayed absorption of water from the digestive tract which, in turn, leads to greater than normal secretion of urine during the hours of sleeping. The apparent mechanism of malabsorption that occurs in celiac sprue results from sensitivity to some component of the protein, gluten, which is present chiefly in wheat but may be present in varying degrees in all grains except rice and corn or maize. This gluten results in a blunting and thickening of the villi of the small bowel and round cell infiltration of the lamina propria. There is a marked decrease in the overall absorptive surface of the bowel mucosa, and in fact, a commensurate decrease in the bowel's ability to absorb almost everything. At the same time, there is diminution in the amount of enzymes formed by or attached to the brush border of the mucosal cells, and a resultant lack of many metabolic functions including hydrolysis, reesterification, and absorption. Protein digestion is likewise inhibited and, of course, protein absorption also suffers. Carbohydrate intolerance can result from lack of enzymatic activity, but even simple sugars are not well absorbed. The combined result is severe progressive malnutrition. In some cases, one type of deficiency may become more apparent than others. For example, protein deficiency may be worse than caloric lack, leading to edema, a potbellied appearance, and other features of kwashiorkor. Anemia is a prominent symptom and may result from deficiency of any of the three major hematopoietic nutrients: iron, vitamin B_{12}, or folic acid. Indeed, any combination of deficiencies of these three may exist, and in one instance of anemia, the author found a deficiency of copper as well as iron. Solomons and others (1976) reported zinc deficiency in patients with celiac sprue, and Reinken and others (1976) found that vitamin B_6 metabolism was affected, even after the acute phase had subsided. Patients who have marked steatorrhea will lose a great many calories as well as fat-soluble vitamins. Although some clinicians have had good results from giving medium-chain triglycerides, the author has not found this form of supplementation to be helpful. The lack of vitamin D contributes to calcium depletion that results from steatorrhea through the formation of insoluble calcium soaps that are excreted in the feces. Deficiencies of vitamins K and A also occur. One would expect deficiencies of vitamin E and of essential fatty acids to occur as well but there are few reports to verify this.

Nutritional management of any patient with malabsorption, or with any other form of malnutrition, must be individualized. The first step is to estimate the patient's normal body weight in kilograms and make an "educated guess" as to the number of kcal/kg/day needed. Basal requirements are about 25 kcal/kg and additional energy is needed on the basis of physical activity and metabolic demands, catabolic state, and estimated nutrient loss. An appropriate figure may be in the range of 35 or 40 kcal/kg/day. Next, the protein requirement can be approximated by multiplying the body weight in kilograms by 0.8 gram (for example, a 70 kg man could be given

$$70 \times 0.8 = 56 \text{ gm protein daily}).$$

Next, the amounts of fat and carbohydrates should be designated. An allowance of 30 per cent of kcal as fats is usually acceptable. And the carbohydrates can be calculated by difference (total kcal − protein and fat). Finally, the physician must determine how to administer these nutrients along with the appropriate Recommended Dietary Allowance (RDA) amounts of all the essential vitamins and minerals. If a severe malabsorption syndrome is evident, there probably will be substantial losses of protein, not only from the food ingested but also from the digestive tract secretions and from the exfoliated cells. Accordingly, a much larger protein allowance may be necessary. An early decision must be made whether to attempt enteral or parenteral feeding. If inadequate digestion is suggested by the presence of steatorrhea, emaciation, edema and specific deficiencies, plus the presence of undigested food particles in the feces, then either an elemental diet or parenteral nutrition should be employed. It is usually wise to make use of the digestive tract whenever possible, and in some instances it is necessary to use *both* enteral and parenteral feedings simultaneously in a severely malnourished patient. This is especially true in the "short-gut" syndrome (Sawyers and Harrington, 1972). Refeeding must be undertaken gradually. Start with a low level of nutrients and increase in modest increments until the target level of nutrients can be safely given. Once a positive balance of calories and of nitrogen has been established, the patient can be given one regular food after another as tolerated. It is important to keep in mind the ubiquitous nature of gluten. A great many processed foods contain wheat or wheat derivatives that will almost certainly expose the patient to some gluten.

Although it is customary to give "therapeutic" doses of those vitamins most likely to be deficient, there is no evidence that recovery occurs any faster in patients given 10 times or 100 times the RDA of vitamins than in those given a normal amount. Of course, depleted stores of some nutrients (vitamin D, vitamin B_{12}, and iron) *can* be replenished more rapidly, but there is no hurry, and overdosage with such nutrients as vitamin D or iron may cause toxic symptoms. If malabsorption is the obvious cause of vitamin deficiencies, then parenteral routes must be used. Since there are relatively few injectable preparations of fat-soluble vitamins available, it is important to read the labels carefully and to give as nearly as possible the recommended dietary allowance of each. An overdose of vitamin D can result in serious hypercalcemia with secondary renal damage. Similarly, an overdose of vitamin A can result in headaches, increased intracranial pressure, and other undesirable or dangerous consequences.

Once the patient with malabsorption has begun to make a good initial recovery, has regained part of the lost weight, and has begun to correct the hypoalbuminemia, anemia, and other manifestations of malnutrition, the physician must initiate measures that will prevent a recurrence. In the case of the patient with tropical sprue, a change of geographic location will usually be of benefit, but continuation of multiple vitamins and folic acid may be wise for six months or more after leaving the tropics. The patient with celiac sprue, however, must be observed carefully and at regular intervals for an indefinite period of time. The first and most important measure is to prohibit the eating of foods that contain gluten, even in small amounts. As mentioned above, the American public has come to rely more and more on convenience foods and "fast foods", almost any of which may contain cereals or cereal byproducts that will introduce gluten into the diet. It is probably wise to give any patient with celiac sprue a single multiple vitamin tablet daily in order to provide the recommended dietary allowances of each vitamin. Many patients will also need iron supplements unless they can be convinced that they should eat liver at least once a week.

The Use of Jejunoileal Bypass in Treatment of Obesity. The almost uniform failure of most methods of treating obesity has led to audacious and radical therapeutic approaches. At present the most popular and most controversial method is the "bowel bypass" or jejunoileal bypass. The objective is to reduce the total absorptive surface of small bowel that comes into contact with the food stream. The digestive juices from the stomach, liver, and pancreas are not prevented from mixing with the food, nor is the essential terminal ileum, which is responsible for absorption of vitamin B_{12}, excluded.

Theoretically, this operation should be safe and effective but clinical experience seems to indicate otherwise (Nutrition Reviews, 1975c). Quite aside from the understandable mortality of a major surgical procedure in a very obese person, the metabolic derangements that follow the bypass operation are only partially understood. Dysfunction of the liver occurs in most of these patients, at least transiently. Mezey and others (1975) observed that some produce ethanol endogenously. Bendezu and others (1976) not only found fatty livers but also observed that carbohydrate intolerance and elevated fasting levels of insulin occurred frequently. And urinary excretion of oxalate increased as a consequence of unabsorbed fats in the bowel that combined with calcium, thus making part of the oxalate load available for absorption (Stauffer, 1977).

Bray and others (1976) made the important observation that patients who had undergone a bowel bypass not only ate less food but also developed new taste preferences, presumably resulting from alterations in sensory perception. If this type of change could be achieved by non-surgical means, the problems of obesity might be managed more safely and effectively.

The mechanism whereby hepatic damage results from the bypass operation is hotly debated. Some suggest that it results from a *relative* deficiency of protein, secondary to impaired absorption of amino acids. Mason (1976) called attention to the large amounts of protein lost in the diarrheal stool of these patients, and Holzbach (1977) believes that hepatic steatosis may contribute to the incidence of cirrhosis in these patients.

Whatever the mechanisms involved, the facts are clear: most patients who undergo the jejunoileal bypass *do* lose a substantial amount of weight, but the risks of developing one or more serious complications are high. The author feels that conservative methods are preferable until the surgical approach is considerably safer.

The Colon

From the nutritional standpoint, the colon serves chiefly as an organ that extracts residual water and electrolytes from the remnants of food in the fecal stream after digestion and absorption have been virtually completed. Undoubtedly, the colonic flora produce many chemical substances that *might* be of use to human economy if they were absorbed. One such example is vitamin K, which is readily produced by microbial action. From rat studies we know that deficiency of vitamin K (prolongation of the prothrombin time) does not occur in healthy rats fed a vitamin K–deficient diet so long as they can eat their own fecal pellets. But if they are placed in a metabolic cage that deprives them of access to their own feces and completely prevents coprophagy they soon become vitamin K–deficient. Furthermore, studies of absorption of vitamin K across the mucosa of rat colons were done in *everted* specimens that were undoubtedly hypoxic and probably devitalized; hence results of questionable value. The very fact that sprue patients who have normal colonic mucosa cannot absorb sufficient vitamin K from their fecal stream to prevent hypoprothrombinemia is suggestive evidence that the colon was *not* designed for absorption of fats or fat-soluble vitamins.

Colonic disorders may be related to diet, at least to some extent. Recent epidemiologic studies which compared Africans with "Western" populations (Burkitt, 1975) have suggested that the amount of undigestible material or "fiber" in the diet plays a role in the causation of a great many common diseases. The theory is that this undigestible material termed "dietary fiber" not only occupies space in the digestive tract, thus decreasing the total food energy consumed, but also interferes with absorption of certain foods such as fats and sterols (Rose et al., 1974). Furthermore, food fiber is thought to be hydrophilic, thus resulting in larger, wetter, and softer stools (Tandon and Tandon, 1975). This, in turn, is supposed to cause increased peristalsis which propels the food stream along more rapidly and shortens the transit time from mouth to anus (Walker, 1975). At the same time, the bacterial flora change substantially (Drasar and Jenkins, 1976). As a consequence of all these events, the alleged benefits result directly from:

1. Decreased straining at stool (Walker, 1974; Wyman et al., 1976): decreased hemorrhoids, decreased varicose veins of the lower extremities, decreased hiatal hernias, decreased gastroesophageal reflux with esophagitis, decreased appendicitis, decreased colonic diverticulae.

2. Decreased food energy intake and decreased absorption of fat and sterols (Heaton, 1973; Trowell, 1976): decreased obesity, decreased diabetes mellitus, decreased hyperlipidemia, decreased atherosclerosis of coronary, cerebral and peripheral arteries.

3. Altered bacterial flora and shortened transit time (MacGregor, 1974; Dorfman et al., 1976): decreased formation of carcinogens, decreased time of contact between potential carcinogens and bowel mucosa.

The practical result of this idea has been a raging controversy over the effect or lack of effect of high fiber diets in a large number of clinical disorders, ranging from irritable bowel syndrome to hyperlipidemia (Eastwood et al., 1974). It is impossible to draw firm conclusions from the varied and contradictory reports currently available. Disorders of colonic motility are mostly allied with those described under "fiber". Most forms of diarrhea result either from enteric infections or infestations, or from some organic lesion such as idiopathic ulcerative colitis. Dietary "therapy" of diarrhea is futile unless the etiology is known. Prescription of a "bland" or low residue diet is largely outmoded. Even the patient with severe ulcerative colitis may tolerate a normal diet better than an insipid amorphous puréed diet. There are no foods that are specifically constipating and none that are "soothing". The important nutritional principles are to provide adequate nutrients in the most acceptable form. There has been one notable advance in the management of severe diarrhea. Physicians in India who did not have sufficient supplies of intravenous fluids available to treat large numbers of patients suffering from cholera found that administration of large volumes of isotonic glucose and saline by mouth was effective in preventing dehydration, ketosis, and severe electrolyte disturbances. This form of therapy has been used successfully in infants and children who had a sudden severe attack of diarrhea (Hirschhorn and Denny, 1975).

Constipation is common among Americans, especially elderly individuals, and may result in part from our customary diet, which is rather low in fiber. Some patients experience welcome relief from constipation as a result of changing to a high fiber diet, but the physician should caution against overenthusiasm. High bulk diets often cause increased gas formation and may result in annoying distress and embarrassing involuntary passage of flatus. In some individuals, the bran of cereals can interfere with absorption of zinc and other essential nutrients. Many patients with diverticulosis are now being told to increase bulk in their diet. Theoretically this should be helpful according to Painter and Burkitt (1971), and many trials are now under way.

Inflammatory diseases of the large bowel can in themselves contribute to malnutrition, because the patient who has a painful peristaltic rush after each meal will soon become conditioned to an inadequate intake of food. Indeed, such conditioning may, in large measure, be responsible for the weight loss manifested by patients who undergo jejuno-ileal bypass in the treatment of massive obesity. Apparently the unpleasant sensations associated with diarrhea have a material effect on the volume of food a patient will eat.

In patients with idiopathic ulcerative colitis and in some patients with radiation colitis, or with Crohn's granulomatous colitis, the problem of reflex stimulation of defecation becomes serious indeed. Under these circumstances, a trial with an elemental diet is worthwhile. Such a diet, if given first in small amounts and diluted to isotonicity may be very well tolerated so that both the quantity and the concentration can be increased progressively. On the other hand, if this is not successful within a short time, such a patient should be given total parenteral nutrition (TPN) without further delay. Avoidance of delay is important because these patients rapidly become depleted of many essential nutrients, and in the process, lose important functions. For example, Ellestad-Sayed and others (1976) found that colonic tissue from such patients was severely depleted of pantothenic acid and coenzyme A, without which the mucosa would soon lose most metabolic functions. The objective is to establish weight gain and protein anabolism (Abbott, 1976). The average duration of TPN therapy will be about one month in patients with ulcerative colitis or Crohn's granulomatous colitis. This form of therapy is entirely nonspecific, but patients benefit from improved strength and sense of well-being, as well as from restoration of their depleted proteins, vitamins, and minerals, correction of their anemia, and improvement in their immune mechanisms. Dudrick's group has expressed the belief that Crohn's disease may subside spontaneously as a result of TPN therapy. It is true that these patients not only gain weight but may also have a reduction in the frequency of defecation, and in those who have fistulas the closure rate is high. They also may regenerate areas of exfoliated mucosa and heal their surgical wounds at a normal rate. Whether TPN therapy provides specific or nonspecific support is of little consequence; most patients with inflammatory disease of the bowel do benefit from TPN therapy.

The Gallbladder and the Liver

Perhaps no other field of medicine has been so divided on the issue of dietary management as that of the liver and the biliary tract. This may result from the apparent association between eating and symptoms in many patients with disease of the biliary tract. And part of the folklore may be traced to primitive pathological studies of diseased livers that contained large amounts of fat. The severe malnutrition and wasting that represent far advanced hepatic disease probably help explain the idea that a low-fat, high-protein diet is needed by such patients. Putting together this melange of partial truths and common beliefs, one might deduce that patients with *any* kind of liver or biliary tract disease should be given a diet that is easy to digest, low in fat, and high in protein. Indeed, this has been the essence of diet therapy for gallbladder disease and liver disease.

The fact is that the types of foods consumed by the patient have very little to do with symptoms. It is true that dietary fats or proteins do stimulate release of cholecystokinin which, in turn, causes the gallbladder to contract. But the elaborate and misguided information that formerly was taught about specific foods and gallbladder symptoms cannot be supported by the evidence. Traditionally, such foods as fried chicken, ice cream, cabbage, and eggs were cited as precipitating factors. Actually, some of these foods, like most others, do cause the gallbladder to contract, but unless a gallstone is located within the duct system, contraction of the gallbladder is unlikely to produce symptoms. And for patients with vague symptoms such as fullness, belching, slight nausea, and dull aching in the right upper quadrant, dietary changes have little or no value. It is wise to tell these patients from the start to begin with a simple diet and introduce one food at a time, keeping a diet-diary of foods eaten and symptoms experienced each day. After a week or two, they can then be advised to avoid the offending foods and still eat a balanced, healthful diet. No doubt this approach is largely psychological, but it often works and it is both harmless and inexpensive. For the patient with parenchymal disease of the liver, whether it results from a viral infection or a toxic chemical (including alcohol) or from malnutrition, certain nutritional principles are important to bear in mind:

The liver is the first organ to process nutrients absorbed from the digestive tract. As such, it is paramount in metabolism of amino acids. This explains the altered plasma amino acid patterns in patients with hepatic failure. Normally the liver removes about 80 per cent of most amino acids from the portal circulation. The major exceptions are the three branch-chain amino acids—leucine, isoleucine, and valine—which are preferentially metabolized by peripheral tissues and are insulin-sensitive. Furthermore, the liver normally extracts much of the insulin secreted by the pancreas, thus regulating the concentration in the peripheral circulation. Tryptophan and other aromatic amino acids are metabolized in the central nervous system to neurotrophic amines. There is some reason to believe that entry of excessive amounts of tryptophan and some of its derivatives into the brain may play a role in the genesis of hepatic encephalopathy. Fischer and others who have studied patients with this disorder have observed that there often are increased amounts of phenylalanine and methionine in the brain (Aguirre et al., 1976). Phenylalanine is normally converted to tyrosine, but this process may be delayed by lack of the enzyme phenylalanine hydroxylase. Higher than normal levels of insulin in the peripheral blood result in lower concentrations of leucine, isoleucine, and valine, which normally compete with the aromatic amino acids for entry into the brain. The brain tissue of such patients has been found to contain increased levels of serotonin and decreased levels of norepinephrine. At the same time, an abnormal substance, octopamine, has been identified in brain tissue and it has been suggested that this competes with dopamine for binding sites. The old concept that increased levels of ammonia account for hepatic encephalopathy no longer seems to be supported by existing evidence. About half of the patients given parenteral nutrition, utilizing the normal amino acid mixture, benefited from this form of management. Fischer has suggested, on the basis of experiments with dogs, that amino acid solutions containing increased amounts of the branched-chain amino acids and lesser amounts of the aromatic amino acids might be beneficial for patients with impending hepatic coma. Additional work in this area will be awaited with great interest.

The best advice for handling the patient with obvious liver disease is to start with a diet of normal, attractive foods, but limit both the protein allowance and the sodium allowance. Unless the patient is already showing evidence of impending hepatic coma, it is reasonable to give 0.5 gm of protein per kilogram of normal body weight per day, or about 35 gm for the average man. The patient should be evaluated daily for signs of confusion, disorientation, and asterixis. The protein allowance can be increased cautiously every three or four days, going up to 40 gm, then to 50 gm, and eventually to 55 gm/day. Larger amounts are probably not wise, nor are they necessary to achieve nitrogen anabolism in the average patient. From the practical standpoint, patients who have little appetite will often tolerate carbohydrates sooner than fats in their diet. Fresh fruits and vegetables may be accepted, whereas meats, eggs, and cheese may not. Fats and proteins have high satiety values and so there is little difficulty in getting patients to agree to a moderate amount of protein restriction.

Many patients with liver disease, and especially those with portal cirrhosis, will have a problem with salt retention. The usual American diet contains about 12 gm of sodium chloride or 205 mEq (note that the virtue of using milliequivalents is that

$$1 \text{ mEq of NaCl} = 1 \text{ mEq of Na}^+ = 1 \text{ mEq of Cl}^-).$$

On the other hand, if one were to calculate the *sodium* content of this diet, one would have to deal with the figure 4.27 gm of sodium/day out of 12 gm of sodium chloride. From the practical standpoint, it is possible to restrict the sodium intake of most patients to about half the usual level without any difficulty. And many patients will tolerate a diet that contains about 40 mEq of sodium per day, but it is important to explain *why* their food is not salted. Severe restriction of sodium (20 mEq) should be imposed only upon those patients who are accumulating ascitic and edema fluid despite moderate salt restriction and judicious use of diuretics.

Patients with liver disease of any kind should not be subjected to starvation. Studies both in normal individuals and in patients with familial abnormalities of the liver, such as the Dubin-Johnson syndrome, have been observed to have a significant rise in bilirubin levels following brief periods of starvation. In addition, glucose is one of the most important detoxifying agents available to the liver in handling not only drugs and medications but also many compounds absorbed from the digestive tract.

Nutritional management of patients with metabolic storage diseases does not play a very important role in medical practice. Patients with hepatolenticular degeneration or Wilson's disease were at one time given diets low in copper as an adjunct to the administration of chelating agents that could remove copper from storage. It seems doubtful that the small amount of copper that could be excluded from their diet was of much importance from a quantitative standpoint.

The second form of storage disease, hemochromatosis, does not usually result from an excessive intake of dietary iron but, instead, from abnormal storage that results from a metabolic error or that follows in the wake of marked and prolonged hemolysis of red blood cells. But such patients are not fed an iron-deficient diet. Instead they undergo repeated blood-letting, or their disease is treated with chelating agents that help remove storage iron.

Pancreatic Diseases

The normal functioning of the pancreas depends upon a cascade of endocrine events as food moves down the digestive tract. In patients with inflammatory or obstructive or hemorrhagic disease of the pancreas, it generally is considered undesirable to stimulate pancreatic secretions because not only will this build up pressure within the acini but, in some instances, secretions will escape from the confines of the ductal system and result either in a pseudocyst or a fistula. Accordingly, it seems logical to do everything possible to prevent or at least to minimize pancreatic secretion in such patients. At present, there is no effective dietary method of inhibiting secretions other than to administer predigested or elemental diets through a tube introduced into the duodenum distal to the opening of the duct of Santorini. Even so, there may be some stimulation of pancreatic secretions. Limited experience with total parenteral nutrition in patients with pancreatic disease has resulted in generally favorable reports (Nutrition Reviews, 1975b). Most of this results from nutritional support consisting of restoration of caloric and nitrogen balance. But in patients with pancreatic fistulas the rate of secretion from the fistula has been observed to decrease progressively as TPN therapy has been continued. The success rate with patients who have developed pancreatitis as a result of trauma or surgical operation seems to be higher than in those resulting from disease of the biliary tract or those associated with excessive use of alcohol. At present, TPN therapy appears to provide some measure of success but wider experience with larger numbers of patients should provide more definitive answers.

Children who have cystic fibrosis suffer from malabsorption that is secondary to inadequate exocrine secretion by the pancreas. These children need the same nutrients that normal children require but, in addition, they will have to be given pancreatic enzymes by mouth in order to permit them to digest and absorb food. Pediatricians have very skillfully achieved this goal despite the many obvious problems that occur in the lives of young people who must do something special in order to survive.

Nutritional therapy coupled with a knowledge of normal and pathological physiology of the digestive tract permits a greater measure of therapeutic success in dealing with patients who have a wide variety of conditions. Many of the old familiar ideas about diet therapy have been abandoned for lack of supporting evidence. New, simplified nutritional principles are proving to be effective in augmenting treatment of most patients. There is no such thing as "therapeutic" starvation.

REFERENCES

Abbott, W. M.: Indications for parenteral nutrition. pp. 3–14 in *Total Parenteral Nutrition*, J. E. Fischer (ed.). Boston, MA, Little, Brown and Company, 1976.

Aguirre, A., Funovics, J., Wesdorp, R. I. C., and Fischer, J. E.: Parenteral nutrition in hepatic failure. pp. 219–230 in *Total Parenteral Nutrition*, J. E. Fischer (ed.). Boston, MA, Little, Brown and Company, 1976.

Anonymous: Cell-mediated immunity to gliadin within the small-intestinal mucosa in celiac disease. *Nutr. Reviews 33*:267, 1975a.

Anonymous: Effects of oral and parenteral feeding on pancreatic enzyme contents. *Nutr. Reviews 33*:187, 1975b.

Anonymous: Intestinal bypass surgery for obesity. *Nutr. Reviews 33*:78, 1975c.

Anonymous: Coffee drinking and peptic ulcer disease. *Nutr. Reviews 34*:167, 1976.

Bendezu, R., Wieland, R. G., Green, S. G., Hallberg, M. C., and Marsters, R. W.: Certain metabolic consequences of jejunoileal bypass. *Amer. J. Clin. Nutr. 29*:366, 1976.

Bray, G. A., Barry, R. E., Benfield, J. R., Castelnuovo-Tedesco, P., and Rodin, J.: Intestinal bypass surgery for obesity decreases food intake and taste preferences. *Amer. J. Clin. Nutr. 29*:779, 1976.

Burkitt, D. P.: Epidemiology and etiology. *J.A.M.A. 231*:517, 1975.

Dorfman, S. H., Ali, M., and Floch, M. H.: Low fiber content of Connecticut diets. *Amer. J. Clin. Nutr. 29*:87, 1976.

Drasar, B. S., and Jenkins, D. J. A.: Bacteria, diet, and large bowel cancer. *Amer. J. Clin. Nutr. 29*:1410, 1976.

Eastwood, M. A., Fisher, N., Greenwood, C. T., and Hutchinson, J. B.: Perspectives on the bran hypothesis. *Lancet 1*:1029, 1974.

Ellestad-Sayed, J. J., Nelson, R. A., Adson, M. A., Palmer, W. M., and Soule, E. H.: Pantothenic acid, coenzyme A, and human chronic ulcerative and granulomatous colitis. *Amer. J. Clin. Nutr. 29*:1333, 1976.

Fordtran, J. S.: Reduction of acidity by diet, antacids, and anticholinergic agents. P. 718 in *Gastrointestinal Disease*, M. H. Sleisenger and J. S. Fordtran (eds.). Philadelphia, W. B. Saunders Company, 1973.

Hartroft, W. S.: The incidence of coronary artery disease in patients treated with Sippy diet. *Amer. J. Clin. Nutr. 15*:205, 1964.

Heaton, K. W.: Food fiber as an obstacle to energy intake. *Lancet 2*:1418, 1973.

Hendrix, T. R.: New concepts in the diagnosis and management of heartburn. *G. I. Tract 1(2)*:4, 1971.

Hirschhorn, N., and Denny, K. M.: Oral glucose-electrolyte therapy for diarrhea: a means to maintain or improve nutrition? *Amer. J. Clin. Nutr. 28*:189, 1975.

Holzbach, R. T.: Hepatic effects of jejunoileal bypass for morbid obesity. *Amer. J. Clin. Nutr. 30*:43, 1977.

Isenberg, J. I.: Facts and habits in duodenal ulcer treatment. *G.I. Tract 5(2)*:15, 1975.

Lebenthal, E., Antonowicz, I., and Shwachman, H.: Correlation of lactase activity, lactose tolerance, and milk consumption in different age groups. *Amer. J. Clin. Nutr. 28*:595, 1975.

Lotz, M., Zisman, E., and Bartter, F. C.: Evidence for a phosphorus-depletion syndrome in man. *New England J. Med. 278*:409, 1968.

MacGregor, I. L.: Carcinoma of the colon and stomach. A review with comment on epidemiologic associations. *J.A.M.A. 227*:911, 1974.

Mainardi, M., Maxwell, V., Sturdevant, R. A. L., and Isenberg, J. I.: Metiamide, an H^2-receptor blocker, as inhibitor of basal and meal-stimulated gastric acid secretion in patients with duodenal ulcer. *New England J. Med. 291*:373, 1974.

Mason, E. E.: Jejunoileal bypass (Letter to the Editor). *Amer. J. Clin. Nutr. 29*:938, 1976.

McMillan, D. E., and Freeman, R. B.: The milk-alkali syndrome. A study of the acute disorder with comments on the development of the chronic condition. *Medicine 44*:485, 1965.

Mezey, E., Imbembo, A. L., Potter, J. J., Rent, K. C., Lombardo, R., and Holt, P. R.: Endogenous ethanol production and hepatic disease following jejunoileal bypass for morbid obesity. *Amer. J. Clin. Nutr. 28*:1277, 1975.

Paige, D. M., Bayless, T. M., and Dellinger, W. S.: Relationship of milk consumption to blood glucose rise in lactose intolerant individuals. *Amer. J. Clin. Nutr. 28*:677, 1975a.

Paige, D. M., Bayless, T. M., Huang, S. S., and Wexler, R.: Lactose hydrolyzed milk. *Amer. J. Clin. Nutr. 28*:818, 1975b.

Painter, N. S., and Burkitt, D. P.: Diverticular disease of the colon: A deficiency disease of Western civilization. *Brit. Med. J. 2*:450, 1971.

Reinken, L., Zieglauer, H., and Berger, H.: Vitamin B_6 nutriture of children with acute celiac disease, celiac disease in remission, and of children with normal duodenal mucosa. *Amer. J. Clin. Nutr. 29*:750, 1976.

Rose, G., Blackburn, H., Keys, A., Taylor, H. L., Kannel, W. B., Paul, O., Reid, D. D., and Stamler, J.: Colon cancer and blood cholesterol. *Lancet 1*:181, 1974.

Rosenzweig, N. S.: Diet and intestinal enzyme adaptation: implications for gastrointestinal disorders. *Amer. J. Clin. Nutr. 28*:648, 1975.

Sawyers, J. L., and Harrington, J. L., Jr.: Short gut syndrome. *Surg. Ann. 4*:273, 1972.

Sigler, M. H.: The Mechanism of the Natriuresis of Fasting, *J. Clin. Invest. 55*:377, 1975.

Solomons, N. W., Rosenberg, I. H., and Sandstead, H. H.: Zinc nutrition in celiac sprue. *Amer. J. Clin. Nutr. 29*:371, 1976.

Stauffer, J. Q.: Hyperoxaluria and calcium oxalate nephrolithiasis after jejunoileal bypass. *Amer. J. Clin. Nutr. 30*:64, 1977.

Tandon, R. K., and Tandon, B. N.: Stool weights in North Indians (Letter to the Editor). *Lancet 2*:560, 1975.

Trowell, H.: Definition of dietary fiber and hypotheses that it is a protective factor in certain diseases. *Amer. J. Clin. Nutr. 29*:417, 1976.

Walker, A. R. P.: Dietary fiber and the pattern of disease (Editorial). *Ann. Intern. Med. 80*:663, 1974.

Walker, A. R. P.: Effect of high crude fiber intake on transit time and the absorption of nutrients in South African negro schoolchildren. *Amer. J. Clin. Nutr. 28*:1161, 1975.

Woteki, C. E., Wesser, E., and Young, E. A.: Lactose malabsorption in Mexican-American children. *Amer. J. Clin. Nutr. 29*:19, 1976.

Wyman, J. B., Heaton, K. W., Manning, A. P., and Wicks, A. C. B.: The effect on intestinal transit and the feces of raw and cooked bran in different doses. *Amer. J. Clin. Nutr. 29*:1474, 1976.

4

DIET, CHOLESTEROL, AND CORONARY HEART DISEASE

Robert E. Hodges, M.D.

The latest statistics available (calendar year 1976) indicate that there were 1,912,000 deaths in the United States, of which more than half resulted from cardiovascular diseases. Ischemic heart disease (coronary heart disease) was responsible for 34 per cent of all deaths, or 649,280 individuals (see Table 4–1). (Vital Statistics *The World Almanac and Book of Facts*, 1978.) Furthermore, 25 per cent of all cardiovascular deaths occurred in persons less than 65 years of age, indicating that heart disease is not limited to the elderly.

Epidemiology of Coronary Heart Disease

In the first two decades of this century, the majority of deaths resulted from infectious diseases, but deaths from heart disease now greatly exceed the *combined total* of deaths from infectious illnesses, cancer, and accidents. Epidemiologists who have devoted a major portion of their time and effort to the problem of coronary heart disease have identified at least ten correlates or "risk factors" in the general population (Table 4–2) (Frantz and Moore, 1969; Gordon and Kannel, 1972; Keys et al., 1972a and b; Stitt et al., 1973; Oliver et al., 1975; Ross and Glomset, 1976; and *Coronary Heart Disease: A New Zealand Report*, 1971). Although each of the factors listed has been found to correlate significantly with death rate from coronary heart

TABLE 4–1   DEATHS FROM HEART DISEASE (1976)
RATES PER 100,000 POPULATION*

Total Deaths, all causes	1,912,000
Major Cardiovascular Diseases	977,410
Heart Disease	726,700
Ischemic Heart Disease	649,280

*Heart disease of all types accounted for 51% of all deaths, and coronary (ischemic) heart disease accounted for 34% of all deaths. Source: Division of Vital Statistics, National Center for Health Statistics. [Provisional data based on 10% sampling of all death certificates for a 12-month (January-December) period.] Cited in *World Almanac and Book of Facts*, 1978, New York, Newspaper Enterprise Association Incorporated.

disease, there are three that occupy a position of preeminence: hypercholesterolemia, high blood pressure, and cigarette smoking. Diabetes mellitus also significantly increases the risk of coronary heart disease. Of course, heredity, age, gender, and personality Type A are also important, but these are factors over which we have no control. The remaining factors — physical inactivity and changing life patterns — have been debated by experts, and although there is some disagreement, the consensus is that they too are important. It is relatively easy to increase physical activity, but not so easy to change one's life style.

Undoubtedly, hypercholesterolemia has received the greatest share of attention, not only by epidemiologists but by clinical investigators as well. Identification of the more specific subgroups of hyperlipidemias (Table 4–3) represents a step forward in our understanding of genetic factors that influence the development of atherosclerosis (Fredrickson, 1971). Type II hyperlipidemia is identical with the old and familiar disorder formerly known as "familial hypercholesterolemia", as well as other descriptive terms. In its homozygous form, this

TABLE 4–2   RISK FACTORS*

A. THOSE AMENABLE TO CHANGE:
Hyperlipidemia (LDL cholesterol, VLDL triglycerides)
High blood pressure
Personal habits (cigarette smoking, abuse of alcohol, coffee)
Physical inactivity
Diabetes mellitus

B. THOSE DIFFICULT OR IMPOSSIBLE TO CHANGE:
Personality, Type A
Heredity (coronary heart disease)
Age
Sex
Changing life patterns

*Statistically, the strongest associations between coronary heart disease and possible risk factors are "the big three": hypercholesterolemia, elevated blood pressure, and cigarette smoking.

TABLE 4-3   THE HYPERLIPIDEMIAS*

TYPE	INCREASED LIPOPROTEIN	APPEARANCE OF PLASMA	PLASMA LIPIDS Cholesterol	Triglycerides	ELECTROPHORETIC PATTERN	INCIDENCE AND CLINICAL FEATURES
I	Chylomicrons	Thick layer of "cream" floating on clear plasma	Normal	Increased	Chylomicrons at origin	Rare; May begin with abdominal pain
II a	LDL	Clear	Increased	Normal	Increased Beta lipoprotein	Common; Tuberous xanthomata
b	LDL + VLDL	Slightly cloudy	Increased	Increased	Same + pre Beta lipoprotein	Thickened tendons; Premature atherosclerosis
III	LDL + abnormal VLDL	Cloudy with layer of "cream"	Increased	Increased	Broad Beta lipoprotein	Uncertain; Eruptive xanthomata; Premature atherosclerosis; Carbohydrate intolerance
IV	VLDL	Cloudy	Normal	Increased	Pre Beta lipoprotein	Common; Obesity; Carbohydrate intolerance; Premature atherosclerosis
V	Chylomicrons + VLDL	Cloudy with layer of "cream"	Normal	Increased	Chylomicrons at origin + pre Beta lipoprotein	Rare; Obesity; Abdominal pain; Eruptive xanthomata; Carbohydrate intolerance

*Of the five major types of hyperlipidemia, only three are associated with an increased incidence of atherosclerotic disease. These are Types II (a and b), III, and IV. Identification of any of these three forms of hyperlipidemia is cause for intervention with appropriate dietary or drug therapy.

syndrome is lethal in a few decades; most of its victims die of coronary heart disease before age 40. Enos and colleagues (1955) studied the incidence of coronary heart disease in United States soldiers killed in action in Korea. Autopsies of 300 soldiers whose average age was 22.1 years disclosed that 77.3 per cent had gross evidence of coronary disease that varied from fibrous thickening to complete occlusion of one or more of the main branches of the coronary tree. This report gave added impetus to the concern of clinicians over the magnitude and severity of coronary heart disease in young men, and led to speculation that heterozygous Type II hyperlipidemia may be very common. A report by Shapiro and others (1969), describing the incidence of coronary heart disease in a population insured for medical care, delineated the magnitude of the problem and the importance of relative risk factors. For example, men were found to have an annual incidence rate of "first myocardial infarction" that was five times that of women of the same age, and male cigarette smokers had twice the risk of comparable non-smokers. Physical inactivity among men greatly elevated their risk of sustaining a first myocardial infarction, and men whose body weight was 15 per cent or more above average had a 50 per cent greater risk. Kannel (1971) described the lipid profiles of potential coronary victims, and Keys and others (1971) reported on the mortality from coronary heart disease among men studied for 23 years. By this time the level of concern over the coronary problem was nearing a peak. McNamara and colleagues (1971) repeated the studies done by Enos and reported that among 105 United States soldiers killed in Vietnam, autopsies that included coronary angiography and dissection of the heart disclosed that 45 per cent had evidence of atherosclerosis. Five per cent had gross evidence of severe coronary atherosclerosis, but angiography failed to demonstrate a single case of severe coronary narrowing. The mean ages of the two series were the same, although the results were different. McNamara's group felt that the degree of obstruction of a coronary vessel could not be judged adequately by gross examination in the post-mortem state, because elastic fibers markedly reduce the size of the lumen and the circumference of the empty vessel. They felt that even angiography might not give a representative picture because of post-mortem changes.

Keys and his group, in a series of studies, evaluated the possibility that ethnic origin might be a factor in the etiology of coronary heart disease. It had long been noted that those Japanese living in Japan were relatively immune to this condition, whereas the white races of Northern and Western European origin had a much greater susceptibility. Epidemiologic studies, coupled with diet histories and measurements of plasma lipid levels, have shown conclusively that Japanese who live in Hawaii not only have modified their diet, but have achieved a greater degree of obesity, higher plasma levels of cholesterol, and a higher incidence of coronary heart disease than Japanese living in their native land. Furthermore, those Japanese who emigrated to California were found to have even more obesity, greater elevation of plasma cholesterol, and a still higher incidence of coronary heart disease than those living in Hawaii. Clearly, this is a problem of environment and not of heredity (Keys et al., 1958; Wen and Gershoff, 1973; Kato et al., 1973; and Rhoads et al., 1976). Furthermore, Yanigihara (1976) described changes that have developed in Japan during the last 20 years. He observed that the number of patients with heart disease has increased fourfold in that period of time and that the mortality from cardiovascular diseases has now reached 47 per cent of total deaths. Although the author does not say so, the implication is that "westernization" of the Japanese diet may have contributed to the changing incidence of cardiovascular disorders. This and other evidence leads to the strong supposition that people of all races are potentially susceptible to developing atherosclerosis, particularly of the coronary arteries. This potential is not developed to any substantial degree in countries where the traditional diet contains very little fat, very little cholesterol, and generally speaking, a scant caloric intake. This is not to minimize other factors, but lifetime dietary practices undoubtedly represent major factors in determining the average plasma cholesterol level in any population group. In the accompanying table (Table 4–4), it can be seen that people living in Southeast Asia, who consume very little fat or cholesterol by American standards, have average plasma-cholesterol levels that are remarkably lower than the average in the United States. (The figures for Southeast Asia are based on survey data collected by the Interdepartmental Committee on Nutrition for National Development [ICNND] and represent an average of several hundred adults. The figures for the United States represent an average of several hundred adult persons employed in industry in the state of Iowa. Data were collected during the 1950's and 1960's).

TABLE 4–4 PLASMA CHOLESTEROL AND DIET IN SOUTHEAST ASIA AND IN IOWA*

COUNTRY	DIETARY INTAKE Cholesterol mg/d	Fat gm/d	PLASMA CHOLESTEROL mg/dl
Thailand	15	18	123
Vietnam	30	32	140
Burma	23	52	162
Malaya	25	62	193
U.S.A. (Iowa)	750	120	240

*Levels of cholesterol in plasma of apparently healthy adults seem to reflect dietary fats more closely than dietary cholesterol. From data collected by the author (Malaya and Iowa) and from data published by the International Committee on Nutrition for National Development.

PREDICTION OF CORONARY HEART DISEASE

The Risk Factors

Until recently, most people believed that coronary heart disease struck down its victims without any warning. It was often said that a man who had just sustained a myocardial infarction had "never been sick a day in his life" until the tragic event. Indeed, the individual often was "a picture of health". We now recognize that these concepts are false. The excessively high death rate from coronary heart disease in the United States and other "westernized" countries has led physicians and other workers to search for methods to identify those individuals who are most likely to develop this disorder. With the information and facilities available to the medical profession it now is possible to identify with a considerable degree of confidence a number of individuals who are at great risk of having a heart attack in the future. Much of this information is based on the meticulous studies conducted at Framingham, Massachusetts during the past quarter century (Gordon and Kannel, 1972). It is, of course, not yet possible for a physician to predict when a given individual will have a heart attack, but it *is* possible to classify an individual as being of low risk, average risk, high risk, or very high risk. Furthermore, the methods for making such classifications are readily available to today's medical practitioners. The classification is based on information of five different types: personal habits, family history, personality, physical examination, and laboratory tests. No doubt the precision and reliability of the many components of these broad categories will become better defined as time goes by and we have accumulated more experience. At present, however, there is reason to believe that predictions based upon the following observations have sufficient reliability to justify specific recommendations to patients.

Personal Habits

The coronary-prone individual is thought to be a restless, nervous person who has acquired certain contemporary habits. Some of these habits can be associated statistically with a greater-than-average risk of developing coronary heart disease. The worst of these is cigarette smoking. There can be no question about the statistical association between the use of cigarettes and the death rate from coronary heart disease (*Coronary Heart Disease. A New Zealand Report*, page 108, 1971). The more cigarettes an individual smokes, the greater his or her risk of having a heart attack.

Another habit that may have significance is the use of alcohol. Despite the old adage that a drink now and then eases tension, there is increasing evidence that more than two drinks may have a significant effect on the plasma lipids, especially the triglycerides, of susceptible individuals. And contrary to the old idea that moderate amounts of alcohol benefit the patient with angina pectoris, there now is evidence that alcohol decreases the stroke volume of the heart of a patient who has coronary artery disease. The net result of alcohol ingestion may be a reduction in exercise tolerance.

The coronary-prone individual is generally considered to be more sedentary, both in occupation and his recreational activities, than his or her counterpart who is apparently normal. Epidemiologic studies are by no means unanimous on this point and must be interpreted with caution. The well-publicized studies of London bus drivers by Morris (1953) suggested that the exercise of climbing up-and-down stairs in double-decker buses afforded some immunity for the conductor, in contrast to the driver who sat at his wheel all day. Some studies in the United States have suggested that farmers are less susceptible to coronary heart disease than are persons in other occupational groups. But today's farmer generally does not engage in strenuous physical activity, depending instead upon an increasingly complex array of machinery to lighten the load.

The recent enthusiasm for jogging, bicycling, tennis, and other sports elicits a variety of reactions from physicians and epidemiologists alike. Exercise is probably important, certainly from the standpoint of increasing caloric expenditure, conditioning skeletal as well as cardiovascular musculature, and providing a general sense of well-being. Exercise may also have a beneficial effect on plasma lipids, especially the triglycerides. The question of whether a program designed to increase physical activity actually lessens death rate from coronary heart disease will no doubt be answered within the next decade or so. Meanwhile, the author believes that it does no harm, is personally gratifying, and may prove to be beneficial.

Family History

A few patients will relate such an incredibly bad history of coronary disease among their relatives that any physician would feel obliged to evaluate the status of all close relatives. For example, if a man 30 years of age sustains a myocardial infarction and there is a history of heart attack or sudden death before age 40 in other male members of his family, it is fair to suspect that his family has an inherited defect of their lipoproteins. In many instances, the patient will be found to have Type II hyperlipidemia. If the family history suggests strongly that the patient is a homozygote and all other male members of his immediate family have hyperlipidemia or atherosclerotic disease, or both, then it is imperative that the lipid patterns of all of his children be evaluated. It also is important to evaluate the lipids of his wife, because if she also has hyperlipidemia, their children may have an even greater problem.

Although coronary heart disease involves many people in our country, the age of onset in a family gives valuable information. It is reasonable to assume that coronary disease that becomes manifest after age 65 or 70 is far less likely to be familial than coronary disease that becomes apparent before age 40. Nonetheless, if a patient relates a family history of coronary disease in both parents, in a number of aunts, uncles, cousins, and in one or more siblings, then the probability of that patient developing this disorder is substantially greater. Conversely, for the individual whose parents, grandparents, aunts, and uncles have survived beyond age 70 without apparent coronary heart disease, it is reasonable to conclude that this person has less-than-average likelihood of having a heart attack. Attempts have been made to classify relatives as having a first-, second-, or third-degree relationship to the patient, and some authorities would further refine the family history on the basis of whether relatives develop coronary disease in the first, middle, or last third of a normal life span. But there is no convincing evidence that this degree of refinement is statistically meaningful, even though the general concept appears to have validity.

Personality

Most people believe that heart attacks are in some way related to overwork, emotional stress, and general discontent. It is difficult to define stress, let alone evaluate it quantitatively. Friedman and his group believe that people can be divided into two broad categories: Type A and Type B. Type A individuals are described as being competitive, restless, driving, impatient, and ambitious. Often they are discontent with their level of achievement, and they tend to regard themselves as failures. Type B individuals are considered to be the opposite in all categories. Medical opinion is sharply divided on the subject of personality and its impact on coronary heart disease. Friedman and Byers (1973) did show that in rats subjected to hypothalamic damage, there was a delay in catabolism of cholesterol into bile acids with resultant hypercholesterolemia. This demonstrates that an organic lesion of the brain can affect cholesterol metabolism, but it certainly does not prove that either personality type or situational stress can have similar effects. Nonetheless, many people believe that stress and personality *do* play a role in the development of coronary heart disease and it seems reasonable for the physician to make some effort to classify patients as Type A or Type B. With all this emphasis on the major risk factor, we may be tempted at times to forget or neglect stressful situations.

Rahe and others (1974) gathered data in Helsinki, Finland about recent changes in life style among 279 survivors of documented myocardial infarctions, compared with 226 cases of abrupt coronary death. They concluded that in all but one group of subjects there had been a marked disruption of the usual life pattern during the six months immediately prior to infarction or death. This was especially true of sudden death victims. The changing events included recent illnesses, a change in employment, family or marital problems, and personal and social problems. In some instances, these problems had a material effect on the eating, drinking, and smoking habits of the subjects, and there may also have been changes in their level of physical activity. Quite probably these nonspecific "stressor effects" contribute materially to the development of overt coronary heart disease.

Physical Examination

As mentioned before, many patients who develop coronary heart disease are generally considered to be "the picture of health" prior to their heart attack. They may be well-developed, somewhat over-nourished and ruddy-cheeked, but there are other characteristics that may lead the physician to suspect coronary heart disease. In men, premature bitemporal grayness of the hair has been named as one factor. A more convincing finding, however, is the appearance of arcus senilis or arcus corneae in relatively young individuals. This phenomenon results from deposition of cholesterol on the posterior surface of the cornea adjacent to the limbus. It appears as a faint blue-gray opacity which may be almost invisible in individuals with blue or green pigmentation of the iris but is readily apparent in those who have dark brown pigmentation of the iris. An arcus senilis is very common in individuals in their seventh or eighth decade of life, but when it is found in a person in the third or fourth decade of life, it has much greater significance (Rosenman et al., 1974).

Another common abnormality is deposition of cholesterol in the soft tissues surrounding the eye, usually referred to as xanthelasma (Fig. 4-1). Although this abnormality may be associated with elevated cholesterol or triglyceride levels, it is not necessarily so. It also has been noted in thyrotoxic individuals who have abnormally low lipid levels. Nonetheless, any patient who has xanthelasma should undergo lipid studies.

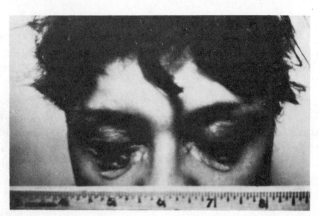

Figure 4–1 Cholesterol deposits in the soft tissues around the eye are called xanthelasma and are an indication for lipid studies. Courtesy Elaine Feldman and *Resident and Staff Physician*.

The lack of specificity of lipid deposits is emphasized by Harlan (1975) in a report of a patient who had extremely high cholesterol and triglyceride levels accompanying a plasma-cell malignancy. In this patient, lipids were carried by a myeloma protein instead of by lipoproteins. There was a "lipid line" on the gums, yet post-mortem examination of vascular tissues demonstrated freedom from atherosclerosis despite these deposits in the gingival mucosa. Other, more common, physical manifestations of hyperlipidemia include tuberous deposits in the skin, especially over such pressure areas as elbows and knees, and deposits of lipid in tendons, particularly the Achilles tendon and the extensor tendons of the hands where they cross the knuckles (Fig. 4–2).

Aside from these evidences of lipid abnormalities, the physician must always be alert for the classical changes in the retinal vessels (increased light reflex, tortuosity and arteriovenous crossing phenomena) which signify arteriosclerosis. In addition, elevation of the arterial blood pressure, left ventricular hypertrophy, and evidence of peripheral vascular disease should lead the physician to consider that atherosclerosis is present. Of course, in younger individuals this would be considered distinctly abnormal, while in elderly persons atherosclerosis and arteriosclerosis may be accepted as common accompaniments of old age.

Although some authorities believe that obesity does not contribute to coronary heart disease specifically, it is well established that obesity may be accompanied by elevation of the arterial blood pressure and by diabetes mellitus, both of which are statistically associated with development of coronary heart disease. Thus, it is highly desirable to determine whether the patient is obese, and the simplest

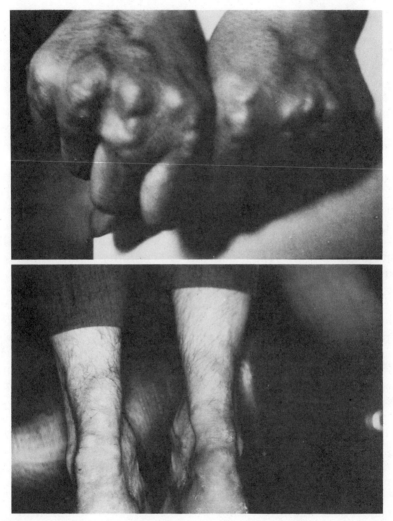

Figure 4–2 Thickening of tendons occurs in patients with hyperlipidemia, especially Type II. Courtesy Elaine Feldman and *Resident and Staff Physician.*

way to do this is to measure height and weight. Any patient whose weight is 20 per cent above his or her normal level may be considered obese. Measurements of skin-fold thickness will provide additional objective information of the degree of obesity.

Laboratory Tests

Appropriate laboratory tests can be very helpful in ascertaining the relative risk of coronary heart disease in any given patient. These tests include both chemical and physiological evaluations.

Biochemical Tests. At the very least, one should measure the concentration of cholesterol and of triglycerides in plasma. If a sample of the patient's anticoagulated blood is placed in the refrigerator overnight, the red cells will settle to the bottom and it will be possible to ascertain whether the supernatant plasma is clear or cloudy. In addition, if there is a substantial degree of hyperchylomicronemia there will be a "cream-layer" at the top of the plasma. This much information will permit reasonably accurate assessment of the probable type of abnormality, if any, in hyperlipidemic patients. Patients who have a simple elevation of cholesterol levels will have clear plasma, assuming that the blood was drawn under fasting conditions. Cloudiness of the plasma generally indicates that there is an increased concentration of triglycerides which are carried by the very low density lipoproteins (VLDLs). And the presence of abnormal numbers of chylomicrons as manifested by the cream-layer suggests a defect in lipoprotein lipase such as that found in Type I hyperlipidemia or the mixed abnormalities found in Type V hyperlipidemia. Types II, III, and IV are of greatest interest because these are associated with an elevated risk of coronary heart disease (see Table 4–3). When a physician finds that a patient has elevated cholesterol or triglyceride levels in his or her plasma, it is necessary to repeat the determination to rule out laboratory error. At the same time, it is desirable to get a lipid profile, easily and inexpensively done by electrophoresis. Even though great emphasis has been placed on the hyperlipidemias it is important to recall that true hyperlipidemia, as defined by Fredrickson, accounts for only about 25 per cent of all coronary deaths in this country. The remaining 75 per cent occur in individuals who have so-called "normal plasma lipids" Obviously we have confused "normal" with "average" values. For example, a popular medical handbook lists the normal cholesterol range as "150 to 280 mg/dl" and the normal triglyceride level as "less than 165 mg/dl". Yet epidemiologic data suggest that individuals who have cholesterol values above 220 or triglyceride values above 120 have a greater risk of developing atherosclerotic lesions than those with values below these levels. And the greater the rise above these levels, the greater the risk of developing coronary heart disease.

More accurate assessment can be achieved by measuring levels of the various lipoprotein fractions: very low density lipoproteins (VLDL), low density lipoproteins (LDL), and high density lipoproteins (HDL). LDL seem to be most harmful, whereas HDL may be somewhat protective (Editorial, Lancet, 1976). Recently published data provide useful information regarding the average lipid values of apparently healthy people of various ages, living in the United States (National Center for Health Statistics, 1978).

Carbohydrate intolerance, as evidenced by finding fasting blood sugar levels above 100 mg/dl or greater, should also be considered as evidence of increased susceptibility to the development of coronary heart disease. Other biochemical findings that are statistically associated with coronary heart disease include elevation in the serum of uric acid levels and of immunoreactive insulin levels. Some cardiologists believe that persons with high levels of hemoglobin and high hematocrit values have an increased risk of coronary heart disease, but others disagree with this conclusion.

Physiologic Tests. Physiologic tests include not only a routine electrocardiogram but some measure of the function of the heart under a workload. The old Master's two-step test has been replaced by a treadmill providing graded levels of exercise, during which an electrocardiogram is recorded continuously. If the patient develops chest pain, shortness of breath, or undue fatigue, the test is terminated. If the electrocardiogram shows a rhythm disturbance or a significant shift in the S-T segment or abnormalities of the T-wave, the test is concluded. Although not all individuals with coronary heart disease will have an abnormal test, a substantial number can be identified by this procedure. In individuals who have evidence of progressive coronary heart disease it is often necessary to perform coronary angiography to determine the presence, location, and severity of atherosclerotic lesions. Patients who have recurrent or severe cardiac arrhythmias should be monitored with a Holter electrocardiographic recorder in order to determine the frequency, type, and duration of the arrhythmias. Ventricular arrhythmias of any kind are more likely to occur in patients who have coronary heart disease.

By employing the techniques available (history, physical examination, and laboratory procedures), today's physicians are able to determine with considerable accuracy whether a given individual is apparently free of coronary disease, has a propensity toward this abnormality, or already has it. This information is valuable in managing both the patient and his family.

Other Factors

Epidemiologists recognize that although the "big three" risk factors are hyperlipidemia, hypertension, and cigarette smoking, there are other factors that must be considered. The gender of the individual has a substantial bearing upon the probability of developing coronary heart disease at any given age. Men are substantially more susceptible, but the reasons are not apparent. Administration of estrogens to men, either with the intent of delaying the rate of growth of carcinoma of the prostate or in an effort to prevent the development of coronary heart disease, not only fails to achieve this purpose but appears to accelerate the onset of coronary disease. The age of the individual is also extremely important. Approximately three-fourths of all patients dying of coronary heart disease are past age 65, with the frequency of heart attacks increasing with advancing age until death.

DIETARY FACTORS

Dietary factors have been discussed at great length and have led to more misunderstanding than perhaps any other topic relating to coronary heart disease. Americans, on the whole, consume a stereotyped diet that contains an abundance of protein, usually of animal origin, and a large amount of fat, much of which is saturated. In addition, we consume relatively large amounts of dietary cholesterol, generous amounts of salt and sugar, and a good deal of coffee. Each of these factors, singly or collectively, has been blamed for the high incidence of coronary heart disease. Epidemiologically, one can make a very good case for several of these factors, but in the opinion of the author, saturated fat and total fat are probably of greatest importance.

Demakis and colleagues (1974) described the cardiomyopathy that occurs in persons who consume large amounts of alcohol. This syndrome is quite different from the hyperlipidemia that follows alcohol ingestion in some individuals. According to Ginsberg and others (1974), some hypertriglyceridemic individuals do have a significant rise in triglycerides following ingestion of even moderate amounts of alcohol. The mechanism, according to Mendelson and Mello (1974), may depend upon such multiple factors as hepatic disease, pancreatic disorders, heavy cigarette smoking, and environmental stress. Wilson and others (1970) also observed enhancement of alimentary lipemia by ethanol in man. Simultaneous ingestion of ethanol and fat, as is customary in our society, leads to a lipemic response that is greater than the sum of the effects of fat given alone and ethanol given alone. Chait and colleagues (1972) found that excessive use of alcohol was remarkably common in hyperlipidemic patients and suggested that alcohol increases hepatic secretion of lipoproteins. Orlando and others (1976) observed that in 12 patients who had angina pectoris, administration of either 2 oz or 5 oz of alcohol by mouth resulted in a reduction in exercise-time-until-angina and an increase in depression of the S-T segment of the electrocardiogram during exertion. They concluded that ethanol aggravates exercise-induced angina pectoris. This leads to the question: what amount of alcohol is excessive? The author believes that habitual ingestion of more than 20 per cent of total calories as ethanol may be harmful.

Coffee has come into the picture as a result of sporadic reports that excessive use of this beverage has an adverse effect on coronary heart disease. The Boston Collaborative Drug Surveillance Program suggested that coffee drinking possibly plays a role in the etiology of acute myocardial infarction. Since that time, a great many reports have appeared in medical journals, as well as in the lay press. Despite much discussion, both pro and con, regarding this issue, there is not a sufficiently well-controlled series to permit a firm conclusion. Jick and Miettinen (1975) call attention to evidence that the prevalence of heavy coffee drinking (7 or more cups per day) decreases by half with each decade of age. This complicates statistical interpretation and may account, in part, for differences of opinion. Gillum (1976) and Hennekens and others (1976) are inclined to a certain degree of skepticism about the role of coffee. Other investigators have been convinced that excessive use of coffee is harmful and that this is a logical finding because caffeine stimulates the central nervous system more than does theophylline, found in tea, or theobromine, found in cocoa. Theophylline is a potent cardiac stimulator and causes coronary dilatation and diuresis, as well as smooth muscle relaxation. Caffeine has much less effect on the cardiac muscle, on the coronary vessels, on the kidneys and on smooth muscle. Some studies indicate that individuals who drink more than two cups of coffee a day have a greater-than-average risk of developing coronary heart disease. Other studies show absolutely no effect. Perhaps the best advice is to tell patients who are coffee drinkers to use it in moderation. An excessive amount of anything may be undesirable.

For more than two decades it has been popular to blame any unexplained illness on our "purified" diet, and sucrose represents one of the most highly purified of foods. Furthermore, it constitutes between 15 and 30 per cent of the caloric intake of the average American and has no nutritional value other than energy. Since most Americans have an excessive intake of energy it is easy to see why sucrose has been a popular target. Epidemiologic studies have been cited as evidence that sucrose may play a role in the causation of coronary heart disease. Indeed, several workers have maintained steadfastly that this contention is valid; yet carefully controlled dietary studies by the author and by others have provided little evidence to support the epidemiologic claims. One of the staunch advocates of the sucrose theory is Walker (1975), who points out, correctly, that no one has conducted a study in a human population wherein the sucrose in the diet has been rigidly restricted for a prolonged period of time. On the other side of the coin, Keys (1971) has attempted to discredit the sucrose theory on the basis that available data are not dependable, either with regard to the accuracy of death certificates or with regard to figures on consumption of sugar. No doubt Keys is correct in these assumptions, but the work by Macdonald and Braithwaite (1964) has shown that sucrose does have a significant effect, albeit rather small, on blood lipids of man. In the author's opinion, sucrose cannot be credited with a major role in the causation of coronary heart disease, yet it probably is wise to advocate moderation in the use of sucrose on the basis of its contribution to an already excessive caloric intake.

Recently, there has been a wave of enthusiasm for dietary fiber. Both epidemiologic and experimental evidence has been cited to indicate that fiber in the diet has a number of potential benefits. One of these is more rapid passage of the food stream with some reduction in absorption of cholesterol and of cholesterol derivatives, such as bile acids. The term "fiber" is not accurate since it really refers to a number of indigestible plant substances, including cellulose, lignin, hemicelluloses, and gelatinous indigestible compounds. Pectin is one such substance, and konjac mannan is another. Studies by Kiriyama and others (1972) showed that purification of konjac mannan had no effect on its ability to lower the plasma cholesterol level of young adult male rats fed a diet containing large amounts of cholesterol plus bile salts. But exposure of konjac mannan to a fungus cellulase for only 30 minutes completely canceled its activity. Although many clinicians have been attracted by the theory that indigestible carbohydrates may be beneficial to their patients, it is only fair to say that the currently available clinical evidence is almost equally divided between positive effects and no effect, especially when patients are advised to use commercial bran as a source of "fiber". Obviously, more experience is needed to evaluate this concept.

From time to time investigators report that certain foods or plant products have some unique and beneficial effect on the heart. Most of these reports eventually prove to be without foundation, but one must remember that digitalis was introduced into medicine as a result of the seemingly illogical concoctions of an old woman in England. Now that we are so concerned about cholesterol and its metabolism, it is inevitable that we will be told that various foods, especially plant foods, have an ability to inhibit absorption, increase destruction or reduce synthesis of this sterol. A provocative review entitled "The Herbs and the Heart" (Nutrition Reviews, 1976) collates recent information on the reported effects of herbs and spices on fibrinolysis and on cholesterol levels. Onions, garlic, and other members of the Allium family have reportedly been shown to have a cholesterol-lowering effect and a fibrinolytic effect. The amount required is somewhere in the neighborhood of 50 gm, and the active principle is heat-stable and water-insoluble. Not all investigators have confirmed the hypocholesterolemic effect, but activation of fibrinolysis has been confirmed. In very large amounts, onions have a hypoglycemic effect, but not enough to be clinically useful in management of diabetic patients. Paprika has a fibrinolytic effect, and the ancient nostrum asafetida has both a hypocholesterolemic and a fibrinolytic effect. Rao and others (1970) observed that tumeric can increase the rate of bile production and secretion. They reasoned that tumeric might contain a substance capable of lowering cholesterol. The hypocholesterolemic effect results principally from the coloring matter, named *curcumin,* which is apparently non-toxic. Curcumin, fed to rats, protected them against the rise in serum and liver levels of cholesterol that follows the feeding of dietary cholesterol. It increased fecal excretion of bile acids and cholesterol in both normal and hypercholesterolemic rats. Curcumin was active when fed as 0.1 per cent of the diet, but the minimum effective dose may be even lower.

Plant sterols, present in foods commonly consumed, have been known for some time to interfere with absorption of dietary cholesterol from the digestive tract. Chemically, these plant sterols have a cyclopentenophenanthrene ring, a Δ^5 and Δ^6 double bond and a 3β-hydroxyl group. The side chain of plant sterols has one or two more carbons than does cholesterol. The three most common plant sterols are campesterol, stigmasterol and β-Sitosterol. Subbiah (1973) studied the metabolism of plant sterols in humans and confirmed the fact that they are absorbed to a certain extent by all animal species. They are catabolized to the same steroid hormones as those formed from cholesterol and they can be converted into bile acids in the liver. The use of plant sterols in attempting to lower cholesterol levels is still in the experimental stages, but this approach does appear to be somewhat promising.

Metabolism of bile acids is intimately linked with cholesterol metabolism because a major portion of cholesterol is converted into these compounds. Hoffman and others (1974) have reported the effects of feeding chenodeoxycholic acid to patients with gallstones in an effort to dissolve them. Bile-acid feeding inhibits synthesis of bile acid from cholesterol, and one might therefore assume that giving chenodeoxycholic acid would expand cholesterol pools and perhaps elevate the plasma level of this sterol. Hoffman's group studied the exchangeable cholesterol pool and cholesterol input in 23 patients with gallstones, seven of whom received cholic acid and eight of whom received chenodeoxycholic acid. Another group of eight patients received a placebo. The exchangeable cholesterol pool and cholesterol input were similar in all three groups. In a large group of patients receiving bile-acid treatment, cholesterol levels in serum did not change significantly. Triglyceride levels decreased modestly in patients receiving chenodeoxycholic acid but remained unchanged in the other two groups. The authors concluded that attempting to dissolve gallstones by this form of bile-acid feeding does not constitute a hazard in terms of cholesterol metabolism.

Among the dietary and environmental factors that have been enumerated as contributors to atherosclerosis, the minerals are not neglected. Several epidemiologic studies have indicated that communities having hard water, usually as a result of a generous content of calcium and magnesium, have less coronary disease than communities where the water is soft (Chipperfield et al., 1976). Yet another relationship has been postulated by Klevay (1975), who calls attention to epidemiologic and metabolic data consistent with the idea that an imbalance between zinc and copper may be a factor in the etiology of coronary disease. This imbalance can occur as a result of abnormal amounts of zinc and copper in human food, or as a lack of ability to absorb copper. According to this theory, either a relative or an absolute deficiency of copper is characterized by a high ratio of zinc to copper. This, in turn, is accompanied by elevation of plasma cholesterol levels.

By far the strongest case can be made for the relationship between fat intake and coronary heart disease (Kromer, 1973; Rizek et al., 1974; and Smith, 1973). It is important to realize that statistical differences have been demonstrated, chiefly in comparisons between groups of people living in different countries where there is a marked dissimilarity not only between diets, but also between many other aspects of everyday life. If one attempts to select any single dietary factor in the United States, it is highly improbable that a statistically significant difference can be shown between the incidence of coronary heart disease in persons who use that particular substance generously and those who use lesser amounts. The explanation for this phenomenon probably rests upon the trend toward similar dietary patterns throughout the United States, which similarity carries through from the lower to the upper socioeconomic groups. Even ethnic minority groups tend, after a couple of generations, to adopt the general dietary pattern of the entire country, and this pattern is one of generous protein intake, relatively high fat consumption, and a relatively low fiber diet. In addition, the dietary cholesterol is high by international standards and the use of both alcohol and sucrose is also relatively high. Recent controversy has arisen regarding the importance or unimportance of dietary cholesterol, particularly with regard to egg yolks. It is widely recognized that dietary cholesterol is high in the diet of people consuming generous amounts of animal protein (Lange, 1950). Although clinical investigative reports are conflicting, the author believes that dietary cholesterol is one of several important factors, and that until further clarification of the controversy, patients would be well advised to use discretion in the amount of cholesterol they consume.

From the discussion of dietary factors above, it should be apparent that physicians are not able to predict on the basis of diet alone the likelihood that a given patient will or will not develop coronary disease. Indeed, it is not unusual to find an individual who has eaten an exemplary diet and has, nonetheless, developed coronary atherosclerosis. Conversely, one may encounter a patient who has partaken generously of all of the foods that are thought to contribute to atherosclerosis, yet this individual may be free of any manifestations of this disease. Unquestionably, the most accurate prediction of coronary heart disease is based on consideration of all factors, including the history, the patient's personal habits, his or her personality characteristics, and the physical examination and laboratory tests (both biochemical and physiological). It is, of course, desirable to elicit information about dietary and such environmental factors as those discussed above, but these are much more difficult to interpret.

MANAGEMENT OF THE PATIENT WITH INCREASED RISK OF CORONARY HEART DISEASE

Academic *versus* Pragmatic

Physicians are sharply divided in their reactions to the deluge of information that has descended upon them during the past 20 years relative to coronary heart disease and its causes. Almost everyone agrees that coronary heart disease is a multifactorial condition and that there is no *single* one of the ten or twelve risk factors the absence of which will absolutely guarantee freedom from coronary disease. On the other hand, epidemiologic studies clearly indicate that there are groups of people in the world who are very nearly immune to this disorder and who have very low scores on one or more of the recognized risk factors. Some authorities argue that, until conclusive proof is available, there is little or no justification for attempting to modify the risk factors of individual patients or of population groups. These individuals have been referred to as the "academics", who seek a cause-and-effect relationship. At the other extreme are the "pragmatics", who feel that epidemiologic studies, bolstered by metabolic studies in both experimental animals and man, are sufficient justification for a determined multifaceted approach to coronary heart disease and its prevention. This is the position taken by the American Heart Association and, indeed, by a majority of cardiologists throughout the country. To the author, it seems reasonable to try to minimize all of the risk factors that are amenable to change, provided, of course, that the methods employed are harmless. Thus, there should be no objection to the concepts of controlling diabetes mellitus and hypertension, of encouraging patients to stop smoking, and of recommending that patients reduce their food intake so as to achieve and maintain normal body weight. The big controversy, however, revolves around hyperlipidemia. Some advocate changes in the American diet so that everyone who might become hyperlipidemic may benefit. Others say that only individuals who have been shown to have abnormal lipids should be given a special diet. Some believe in a unilateral view of diet, whereas others would prescribe a diet tailored to each type of hyperlipidemia encountered in a patient. These and other concepts will be explored in the following paragraphs.

In the opinion of the author, dietary modifications *are* indicated, not only for individuals who are clearly identifiable as "hyperlipidemic" but also for the large number of persons who have lipid values in the so-called "normal range" but who statistically have at least a moderate risk of developing coronary heart disease. The Framingham study has shown that individuals who have a cholesterol level of 220 mg/dl have only a slightly greater risk than those with considerably lower values. On the other hand, individuals with levels only a little above 220 have a substantial increase in their risk of developing coronary heart disease within a decade or so (Kannel, 1971). Accordingly, a level of 220 seems reasonable as a "desirable" value. Data on triglycerides are not as sharply defined, but a value below 120 mg/dl probably is to be desired. Of course, patients who have the familiar triad of obesity, carbohydrate intolerance, and elevated triglyceride levels in their serum are recognized as being at greater-than-normal risk, but it is difficult to ascribe the increased risk to any one of the three factors. In managing a patient who has hyperlipidemia of any kind, it is wise to advise him or her of the objectives, describe the methods to be used, and then make every effort to retain as many of the characteristics of the patient's normal diet as possible. The objectives are simple and can be compatible with a very acceptable diet that provides all essential nutrients and is, at the same time, safe and economical.

The first step is to determine the patient's normal weight and prescribe an appropriate diet on this basis. The normal weight can be estimated from the patient's height or can be obtained from such standard insurance tables as the one reproduced in Tables 4–5 and simplified in Table 4–6. If the patient is considerably overweight— for example, more than 20 per cent above ideal—it is reasonable to reduce calories to the basal level, which is about 25 kcal/kg of *normal* body weight. Thus, a man who normally should weigh 70 kg but who weighs 90 kg at the time of his first visit, might be started on 25 kcal/kg or 25 × 70 = 1750 kcal/day. This figure is accurate if this patient is relatively inactive. In the event he expends considerable amounts of energy in performing his everyday work, it may be necessary to increase the caloric allowance to 30 kcal/kg for a total of 2100 kcal/day. The protein allowance is equally easy to estimate. The recommended allowance of protein is 0.8 gm/kg, but Americans characteristically consume larger amounts, so it may be desirable to give 1.0 gm/kg. Accordingly, for our hypothetical 70 kg person, we would allow 70 gm of protein. Since protein furnishes four kcal/gm, this would provide 280 of his 1750 kcal total. The fat allowance should not exceed 30 per cent of the energy in the diet, or 525 kcal/day. Since each gram of fat provides 9 kcal of energy, our patient would be allowed 525 ÷ 9, or 58 gm of fat per day. The balance of calories is 945, which will be provided by carbohydrates; 945 ÷ 4 = 236 gm of carbohydrate per day. This can be summarized:

Sample Diet for a 70 kg Man

Allow 25 kcal/kg = 1750 kcal
This is apportioned as follows:

		kcal
Protein:	1 gm/kg = 70 gm × 4 =	280
Fat:	30% of 1750 kcal =	525
	525 kcal ÷ 9 kcal = 58 gm	
Carbohydrate:	by difference	
	1750 kcal − (280 kcal + 525 kcal) =	945
	945 kcal ÷ 4 = 236 gm	
	Total	1750

The diet contains: 70 gm Protein
58 gm Fat
236 gm Carbohydrate

TABLE 4–5   DESIRABLE WEIGHTS FOR MEN AND WOMEN
(According to Height and Frame, Ages 25 and Over)*

HEIGHT (Wearing Shoes)†	WEIGHT IN POUNDS (IN INDOOR CLOTHING)		
	Small Frame	Medium Frame	Large Frame
MEN			
5' 2"	112–120	118–129	126–141
3"	115–123	121–133	129–144
4"	118–126	124–136	132–148
5"	121–129	127–139	135–152
6"	124–133	130–143	138–156
7"	128–137	134–147	142–161
8"	132–141	138–152	147–166
9"	136–145	142–156	151–170
10"	140–150	146–160	155–174
11"	144–154	150–165	159–179
6' 0"	148–158	154–170	164–184
1"	152–162	158–175	168–189
2"	156–167	162–180	173–194
3"	160–171	167–185	178–199
4"	164–175	172–190	182–204
WOMEN			
4' 10"	92– 98	96–107	104–119
11"	94–101	98–110	106–122
5' 0"	96–104	101–113	109–125
1"	99–107	104–116	112–128
2"	102–110	107–119	115–131
3"	105–113	110–122	118–134
4"	108–116	113–126	121–138
5"	111–119	116–130	125–142
6"	114–123	120–135	129–146
7"	118–127	124–139	133–150
8"	122–131	128–143	137–154
9"	126–135	132–147	141–158
10"	130–140	136–151	145–163
11"	134–144	140–155	149–168
6' 0"	138–148	144–159	153–173

*This widely quoted table of desirable weights is still very popular; but for practical purposes, this table can be simplified as shown in Table 4–6, in which height and weight are also shown in metric values. Prepared by the Metropolitan Life Insurance Company. Derived primarily from data of the *Build and Blood Pressure Study, 1959,* Society of Actuaries.

†1-inch heels for men and 2-inch heels for women.

TABLE 4–6 APPROXIMATE "DESIRABLE" WEIGHTS FOR HEIGHT OF "MEDIUM FRAME" MEN AND WOMEN (in Indoor Clothing)*

Height		Men (With Shoes, 1" Heels)		Women (With Shoes, 2" Heels)	
Inches	Cm	Lbs.	Kg	Lbs.	Kg
58	147	—	—	101	46
59	150	—	—	104	47
60	152	—	—	107	48
61	155	—	—	110	50
62	157	123	56	113	51
63	160	126	57	116	53
64	163	130	59	119	54
65	165	133	60	123	56
66	168	136	62	127	58
67	170	140	64	131	59
68	173	145	66	135	61
69	175	149	68	139	63
70	178	153	69	143	65
71	180	157	71	147	67
72	183	162	73	151	69
73	185	166	75	—	—
74	188	171	78	—	—
75	190	176	80	—	—
76	193	181	82	—	—

*Modified from Metropolitan Life Insurance Company tables (1960). Data have been averaged for simplification. Courtesy Metropolitan Life Insurance Company.

Dietary Cholesterol

Dietary cholesterol is of concern to some individuals and initially should be reduced to less than 300 mg/day. Since the average egg yolk contains about 250 mg, and since one small serving of meat contains around 80 mg, it is obvious that the patient cannot be allowed *both* eggs and meat on the same day.

Dietary Fats

Furthermore, the 58 gm of fat that we have allowed this hypothetical patient should be carefully selected so as to minimize the intake of saturated fats. It was mentioned above that most saturated fats are of animal origin. Most vegetable fats, which are provided by nuts, grains, and other plant seeds, contain generous amounts of polyunsaturated fats and lesser amounts of saturated fats. There are, however, two exceptions to this general rule: coconut oil contains rather large amounts of saturated fats, and any vegetable oil may be hydrogenated in processing so as to make a saturated fat product that has a higher melting point. In general, liquid oils are polyunsaturated and solid fats are saturated. Patients are well advised to read the labels of margarine, shortenings and any other processed food item that may contain considerable fat. The law requires that the label list the *most abundant substance first* and other substances in decreasing order of content.

The dietary goal is to reduce the intake of fat to only 30 per cent of total calories, with about one-third of this as polyunsaturated oils, one-third as monounsaturated fat, and one-third as saturated fat. This is a reasonable compromise in that it allows people to eat familiar foods in small quantities and it avoids overloading the diet with vegetable oils in an effort to achieve a very high intake of polyunsaturated fats.

"Toxicity" and Side Effects

There have been unsubstantiated claims that large amounts of polyunsaturated fats in the diet may have adverse effects. Dayton and others (1969, 1970) conducted studies in which elderly inmates of a Veterans Administration domiciliary hospital consumed either the usual hospital cafeteria diet or a modified diet that contained generous amounts of polyunsaturated fats and oils. They demonstrated that the serum cholesterol levels of those men on the modified diet declined significantly and that the combined total of deaths from heart attack and stroke was significantly reduced. Subsequently, Pearce and Dayton (1971) presented evidence of more cancer in the subjects who had received the polyunsaturated diet than in those who ate the conventional diet. There are several reasons for the author to feel that Pearce's interpretation of the data may not be correct. The first is the fact that a number of the subjects who developed malignant disease had consumed the polyunsaturated fat diet for only a short period of time or had been rather poor compliers; i.e., they had eaten a majority of meals away from the domiciliary. If individuals who fell into these two categories were disqualified from statistical consideration, the significance of cancer in the experimental group would disappear.

Other clinical trials (Leren, 1966, 1970) failed to show an increase in malignant disease among subjects who consumed a polyunsaturated fat diet. But perhaps a more convincing argument is the fact that if a given population is susceptible to two potentially fatal diseases, "A" and "B", and if one employs a preventive measure that lessens the death rate from disease A, then inevitably the death rate from disease B will increase, because the additional survivors who would have died from A are still living and are at risk of dying of B. In any event, the diet we are recommending for reduction of plasma lipid levels does *not* contain large amounts of polyunsaturated fats and so the question is a moot one. Furthermore, Ederer (1971) reviewed the experience from five clinical trials (one of which was the trial by Dayton and Pearce), in which polyunsaturated fats were fed to patients, and found that only one of the other four trials seemed to show an increased incidence of cancer in the experimental group, whereas the other three showed opposite results. In two studies by Schramm (Part I, 1961 and Part II, 1961), female rats were given a carcinogen, 3'-methyldimethylaminoazobenzene, along with small amounts of various fatty acids and esters, by pharyngeal tube. Feeding linolenic acid resulted in complete freedom from neoplastic changes in the liver, whereas administration of other fats resulted in pathological changes consistent with early neoplasia. In other studies, both male and female rats were fed either 0.2 mg or 0.3 mg of 4-dimethylaminostilbene up to a total dose of 100 mg per animal and the animals were also given 0.2 mg of linolenic acid ester, which resulted in a lowering of the tumor rate from 78.3 per cent in the controls to 14.3 per cent in the group receiving polyunsaturated fats.

There are, however, certain abnormalities that result from feeding large amounts of polyunsaturated fatty acids. One of these is a rise in serum uric acid level. Ogryzlo (1965) reported that starvation and administration of polyunsaturated fats had similar effects. He noted a correlation between accumulation of ketones in the blood and their excretion in the urine on one hand, and the excretion of uric acid on the other. The rate and amount of uric acid excreted were the reciprocal of the rate and amount of ketones excreted in the urine. This effect occurred only when a high-fat diet was given.

One of the most ardent opponents of polyunsaturated fats is Pinckney (1973), who paints a dismal picture of what may happen to individuals who choose to follow the recommendations of the American Heart Association. Not only does he claim that cancer may result, but he also suggests that there is premature aging of the skin and, perhaps, premature aging of the entire body. There are few clinicians who agree with all the conclusions drawn by Pinckney, and indeed most cardiologists are convinced that a prudent diet is both effective and safe. It is important to keep in mind that we are talking about a diet that contains only 10 per cent of total calories as polyunsaturated fat, as opposed to some of the extreme diets that might contain as much as 50 per cent of calories as polyunsaturated fats. But some skeptics persist in their view that polyunsaturated fats in the human diet are potentially harmful and that the whole idea of lowering blood cholesterol is unproven (West and Redgrave, 1975).

Alterations in the fat content of the diet may have an important effect upon the solubility of bile. Indeed, several investigators have reported that diets containing generous amounts of polyunsaturated fats may result in cholelithiasis. Sturdevant, working with Pearce and Dayton (1973), reviewed the data from the Veterans Administration study, and found autopsy evidence that men who ate more than a third of their meals in the special diet area were more likely to have gallstones (34 per cent) than control subjects who ate regular food (14 per cent). The mechanism is not entirely clear, but it is well known that any factor that causes an increased loss of bile acids from the digestive tract — whether the cause is surgical removal of a portion of the small bowel or administration of a sequestering agent such as cholestyramine — may result in cholelithiasis. It is tempting to speculate that the liver is forming bile acids at an abnormally rapid rate in order to compensate for the loss, but this is probably an oversimplification. In any event, diets containing large amounts of polyunsaturated fatty acids can cause an increased incidence of cholelithiasis.

Some patients will have only a modest response to a change in their dietary fats although, fortunately, those with the highest levels of cholesterol in their plasma generally have the best response (Hodges et al., 1975). Nonetheless, it is sometimes desirable to give both diet and medications to patients who have abnormally high lipid levels. Some authorities believe that patients with the various types of familial hyperlipidemia should have not only different diets but also different medications (Lees, 1973; and Levy et al., 1974). But more and more, physicians prefer to give their hyperlipidemic patients a trial with a "prudent diet" and reevaluate them after a period of several months. If this results in an inadequate response the physician may further modify the diet or prescribe drug therapy, or both. The specifics of drug treatment of hyperlipidemias will not be reviewed here, but drug therapy does appear to have a place in the management of markedly hyperlipidemic patients (Levy et al., 1972; Levy, 1976; Parsons et al., 1956; and Tolman et al., 1969).

Clinicians who are not highly knowledgeable about the details of recent chemical developments tend to use broad or generic terms when dealing with complex nutritional problems. For the past two decades, it has been popular to refer to food fats as being "saturated" or "unsaturated". It has generally been assumed that saturated fats result in higher levels of cholesterol in plasma, while polyunsaturated fats have the opposite effect.

The effects of saturated *versus* polyunsaturated fats are more specific than was once thought. Keys and his colleagues (1965) reported on serum cholesterol responses to changes in the diet, with particular reference to the saturated fatty acids, but this was largely ignored by the medical profession. Keys' careful tabulation of many diet studies permitted him to derive information regarding the relative impact of many different fatty acids on cholesterol metabolism in humans. A surprising finding at that time was the revelation that stearic acid, which is one of the major saturated fats of beef, has little or no effect on serum cholesterol levels in humans. Neither do the shorter chain fatty acids with 12 or fewer carbons. That leaves the two saturated fatty acids with 14 or 16 carbons, namely, myristic acid and palmitic acid, as the major contributors to hypercholesterolemia. Subsequent observations have fully confirmed Keys' prediction that these two fatty acids have the greatest impact in elevating cholesterol levels.

Intervention Studies

Intervention studies by Hood and others (1965), in a group of men and women who survived a myocardial infarction, demonstrated that over a period of 5 to 17 years, 112 patients who followed a rigid dietary regimen had a lower mortality than did a control group of 112 patients matched according to age, sex, blood pressure, degree of vascular symptoms, and cholesterol levels. In the fat-controlled-diet group of 112 subjects, there were 12 deaths, but in the unmodified control group of 112 subjects, there were 38 deaths. Most dietary intervention studies have included middle-aged or older subjects, with or without coronary heart disease. Bierenbaum and others (1973) reported a group of 100 "younger men", aged 30 to 50 years, with confirmed coronary heart disease and previous myocardial infarction. In general, one could assume that individuals who had a heart attack at a younger age may have had a more severe degree of lipid abnormality than older coronary patients. These 100 men were given a fat-restricted diet (28 per cent of calories) and were required to lose weight. Over a period of ten years they had significant reductions in their serum lipids. These experimental subjects had a 17 per cent greater survival rate than did the control group.

Dietary Recommendations

A recent publication (Special Report, *Nutrition Reviews*, 1976) presents an article, "Prevention of Coronary Heart Disease", as outlined by a Joint Working Party of the Royal College of Physicians of London and the British Cardiac Society. Dietary recommendations include reduction in the amount of saturated fats and partial substitution by polyunsaturated fats. This report also recommends correction of obesity, a decrease in consumption of sugar and alcohol as common sources of excess energy, and a regular exercise program. Along with this, it is recommended that smoking be discontinued, that elevated blood pressure or diabetes mellitus be controlled, and that stress be minimized or appropriately managed. Finally, an educational program to change behavior patterns in relation to diet, physical activity, and cigarette smoking is advocated.

Lipoprotein Metabolism

When Fredrickson and his group first described the various forms of hyperlipidemia, it was assumed that Type II was most prevalent and accounted for the most deaths. More and more reports show that Type IV is as common as or even more common than Type II, but that it responds to dietary treatment quite well. Smith and colleagues (1976), and others (Special Report, *Nutrition Reviews*, 1976), demonstrated that weight reduction was the most important aspect of dietary therapy in Type IV hyperlipidemic subjects. Furthermore, it was possible to get a large group of asymptomatic young people to establish a program to which they could adhere on a long-term basis. Whether lowering serum triglyceride levels in Type IV hyperlipoproteinemia actually decreases the risk of heart attack has not yet been decided conclusively, but it seems reasonable to assume that it may. Although several investigators have postulated that the very low density lipoproteins (VLDL), which contain 13 per cent of the cholesterol and 55 per cent of the triglycerides in plasma, can be converted to low density lipoproteins (LDL), which contain 70 per cent of the circulating cholesterol and only 29 per cent of the triglycerides, this mechanism was not firmly established until the work of Sigurdsson and others (1975). They labeled the apolipoprotein B portion of VLDL and showed that in both normal and hyperlipidemic individuals, the labeled apolipoprotein was rapidly and almost completely incorporated into LDL lipoproteins. Evidently, most, if not all, VLDL-B is converted to LDL-B peptide. This provides a firm rationale for controlling obesity in hyperlipidemic subjects who have elevation of their VLDL fraction. In practical terms, this means that most individuals who have elevation of their triglycerides also have elevation of the LDL fraction of their lipoproteins. Since LDL cholesterol is thought to be the form in which lipids are most readily conveyed to the tissues that make up the walls of arteries, it seems logical that control of obesity should indeed be a part of dietary control of any hyperlipidemia that may be associated with an increased incidence of coronary heart disease.

In addition to the growing evidence that one form of lipoprotein can be converted to another, there now is additional evidence that high density lipoprotein (HDL) in plasma may also be affected by diet and physical activity. Exercise programs may induce a significant rise in HDL, and control of obesity may have a similar effect. Several reports have indicated that HDL may have a reciprocal relationship to atherosclerosis; the higher the concentration of HDL in the plasma, the less the extent of atheromatous deposits. HDL contains only 17 per cent of the circulating cholesterol in the plasma and only 11 per cent of the triglycerides (*Lancet*, 1976). The size of cholesterol pools in patients with hypercholesterolemia has been negatively correlated with the concentration of HDL in plasma, and incubating smooth muscle cells derived from arterial walls with HDL has been shown to reduce the accumulation of LDL in these cells, possibly as the result of competition between HDL and LDL for lipoprotein receptors on the cell surface. In any event, it seems desirable to measure HDL in clinical situations so as to generate sufficient data to permit accurate interpretation of these apparent associations.

Practical Management

The management of patients with evidence of increased risk of developing coronary heart disease can be summarized as: "The first rule is *start early*". It is important not only to identify the individual who has coronary disease, but to examine his or her children to determine whether they have familial hyperlipidemia, whether their blood pressure is normal, and whether there is any evidence of obesity, diabetes, or other metabolic disorder. The incidental finding of elevated blood pressure, abnormal plasma lipids, or an elevated fasting blood sugar level in an individual who has requested a routine physical examination for insurance purposes or for employment may allow that person to escape the development of serious cardiovascular disease in the future. The mean levels of cholesterol in plasma change with age. Knowledge of these changes, which are different for men and women, will permit the physician to evaluate individual patients more accurately (see Figure 4–3). In any patient who is found to be abnormal, it is advisable to employ *all* measures simultaneously in an effort to avoid coronary heart disease. These measures include diet, personal habits, physical activity, emotional factors, and existing diseases. The best dietary advice is to regulate calories so as to correct obesity and maintain normal body weight. This program should be accompanied by reduction in the total amount of dietary fat to 30 per cent of total

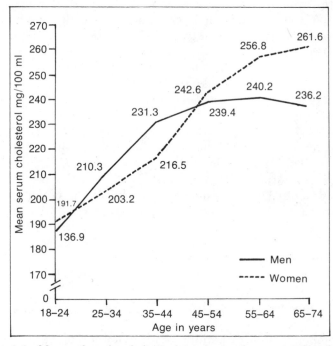

Figure 4–3 Mean values for cholesterol in plasma change significantly with advancing age. For men the peak is reached by about age 55, but for women the peak may occur 10 or more years later. Figure courtesy of National Center for Health Statistics, U.S. Dept. HEW, Public Health Service.

calories, with special attention to lowering saturated fats. At the same time, lowering dietary cholesterol is probably advisable, although this point is currently disputed. Control of habits, especially cigarette smoking and excessive use of coffee and alcohol, should be enforced. Physical activity should be increased by provision of some form of regular vigorous excercise. This may consist of jogging, swimming, bicycling, tennis, or any other activity compatible with the patient's physical condition and personal wishes. It is also desirable to help a patient combine a productive career with enjoyable recreation. Frequently, a patient can reexamine his or her pattern of behavior and achieve success without sacrificing peace of mind. Lastly, the physician can employ appropriate measures to control elevated blood pressure, diabetes mellitus, or hyperlipidemia that does not respond to diet alone.

PUBLIC HEALTH MEASURES IN PREVENTING CORONARY HEART DISEASE

Reducing Risk Factors

Despite an abundance of epidemiologic evidence linking deaths from coronary heart disease with certain risk factors, especially hypercholesterolemia, high blood pressure, and cigarette smoking, there has been an amazing amount of resistance on the part of some individuals to advice from the American Heart Association and from others who suggest that dietary modifications of the *entire* American population could result in lower plasma cholesterol levels and might diminish the death rate from coronary heart disease.

Dietary Changes

Numerous studies of limited population groups have demonstrated the feasibility of lowering cholesterol in the plasma and, in several instances, have shown a significant reduction either in cardiovascular deaths or in new events of cardiovascular disease. Indeed, the studies by Dayton and others (1969, 1970) demonstrated a significant reduction not only in plasma lipids but also in deaths from cardiovascular events. It is true that not all clinical trials have demonstrated a beneficial effect. The study conducted by the Medical Research Council of Great Britain (1968) employing a soybean-oil diet failed to provide evidence of a change in the relapse rate of myocardial infarction for men having had previous heart attacks. By contrast, a controlled clinical trial by Leren (1970) compared the effect of a plasma cholesterol-lowering diet on the coronary heart disease relapse rate of 206 men who had experienced a previous myocardial infarction, with the results obtained in a control group of 200 similar men who ate a conventional diet. In the experimental group there was not only a significant decrease in the average level of cholesterol in the plasma but also a reduction in the total incidence of coronary heart disease relapses. The significance of this difference was much greater in younger men than it was in older men. Sudden death occurred at an identical rate in both the experimental and the control groups. Christakis (1966) conducted studies of New York men who were given a "prudent diet" to lower the level of cholesterol in their plasma. By the end of seven years, it was evident that adherence to the experimental diet effectively lowered the serum cholesterol within the first year. By six years, the average values had changed from 260 to 228 mg/dl, compared with the control group, which had an average value of 250 mg/dl. A significantly lower incidence of coronary heart disease was observed in the experimental group, yielding incidence rates of 196 per 100,000 person years for the experimental, and 642 for the control groups. Both groups ranged in age from 40 to 49 years at the start of the study. In another study conducted in two separate mental hospitals, a team of Finnish investigators, Turpeinen (1968) and Miettinen (1972) and their colleagues, observed the effects of feeding a modified fat diet to the inmates of one mental hospital while those in a second hospital were given a regular diet. After six years, the diets served in these were reversed and the effects were followed for another six years to observe changes in lipid levels and in cardiovascular events. In 327 male subjects in the first hospital, who were 34 to 64 years of age at the start of the study, there was a significant fall in serum cholesterol levels following the dietary change. In the control hospital, 254 patients of comparable ages demonstrated no significant change in lipid levels. The difference between the averages in the experimental and control hospitals was 51 mg/dl for serum cholesterol. There were lesser changes in triglycerides. The incidence of electrocardiographic patterns indicative of coronary heart disease was markedly and significantly lower in the experimental hospital, but the numbers of deaths were too small to give statistically valid comparisons. After twelve years had elapsed the investigators reviewed their overall experience, comparing the first half of the study with the second half. In men, the use of the cholesterol-lowering diet was associated with reduction in mortality from coronary heart disease. Total mortality also was consistently lower, although the differences were too small to be of statistical significance. Similarly, in women, the differences were small and not statistically significant.

The American Heart Association (Mass Field Trials, 1969) attempted to evaluate the significance, timeliness, feasibility, and applicability of various experimental designs that might, in their opinion, answer the question of whether primary prevention of coronary heart disease by means of dietary methods is feasible. The panel emphasized that several important points remain unproven, including the question of whether dietary modification can prevent atherosclerotic heart disease in humans and whether demonstration of such an effect could or would result in general applicability to our society. They also attempted to project the numbers of observations necessary to give meaningful results under each of seven proposed schemes. The eventual result of this assessment was the design and conduct of studies, under way at the time of this writing (1977), to evaluate the effects of multiple risk factor intervention trials on participating subjects. It should be pointed out, however, that when an investigation involves large groups of scientists, it is inevitable that substantial, even unreconcilable differences of opinion will arise. Accordingly, it seems unlikely that this study will answer the question of whether a nationwide change in diet would have an appreciable effect on the high incidence of coronary heart disease in the United States.

It is remarkable that efforts to reduce death rates from coronary disease by means of dietary manipulation have been made for more than 20 years. One of the earliest to study the effects of diet on the incidence of coronary heart disease was Nelson (1956), who reduced the fat intake of 88 men and women, between ages 31 and 75 years, who had shown evidence of coronary disease. There were 154 subjects who were divided into a reduced-fat group and an unmodified group. The endpoint for comparison was death ascribable to atherosclerotic disease. After 13 years, only 35 per cent of the fat controlled group had died, whereas 79 per cent of the unmodified diet group had died.

Even in diabetic subjects, it has been shown that modification of the diet so as to reduce the total fat and saturated fat content not only will reduce cholesterol levels but also will reduce triglycerides without having an adverse effect upon insulin requirements or level of diabetic control (Stone and Connor, 1963).

Physical Activity

A great deal of interest has been focused on the level of physical activity and its role in preventing or modifying coronary heart disease. The early studies by Morris and others (1953) of London bus drivers suggested that a sedentary occupation had an adverse effect upon the cardiovascular system. Most efforts at reducing plasma lipid levels by means of exercise alone have been disappointing, although when exercise results in weight loss there usually is an accompanying lowering of plasma triglyceride levels. Cholesterol levels have been more resistant to change but combinations of diet and exercise have been shown to be quite effective in lowering the lipids of free-living men (Shorey et al., 1976). It is particularly interesting to note that these investigators felt restriction of dietary cholesterol as well as fat was worthwhile in controlling hypercholesterolemia in Type II individuals, whereas there was no added advantage to this dietary restriction in Type IV individuals. This study lends additional support to the concept (which is shared by the author) that a majority of persons who are hyperlipidemic can be managed quite effectively by restriction of total dietary fat, total saturated fat, total cholesterol, and total calories. Nonetheless, there are some patients who will require not only special attention to their diet but also some form of drug therapy. A good example of this is the individual (see "Type III hyperlipoprotein-emia," 1975) who has elevated plasma levels of cholesterol and triglycerides as well as elevation of very low density lipoproteins. Xanthomas are often present and ischemic heart disease commonly occurs in these individuals. Fortunately, this type of hyperlipidemia responds well to dietary and drug therapy, but best of all to weight loss. A suitable diet will allow 40 per cent of calories from fats, 40 per cent from carbohydrates and 20 per cent from protein. Of course, emphasis is placed upon reducing saturated fats and replacing them with polyunsaturated fats. It may be necessary to initiate drug therapy: for this purpose, clofibrate* may be effective. Following successful reduction of hyperlipidemia, patients may have regression of xanthomas and improvement of their abnormal glucose tolerance.

Patients who are found to be homozygous familial Type II hyperlipidemics are at great risk of developing coronary heart disease at a young age. Many do not survive beyond age 30 to 40 years. For this reason, extreme measures have been considered by some clinicians. These measures include jejunoileal bypass in order to cause malabsorption, total parenteral nutrition to avoid the digestive tract completely, and even establishment of a portocaval shunt (Ahrens, 1974).

The Results to Date

What is the meaning of all of this discussion when the leading scientists in the country openly admit that they have no proof that dietary changes, or indeed, that lowering of cholesterol itself will reduce the heavy toll from coronary heart disease? Little wonder that many practicing physicians and a majority of the American public have developed a neurotic uncertainty about the food they eat and the future

---

*Recent information suggests that this drug may be ineffective and perhaps harmful. (Editorial, *Lancet* 2:1131, 1978.)

health of their families, as well as themselves. Words of reassurance are welcome and some have been provided by Walker (1974, 1976), who points out that in the American populace there has been a major reduction in smoking in men, a major reduction in the intake of saturated fat, and a lower intake of dietary cholesterol, especially from eggs. Walker refers to age-adjusted death rates for cerebral vascular diseases and for ischemic heart disease in the United States, and calls attention to the 18.4 per cent decrease in deaths between 1963 and 1973. Hospital admissions for persons 45 through 64 years who have had a heart attack declined 16 per cent between 1968 and 1971. Walker believes that the decrease in death rate is a direct result of reduction in the risk factors among the general population in our country. He suggests that meaningful current health statistics must be obtained and widely distributed to encourage this promising trend. It is interesting to note that in "Vital Statistics" of the World Almanac and Book of Facts (1978), the vital statistics on leading causes of death in the United States (1976 estimates) confirm Walker's report and, furthermore, indicate that civilian consumption of butter is down sharply, whereas consumption of margarine has risen progressively over the past 15 years. At the same time, consumption of eggs is down from 356 to 286 per person per year and consumption of grains, which had been falling, is now on the rise.

The incontrovertible evidence of enormous differences in the incidence of cardiovascular diseases from one country to another, and the much lower incidence among American Seventh Day Adventists who are largely vegetarian, lends further credence to Walker's optimistic forecast.

Recently, Whyte and Havenstein (1976) published a Guide to Dieting in an effort to lower plasma cholesterol levels. According to them, the major contributors to dietary cholesterol in the American diet, each adding more than 10 mg/dl of cholesterol to the plasma, are brains, double servings of meat, one egg per day, and butter. At the other extreme, polyunsaturated oils and margarines actively lower the cholesterol level, whereas other foods have little or no effect. There is, of course, some evidence to dispute the value of limiting dietary cholesterol but in the experience of the author, reducing dietary cholesterol is compatible with a healthful, attractive diet and it probably is a worthwhile accompaniment of caloric and fat restriction.

A Recommendation for All

The American Heart Association fat-controlled diet (Wilson et al., 1971) is not only sensible, palatable, inexpensive, and easily prepared, but also effective in lowering lipid and lipoprotein concentrations in plasma. In a group of 59 non-obese men, both normal and hyperlipidemic, Wilson's group observed similar responses in the 31 "normal" individuals, the 8 "Type II" hyperlipidemics and the 11 "Type IV" hyperlipidemics, as well as the 9 "mixed type" hyperlipidemic individuals. There was a tendency for serum urate levels to rise, but not significantly. Further reduction of carbohydrate intake causes a greater decrease in triglyceride levels of Type IV hyperlipidemics.

The author favors this diet for the general public: (1) reduce calories sufficiently to correct obesity and to maintain normal body weight; (2) reduce fats to around 30 per cent of total calories; (3) minimize consumption of saturated fats, which are chiefly of animal origin or from hydrogenated vegetable oils; (4) regulate cholesterol intake to less than 300 mg/day; and (5) avoid abuses of alcohol, sugar, and other sweets.

Infants and Children

What Should the Pediatrician Tell Parents? Both internists and pediatricians are becoming ever more aware that atherosclerosis begins in the early years of life, although it may not become apparent until middle age or later. Numerous studies have been undertaken to determine whether or not the diet of infants and children has an appreciable impact on their plasma lipids. The answer is conclusive: it does. Investigations over a span of more than 50 years have established a firm relationship between hypercholesterolemia and atherosclerosis. Ordinarily, the rat is remarkably resistant to the development of atherosclerosis unless some major changes are made in its physiology, such as induction of hypothyroidism or blocking bile acid synthesis by feeding bile salts. Bajwa and colleagues (1971) demonstrated that feeding excessive doses of vitamin D to young adult male rats rendered them much more susceptible to the atherogenic effects of a diet containing large amounts of cholesterol and cholic acid. Apparently, vitamin D gave the arterial tissues a much greater affinity for deposition of cholesterol.

The endothelial lining of the vascular tree of any young, rapidly growing mammal seems to be susceptible to deposition of lipids. The "fatty streak" has been observed in the aorta of a wide variety of experimental animals fed diets designed to induce hyperlipidemia. Indeed, the intima of many human infants who die suddenly without a prolonged illness may show similar fatty streaks. It is doubtful that these fatty streaks represent an abnormality or that they necessarily lead to elevated cholesterol plaques, but there does seem to be some relationship between the two types of lipid deposits. Fomon (1971) expressed a conservative view about altering feeding practices to avoid atherosclerosis. He called attention to the possibility that formula feeding may lead to overfeeding of infants and that excess food may contribute to obesity in later life. Fomon has shown that the serum cholesterol concentration of infants is influenced by the type of milk they are given in the first two months of life. When fat in the diet was provided by either human milk or cow's milk, the cholesterol concentrations were relatively high, but when dietary fat was derived from corn, coconut, or soy oil, the concentrations of cholesterol in the infant's plasma were significantly lower. Fomon called attention to two potential hazards in attempting to maintain low serum concentrations of cholesterol during early infancy. The first is that cholesterol may be necessary to stimulate development of those metabolic systems responsible for degradation of this sterol. The second is that the rate of myelination of the brain has been found to be somewhat retarded in immature rats fed drugs that inhibit biosynthesis of cholesterol. Accordingly, Fomon opposes efforts to maintain low cholesterol levels in infants during the early weeks and months of life.

Bartov and others (1973) demonstrated that feeding egg yolks or crystalline cholesterol dissolved in lard to female rats resulted in higher serum and liver cholesterol levels that in turn caused a great increase in fecal bile acids. Apparently, part of the homeostatic mechanism for maintaining plasma levels of cholesterol within a normal range entails an increase in the fecal excretion of cholesterol derivatives, especially bile acids. Reiser and Sidelman (1972) postulated that newborn mammals may develop mechanisms for metabolizing dietary cholesterol if they are exposed to this substance early in life. Suckling male rats were allowed to nurse from mothers that had varying cholesterol concentrations in their milk as a result of manipulation of the maternal diets. Rat pups that consumed milk with the highest concentrations of cholesterol were found, by the time they became adults, to have serum cholesterol levels inversely related to the amount of cholesterol in their mother's milk. In other words, exposure to a large amount of cholesterol during early life apparently resulted in development of mechanisms that permitted test animals to metabolize this sterol more effectively than litter mates that had less exposure to dietary cholesterol. This phenomenon, strangely enough, was not evident in female rats.

At the clinical level, Mitchell and others (1972), representing a subcommittee on atherosclerosis, Council of Rheumatic Fever and Congenital Heart Disease of the American Heart Association, considered the problem of pediatric diets as they may influence adult atherosclerotic disease and stated, "The subcommittee decided that on the basis of data available there is no scientific justification at this time for recommending to the population at large that diets of all children be radically altered in the hope of preventing premature heart disease. However, the child at high risk (in particular, Type II hyperlipoproteinemia) can be identified and should be placed on an appropriate diet." It was further suggested that children over the age of five years and with a family history of premature coronary disease should have measurements of fasting serum cholesterol and triglyceride levels. If abnormal values are found, then a careful medical examination should be conducted to determine whether secondary or primary hyperlipidemia exists. If familial hyperlipidemia is confirmed, then appropriate dietary and drug therapy should be introduced. A somewhat more liberal viewpoint was expressed by participants in a two-day symposium held in Britain (Brook and Ball, 1977). They felt that pediatricians should take an active role in identifying children at special risk from premature atherosclerosis. Glueck and Tsang (1972) studied the effects of diet on the plasma cholesterol levels of infants with neonatal hypercholesterolemia. They found that the level of cholesterol in cord blood aided in identification of hyperlipidemic babies in some but not all instances. Changing from one diet to another during the first year of life led to abrupt changes in plasma cholesterol levels. Familial Type II hypercholesterolemia may be diagnosed by measurement of cholesterol or beta-lipoprotein cholesterol in the cord blood. In seven infants with familial Type II hyperlipoproteinemia, mean plasma cholesterol levels increased from 114 to 224 mg/dl at six months of age when a normal cow's milk formula was fed. Seven other infants fed a diet containing very little cholesterol and increased amounts of polyunsaturated fats had a fall in serum cholesterol levels from 155 to 130 mg/dl by six months of age. The authors emphasized that evidence documenting the efficacy or lack of efficacy of early normalization of cholesterol in the prevention of atherosclerosis remains to be demonstrated.

The sterol content of milk fat and of vegetable oils has taken on added significance because of the growing emphasis on dietary sterols as well as the type of fat in the diet. Parodi (1973) published data on the sterol content of a wide variety of fatty foods, including milk fat, beef fat, lard, several types of margarine, and seven different vegetable oils. This information is of value to those who may wish to manipulate the sterol content of experimental diets.

Friedman and Goldberg (1975) attempted to test Reiser's theories in infants who had been fed either breast milk or formula diets. They compared the serum cholesterol levels of children, ages two to four months, twelve months, 18 to 24 months, and 15 to 19 years, who had been breast-fed with those of children who had been bottle-fed. The same child was not necessarily followed longitudinally. They concluded that breast-fed children had significantly higher serum cholesterol levels than bottle-fed children at ages two to four months and at twelve months, but after one year no significant difference could be found between cholesterol levels of children in the two groups.

Harrison and Peat (1975) have studied the relationship between bacterial flora in the bowels of newborn children and the level of cholesterol in their serum. They found this level to be 140 mg/dl in bottle-fed infants five days old and they observed that the stools of these infants had more *Escherichia coli* than lactobacilli. The ratio of these two organisms could be reversed by adding either bicarbonate or lactobacilli to their formula. This change was associated with a fall in cholesterol to a mean level of 119 mg/dl over a period of three days. Lactobacilli predominate in the stool when cholesterol is low and may play a role in its metabolism.

Other aspects of lipid metabolism in breast-fed infants were studied by Potter and Nestel (1976), who observed that they could change the plasma cholesterol concentration in each of ten lactating women by modifying their diets. In milk taken by eight infants, changes in maternal plasma cholesterol levels were not closely reflected in the cholesterol concentration in their milk. The cholesterol content of milk was closely correlated with the concentration of other milk lipids, presumably reflecting a functional role for cholesterol in the secretion of milk fat. In the maternal milk consumed by the eight infants the linoleic acid content rose from 9.4 to 15.5 per cent of total fatty acids as a result of a moderate increase in the polyunsaturated fat of the maternal diets. This in turn was reflected in a fall in the infants' plasma cholesterol levels from 185 to 157 mg/dl.

Further studies by Potter and Nestel (1976) evaluated fecal excretion of bile acids as a result of feeding either soybean milk or cow's milk to human infants. The average rate of excretion of bile acids was 6.8 mg/kg/day when soybean milk was fed, but only 3.6 mg/kg/day when cow's milk was given. The net excretion of cholesterol remained higher when soybean milk was fed instead of cow's milk, even when egg yolk cholesterol was added to the soybean milk. It appears that substitution of soybean milk for cow's milk results in an increase in bile-acid excretion and probably also in cholesterol excretion in young infants. It remains to be seen whether this mechanism will have clinical utility in the management of infants found to have familial Type II hyperlipidemia.

Soft *versus* Hard Water

The relationships between soft-water regions and total cardiovascular disease have been discussed since the mid 1950's. For example, the age-adjusted annual death rate varied from a maximum of 983 per 100,000 people in South Carolina where the water is "soft" to a minimum of 712 in Nebraska where the water is "hard". Division of deaths into cardiovascular and "others" seems to exaggerate the difference between hard-water and soft-water states. Thus, in ten hard-water states, the total death rate was 782.9 per 100,000 people compared to 852.7 for the ten soft-water states. But cardiovascular deaths in these hard-water states occurred at a rate of 358.3 per 100,000 compared with 431.8 in soft-water states. This was a difference of seventeen per cent.

Kidneys from hypertensive patients who came to autopsy were found to contain more cadmium than those of normotensive subjects, but the significance of cadmium is not yet apparent. There is no doubt that high intakes of sodium have been statistically associated with a high incidence of cardiovascular disease, particularly hypertension. These and other factors are of interest to the practicing physician, chiefly because of the notoriety that cardiovascular disease receives through the daily media. Citizens groups, municipal councils, and others may call upon a physician to give advice concerning the quality of drinking water or the potential impact of water softeners on health. At present, it appears that hard water may be preferable to soft water for drinking and that excessive intakes of salt may be harmful to some people. Patients should be advised to avoid drinking water that has been softened by the usual zeolite resin exchange method.

The entire field of cardiovascular disease is related epidemiologically, pharmacologically, and therapeutically to nutrition. The rapidly accumulating information linking nutritional factors to cardiovascular disease has stimulated the interest of many physicians and paramedical persons. Some of the available data provide confusing and conflicting interpretations. Other bits of information seem trivial or even foolish; yet the practicing physician needs to have some familiarity with all of these topics to be able to give informed advice to patients and to their relatives. But more importantly the physician who has a broad knowledge of nutrition as it affects the health and disease of his or her patients is in a much better position to provide them with the greatest possible therapeutic benefit and the lowest level of risk.

The author believes that a sensible approach to the problem of coronary heart disease includes a constant search for unusually susceptible persons and a broad program to minimize the magnitude of the major risk factors: hypercholesterolemia, hypertension, and cigarette smoking. There is reason to believe that preventive efforts work. This was well stated in a very recent editorial review (Glueck et al., 1978).

REFERENCES

Ahrens, E. H., Jr.: Homozygous hypercholesteraemia and the portocaval shunt. *Lancet* 2:449, 1974.

Alexander, J. K.: Interactions of hyperlipidemia, hypertension, and obesity as coronary risk factors. *Triangle 14*:1, 1975.

Anderson, J. T., Grande, F., and Keys, A.: Cholesterol-lowering diets. *J. Am. Dietet. A.* 62:133, 1973.

Bajwa, G. S., Morrison, L. M., and Ershoff, B. H.: Induction of aortic and coronary athero-arteriosclerosis in rats fed a hypervitaminosis D, cholesterol-containing diet. *Proc. Soc. Exper. Biol. Med. 138*:975, 1971.

Balfour, J. F., and Kim, R.: Homozygous Type II hyperlipoproteinemia treatment. Partial ileal bypass in two children. *J.A.M.A. 227*:1145, 1974.

Bartov, I., Reiser, R., and Henderson, G. R.: Hypercholesterolemic effect in the female rat of egg yolk *versus* crystalline cholesterol dissolved in lard. *J. Nutrition 103*:1400, 1973.

Berg, K., Borresen, A. L., and Dahlen, G.: Serum-high-density-lipoprotein and athero-sclerotic heart-disease. *Lancet 1*:499, 1976.

Bierenbaum, M. L., Fleischman, A. I., Raichelson, R. I., Hayton, T., and Watson, P. B.: Ten-year experience of modified-fat diets on younger men with coronary heart-disease. *Lancet 1*:1404, 1973.

Brook, C. G. D., and Ball, K. P.: Prevention of coronary heart disease starts in childhood. *Arch. Dis. Child. 52*:904, 1977.

Carew, T. E., Koschinsky, T., Hayes, S. B., and Steinberg, D.: A mechanism by which high-density lipoproteins may slow the atherogenic process. *Lancet 1*:1315, 1976.

Chait, A., Mancini, M., February, A. W., and Lewis, B.: Clinical and metabolic study of alcoholic hyperlipidaemia. *Lancet 2*:62, 1972.

Chase, H. P., O'Quin, R. J., and O'Brien, D.: Screening for hyperlipidemia in childhood. *J.A.M.A. 230*:1535, 1974.

Chipperfield, B., Chipperfield, J. R., Behr, G., and Burton, P.: Magnesium and potassium content of normal heart muscle in areas of hard and soft water. *Lancet 1*:121, 1976.

Christakis, G., Rinzler, S. H., Archer, M., Winslow, G., Jampel, S., Stephenson, J., Friedman, G., Fein, H., Kraus, A., and James, G.: The Anti-coronary Club. A dietary approach to the prevention of coronary heart disease — a seven-year report. *Am. J. Public Health 56*:299, 1966.

Committee on Nutrition: Childhood diet and coronary heart disease. *Pediatrics 49*:305, 1972.

Connor, W. E., Stone, D. B., and Hodges, R. E.: The interrelated effects of dietary cholesterol and fat upon human serum lipid levels. *J. Clin. Invest. 43*:1691, 1964.

Connor, W. E., and Connor, S. L.: The key role of nutritional factors in the prevention of coronary heart disease. *Preventive Medicine 1*:49, 1972.

Coronary Heart Disease. A New Zealand Report. National Heart Foundation of New Zealand. Dunedin, John McIndoe, Ltd., 1971.

Dayton, S., Pearce, M. L., Hashimoto, S., Dixon, W. J., and Tomiyasu, U.: A controlled clinical trial of a diet high in unsaturated fat in preventing complications of athero-sclerosis. *Circulation XL (no. 1) Supplement no. II*, II-1 to II-63, 1969.

Dayton, S., Chapman, J. M., Pearce, M. L., and Popják, G. J.: Cholesterol, atherosclerosis, ischemic heart disease, and stroke. *Ann. Intern. Med.72*:97, 1970.

de Haas, J. H.: Primary prevention of coronary heart disease. A socio-pediatric problem. *Overdruk Hart Bulletin 4*:3, 1973.

Demakis, J. G., Proskey, A., Rahimtoola, S. H., Jamil, M., Sutton, G. C., Rosen, K. M., Gunnar, R. M., and Tobin, J. R., Jr.: The natural course of alcoholic cardiomyopathy. *Ann. Intern. Med. 80*:293, 1974.

Dietary Management of Hyperlipoproteinemia. A Handbook for Physicians and Dieti-tians. Prepared and compiled under the direction of: Fredrickson, D. S., Bonnell, M., Levy, R. I., and Ernst, N. Bethesda, National Heart and Lung Institute, 1974. DHEW Publ. No. (NIH) 75–110.

Dietschy, J. M., and Wilson, J. D.: Regulation of cholesterol metabolism. *New England J. Med. 282*:1128, 1179, 1241, 1970.

Ederer, F., Leren, P., Turpeinen, O., and Frantz, I. D., Jr.: Cancer among men on cholesterol-lowering diets: Experience from five clinical trials. *Lancet 2*:203, 1971.

Editorial: A bit of good news — coronary death rate seems to have peaked. *J.A.M.A. 231*:691, 1975.

Editorial: Free fatty acids and arrhythmias after acute myocardial infarction. *Lancet* *1*:313, 1975.

Editorial: H.D.L. and C.H.D. *Lancet* 2:131, 1976.

Enos, W. F., Holmes, R. H., and Beyer, J.: Coronary disease among United States soldiers killed in action in Korea. *J.A.M.A. 152*:1090, 1955.

Epstein, F. H.: Predicting coronary heart disease. *J.A.M.A. 201*:795, 1967.

Fomon, S. J.: A pediatrician looks at early nutrition. *Bull. New York Acad. Med. 47*:569, 1971.

Frantz, I. D., and Moore, R. B.: The sterol hypothesis in atherogenesis. *Amer. J. Med. 46*:684, 1969.

Fredrickson, D. S.: Mutants, hyperlipoproteinaemia, and coronary artery disease. *Brit. Med. J.* 2:187, 1971.

Friedman, G., and Goldberg, S. J.: Normal serum cholesterol values. Percentile ranking in a middle-class pediatric population. *J.A.M.A. 225*:610, 1973.

Friedman, G., and Goldberg, S. J.: Concurrent and subsequent serum cholesterols of breast- and formula-fed infants. *Amer. J. Clin. Nutr. 28*:42, 1975.

Friedman, M., and Byers, S. O.: The pathogenesis of neurogenic hypercholesterolemia: V. Relationship to hepatic catabolism of cholesterol. *Proc. Soc. Exper. Biol. Med. 144*:917, 1973.

Gillum, R. F.: Myocardial infarction and coffee drinking. *New England J. Med. 295*:104, 1976.

Ginsberg, H., Olefsky, J., Farquhar, J. W., and Reaven, G. M.: Moderate ethanol ingestion and plasma triglyceride levels. A study in normal and hypertriglyceride-mic persons. *Ann. Intern. Med. 80*:143, 1974.

Glueck, C. J., Mattson, F., and Bietman, E. L.: Diet and coronary heart disease: another view. *New Engl. J. Med. 298*:1471, 1978.

Glueck, C. J., and Tsang, R. C.: Pediatric familial Type II hyperlipoproteinemia: effects of diet on plasma cholesterol in the first year of life. *Amer. J. Clin. Nutr. 25*:224, 1972.

Goldstein, J. L., and Brown, M. S.: Hyperlipidemia in coronary heart disease: a biochemical genetic approach. *J. Lab. Clin. Med. 85*:15, 1975.

Gordon, T., and Kannel, W. B.: Predisposition to atherosclerosis in the head, heart, and legs. *J.A.M.A. 221*:661, 1972.

Harlan, W. R.: Gingival "lipid line" and discordant development of xanthomas and arteriosclerosis. *Ann. Intern. Med. 82*:227, 1975.

Harrison, V. C., and Peat, G.: Serum cholesterol and bowel flora in the newborn. *Amer. J. Clin. Nutr. 28*:1351, 1975.

Hazzard, W. R., O'Donnell, T. F., and Lee, Y. L.: Broad β disease (Type III hyperlipoproteinemia) in a large kindred. Evidence for a monogenic mechanism. *Ann. Intern. Med. 82*:141, 1975.

Hennekens, C. H., Drolette, M. E., Jesse, M. J., Davies, J. E., and Hutchison, G. B.: Coffee drinking and death due to coronary heart disease. *New England J. Med. 294*:633, 1976.

The herbs and the heart. *Nutr. Reviews 34*:43, 1976.

Hodges, R. E., Salel, A. F., Dunkley, W. L., Zelis, R., McDonagh, P. F., Clifford, C., Hobbs, R. K., Smith, L. M., Fan, A., Mason, D. T., and Lykke, C.: Plasma lipid changes in young adult couples consuming polyunsaturated meats and dairy products. *Amer. J. Clin. Nutr. 28*:1126, 1975.

Hoffman, N. E., Hofman, A. F., and Thistle, J. L.: Effect of bile acid feeding on cholesterol metabolism in gallstone patients. *Mayo Clin. Proc. 49*:236, 1974.

Hood, B., Sanne, H., Orndahl, G., Ahlstrom, M., and Welin, G.: Long-term prognosis in essential hypercholesterolemia. The effect of strict diet. *Acta Med. Scand. 178*:161, 1965.

Hulley, S. B., Wilson, W. S., Burrows, M. I., and Nichaman, M. Z.: Lipid and lipoprotein responses of hypertriglyceridaemic outpatients to a low-carbohydrate modification of the A.H.A. fat-controlled diet. *Lancet* 2:551, 1972.

Intervention in Type IV hyperlipoproteinemia. *Nutr. Reviews 34*:204, 1976.

Jick, H., and Miettinen, O.S.: Statistics of coffee drinking and myocardial infarction. *New England J. Med. 292*:265, 1975.

Kannel, W. B.: Lipid profile and the potential coronary victim. *Amer. J. Clin. Nutr.* 24:1074, 1971.

Kato, H., Tillotson, J., Nichaman, M. Z., Rhoads, G. G., and Hamilton, H. B.: Epidemiologic studies of coronary heart disease and stroke in Japanese men living in Japan, Hawaii, and California. Serum lipids and diet. *Amer. J. Epidemiol.* 97:372, 1973.

Keys, A., Kimura, N., Kusukawa, A., Bronte-Stewart, B., Larsen, N., and Keys, M. H.: Lessons from serum cholesterol studies in Japan, Hawaii and Los Angeles. *Ann. Intern. Med.* 48:83, 1958.

Keys, A., Anderson, J. T., and Grande, F.: Serum cholesterol responses to changes in the diet. IV. Particular saturated fatty acids in the diet. *Metabolism 14*:776, 1965.

Keys, A: Sucrose in the diet and coronary heart disease. *Atherosclerosis 14*:193, 1971.

Keys, A., Taylor, H. L., Blackburn, H., Brozek, J., Anderson, J. T., and Simonson, E.: Mortality and coronary heart disease among men studied for 23 years. *Arch. Intern. Med. 128*:201, 1971.

Keys, A., Aravanis, C., Blackburn, H., Van Buchem, F. S. P., Buzina, R., Djordjevic, B. S., Fidanza, F., Karvonen, M. J., Menotti, A., Puddu, V., and Taylor, H.L.: Coronary heart disease: overweight and obesity as risk factors. *Ann. Intern. Med.* 77:15, 1972a.

Keys, A., Aravis, C. , Blackburn, H., van Buchem, F. S.P., Buzina, R., Djordjevic, B. S., Fidanza, F., Karvonen, M. J., Menotti, A., Puddu, V., and Taylor, H. L.: Probability of middle-aged men developing coronary heart disease in five years. *Circulation XLV*:815, 1972b.

Khachadurian, A. K., and Kawahara, F. S.: Cholesterol synthesis by cultured fibroblasts: decreased feedback inhibition in familial hypercholesterolemia. *J. Lab. Clin. Med.* 83:7, 1974.

Kiriyama, S., Ichihara, Y., Enishi, A., and Yoshida, A.: Effect of purification and cellulose treatment on the hypocholesterolemic activity of crude konjac mannnan.*J. Nutrition 102*:1689, 1972.

Klevay, L. M.: Coronary heart disease: the zinc/copper hypothesis. *Amer. J. Clin. Nutr.* 28:764, 1975.

Kromer, G. W.: Food fat consumption: more now and in the future. Presented at Symposium on fats and carbohydrates in processed foods. Sponsored by the American Medical Association, Chicago, Ill., October 1, 1973.

Lange, W.: Cholesterol, phytosterol, and tocopherol content of food products and animal tissues. *J. Amer. Oil Chem. Soc.* 27:414, 1950.

Lees, R. S., and Wilson, D. E.: The treatment of hyperlipidemia. *New England J. Med.* 284:186, 1971.

Lees, R. S.: Editorial: A progress report on lipoprotein phenotyping. *J. Lab. Clin. Med.* 82:529, 1973.

Lehman, H., and Lines, J. G.: Hyperlipoproteinaemia classification: The optimum routine electrophoretic system and its relevance to treatment. *Lancet 1*:557, 1972.

Leren, P.: The effect of plasma cholesterol lowering diet in male survivors of myocardial infarction. A controlled clinical trial. *Acta Medica Scandinavica, Supplementum 466*, Oslo 1966, pp. 1–92.

Leren, P.: The Oslo diet-heart study. Eleven-year report. *Circulation XLII*:935, 1970.

Levy, R. I., Fredrickson, D. S., Shulman, R., Bilheimer, D. W., Breslow, J. L., Stone, N. J., Lux, S. E., Sloan, H. R., Krauss, R. M., and Herbert, P. N.: Dietary and drug treatment of primary hyperlipoproteinemia. *Ann. Intern. Med.* 77:267, 1972.

Levy, R. I., Morganroth, J., and Rifkind, B. M.: Drug therapy: Treatment of hyperlipidemia. *New England J. Med.* 290:1295, 1974.

Levy, R. I.: Drug therapy of hyperlipoproteinemia. *J.A.M.A. 235*:2334, 1976.

Levy, R. I.: Hyperlipoproteinemia: Some basic concepts on diagnosis and management. *J.A.M.A. 226*:648, 1973.

Lew, E. A., and Entmacher, P. S.: Mortality in cardiovascular disease. (Metropolitan Life Insurance Company). Presented at the Skandia International Symposium on Early Phases of Coronary Heart Disease. Stockholm, Sweden, September 19–21, 1972.

Lewis, L. A., Brown, H. B., and Page, I. H.: Ten years' dietary treatment of primary hyperlipidemia. *Geriatrics 12*:64, 1970.

Macdonald, I., and Braithwaite, D. M.: The influence of dietary carbohydrates on the lipid pattern in serum and in adipose tissue. *Clin. Sci.* 27:23, 1964.

Mass Field Trials of the Diet-Heart Question. *Amer. Heart Assn. Monograph No. 28,* New York, 1969.

McIntyre, N., and Isselbacher, K. J.: Role of the small intestine in cholesterol metabolism. *Amer. J. Clin. Nutr.* 26:647, 1973.

McNamara, J. J., Molot, M. A., Stremple, J. F., and Cutting, R. T.: Coronary artery disease in combat casualties in Vietnam. *J.A.M.A.* 216:1185, 1971.

Medical Research Council of Great Britain. Morris, J. N. (Chairman of Research Committee): Controlled trial of soya-bean oil in myocardial infarction. *Lancet* 2:693, 1968.

Mendelson, J. H., and Mello, N. K.: Significance of alcohol-induced hypertriglyceridemia in patients with Type IV hyperlipoproteinemia. *Ann. Intern. Med.* 80:270, 1974.

Miettinen, M., Turpeinen, O., Karvonen, M. J., Elosuo, R., and Paavilainen, E.: Effect of cholesterol-lowering diet on mortality from coronary heart-disease and other causes. A twelve-year clinical trial in men and women. *Lancet* 2:835, 1972.

Miller, G. J., and Miller, N. E.: Plasma-high-density-lipoprotein concentration and development of ischaemic heart-disease. *Lancet* 1:16, 1975.

Mitchell, S., Blount, S. G., Jr., Blumenthal, S., Jesse, M. J., and Weidman, W. H.: Commentary: The pediatrician and atherosclerosis. *Pediatrics* 49:165, 1972.

Morris, J., Heady, J., Raffle, P., Roberts, C., and Parks, J.: Coronary heart disease and physical activity of work. *Lancet* 2:1053, 1953.

Motulsky, A. G.: Current concepts in genetics: the genetic hyperlipidemias. *New England J. Med.* 294:823, 1976.

Murphy, B. F.: Management of hyperlipidemias. *J.A.M.A.* 230:1683, 1974.

National Center for Health Statistics. Total serum cholesterol levels of adults 18–74 years, United States, 1971–74. *Vital Health Statistics, series II,* no. 205; U.S. Department of Health, Education, and Welfare, Public Health Service, 1978.

Nelson, A. M.: The effect of a fat-controlled diet on patients with coronary disease. *Northwest Med.* 55:643, 792, 874, 1956.

Nestel, P. J., Whyte, H. M., and Goodman, D. W. S.: Distribution and turnover of cholesterol in humans. *J. Clin. Invest.* 48:982, 1969.

Ogryzlo, M. A.: Hyperuricemia induced by high fat diets and starvation. *Arthritis and Rheumatism* 8:799, 1965.

Oliver, M. F., Nimmo, I. A., Cooke, M., Carson, L. A., and Olsson, A. G.: Ischaemic heart disease and associated risk factors in 40-year-old men in Edinburgh and Stockholm. *Europ.J. Clin. Invest.* 5:507, 1975.

Orlando, J., Aronow, W. S., Cassidy, J., and Prakash, R.: Effect of ethanol on angina pectoris. *Ann. Intern. Med.* 84:652, 1976.

Parodi, P. W.: The sterol content of milkfat, animal fats, margarines, and vegetable oils. *Australian J. Dairy Tech.* 28:135, 1973.

Parsons, W. B., Achor, R. W. P., Berge, K. G., McKenzie, B. F., and Barker, N. W.: Changes in concentration of blood lipids following prolonged administration of large doses of nicotinic acid to persons with hypercholesterolemia: Preliminary observations. *Proc. Staff Meetings of Mayo Clinic* 31:377, 1956.

Pearce, M. L., and Dayton, S.: Incidence of cancer in men on a diet high in polyunsaturated fat. *Lancet* 1:464, 1971.

Perry, H. M., Jr.: Minerals in cardiovascular disease. *J. Am. Dietet. A.* 62:631, 1973.

Pinckney, E. R.: The biological toxicity of polyunsaturated fats. *Med. Counterpoint (Feb.)*:53, 1973.

Potter, J. M., and Nestel, P. J.: The effects of dietary fatty acids and cholesterol on the milk lipids of lactating women and the plasma cholesterol of breast-fed infants. *Amer. J. Clin. Nutr.* 29:54, 1976a.

Potter, J. M., and Nestel, P. J.: Greater bile acid excretion with soy bean than with cow milk in infants. *Amer. J. Clin. Nutr.* 29:546, 1976b.

Rahe, R. H., Romo, M., Bennett, L., and Siltanen, P.: Recent life changes, myocardial infarction, and abrupt coronary death. *Arch. Intern. Med.* 133:221, 1974.

Rao, D. S., Sekhara, N. C., Satyanarayana, M. N., and Srinivasan, M.: Effect of curcumin in serum and liver cholesterol levels in the rat. *J. Nutrition* 100:1307, 1970.

Reiser, R., and Sidelman, Z.: Control of serum cholesterol homeostasis by cholesterol in the milk of the suckling rat. *J. Nutrition* 102:1009, 1972.

Rhoads, G. G., Gulbrandsen, C. L., and Kagan, A.: Serum lipoproteins and coronary heart disease in a population study of Hawaii Japanese men. *New England J. Med.* 294:293, 1976.

Rizek, R. L., Friend, B., and Page, L.: Fat in today's food supply — of use and sources. *J. Amer. Oil Chem. Soc.* 51:244, 1974.

Rosenman, R. H., Brand, R. J., Sholtz, R. I., and Jenkins, C. D.: Relation to corneal arcus to cardiovascular risk factors and the incidence of coronary disease. *New England J. Med.* 291:1322, 1974.

Ross, R., and Glomset, J. A.: The pathogenesis of atherosclerosis (Part I). *New England J. Med.* 295:369, 1976. (Part II) ibid. 420, 1976.

Rowe, M. J., Neilson, J. M. M., and Oliver, M. F.: Control of ventricular arrhythmias during myocardial infarction by antilipolytic treatment using a nicotinic acid analogue. *Lancet* 1:295, 1975.

Samuel, P., and Perl, W.: Long-term decay of serum cholesterol radioactivity: Body cholesterol metabolism in normals and in patients with hyperlipoproteinemia and atherosclerosis. *J. Clin. Invest.* 49:346, 1970.

Schonfeld, G., and Kudzma, D. J.: Type IV hyperlipoproteinemia. *Arch. Intern. Med.* 132:55, 1973.

Schramm, T.: Einfluss von Fettsäuren auf die Carcinogenese. II. Einfluss von Fettsäuren auf die durch 3'-methyl-4-dimethylaminazobenzol induzierte Carcinogenese bei der Ratte. *Acta Biol. Med. Germ.* 6:322, 1961a.

Schramm, T.: Einfluss von Fettsäuren auf die Carcinogenese. II. Einfluss von Fettsäuren auf die durch 4-Dimethylaminostilben induzierte Carcinogenese bei der Ratte. *Acta Biol. Med. Germ.* 6:428, 1961b.

Schreibman, P. H., and Dell, R. B.: Human adipocyte cholesterol: Concentration, localization, synthesis, and turnover. *J. Clin. Invest.* 55:986, 1975.

Schrott, H. G., Goldstein, J. L., Hazzard, W. R., McGoodwin, M. M., and Motulsky, A. G.: Familial hypercholesterolemia in a large kindred. Evidence for a monogenic mechanism. *Ann. Intern. Med.* 76:711, 1972.

Shapiro, S., Weinblatt, E., Frank, C. W., and Sager, R. V.: Incidence of coronary heart disease in a population insured for medical care (HIP). *Am. J. Public Health* 59:1, 1969.

Shorey, R. A. L., Sewell, B., and O'Brien, M.: Efficacy of diet and exercise in the reduction of serum cholesterol and triglyceride in free-living adult males. *Amer. J. Clin. Nutr.* 29:512, 1976.

Sigurdsson, G., Nicoll, A., and Lewis, B.: Conversion of very low density lipoprotein to low density lipoprotein. A metabolic study of apolipoprotein B kinetics in human subjects. *J. Clin. Invest.* 56:1481, 1975.

Smith, L. K., Luepker, R. V., Rothchild, S. S., Gillis, A., Kochman, L., and Warbasse, J. R.: Management of Type IV hyperlipoproteinemia. Evaluation of practical clinical approaches. *Ann. Intern. Med.* 84:22, 1976.

Smith, L. M.: Introduction to the symposium on milk lipids. *J. Amer. Oil Chem. Soc.* 50:175, 1973.

Sodhi, H. S., and Kudchodkar, B. J.: Correlating metabolism of plasma and tissue cholesterol with that of plasma lipoproteins. *Lancet* 1:513, 1973.

Sodhi, H. S., Kudchodkar, B. J., Varughese, P., and Duncan, D.: Validation of the ratio method for calculating absorption of dietary cholesterol in man. *Proc. Soc. Exper. Biol. Med.* 145:107, 1974.

Special Report: Prevention of coronary heart disease. *Nutr. Reviews* 34:220, 1976.

Stein, E. A., Mendelsohn, D., Fleming, M., Barnard, G. D., Carter, K. J., du Toit, P. S., Hansen, J. D. L., and Bersohn, I.: Lowering of plasma cholesterol levels in free-living adolescent males: Use of natural and synthetic polyunsaturated foods to provide balanced fat diets. *Amer. J. Clin. Nutr.* 28:1204, 1975.

Stern, M. P., Kolterman, O. G., McDevitt, H., and Reaven, G. M.: Acquired Type 3 hyperlipoproteinemia. *Arch. Intern. Med.* 130:817, 1972.

Stitt, F. W., Clayton, D. G., Crawford, M. D., and Morris, J. N.: Clinical and biochemical indicators of cardiovascular disease among men living in hard and soft water areas. *Lancet* 1:122, 1973.

Stone, D. B., and Connor, W. E.: The prolonged effects of a low cholesterol, high carbohydrate diet upon the serum lipids in diabetic patients. *Diabetes* 12:127, 1963.

Sturdevant, R. A. L., Pearce, M. L., and Dayton, S.: Increased prevalence of cholelithiasis in men ingesting a serum-cholesterol-lowering diet. *New England J. Med. 288*:24, 1973.

Subbiah, M. T. R.: Dietary plant sterols: current status in human and animal sterol metabolism. *Amer. J. Clin. Nutr. 26*:219, 1973.

Taylor, C. B., and Ho, K. J.: Studies on the Masai. *Amer. J. Clin. Nutr. 24*:1291, 1971.

Tolman, E. L., Tepperman, J., and Tepperman, H. M.: Effects of ethyl-α-p-chlorophenoxybutyrate (CPIB) on total cholesterol concentrations of rat aorta. *Proc. Soc. Exper. Biol. Med. 132*:936, 1969.

Turpeinen, O., Miettinen, M., Karvonen, M. J., Roine, P., Pekkarinen, M., Lehtosuo, E. J., and Alivirta, P.: Dietary prevention of coronary heart disease: Long-term experiment. I. Observations on male subjects. *Amer. J. Clin. Nutr. 21*:255, 1968.

Type III hyperlipoproteinemia. *Nutr. Reviews 33*:173, 1975.

Vital Statistics: Leading Causes of Death. United States 1976 Estimates. *The World Almanac and Book of Facts, 1978.* New York, Newspaper Enterprise Assoc., Inc.

Walker, A. R.P.: Sucrose, hypertension, and heart disease. *Amer. J. Clin. Nutr. 28*:195, 1975.

Walker, W. J.: Special Communication: Coronary mortality: what is going on? *J.A.M.A. 227*:1045, 1974.

Walker, W. J.: Curbing risk factors *has* helped reduce U.S. coronary deaths. *Modern Medicine,* June 1, 1976, pp. 33–47.

Wen, C-P, and Gershoff, S.: Changes in serum cholesterol and coronary heart disease mortality associated with changes in the postwar Japanese diet. *Amer. J. Clin. Nutr. 26*:616, 1973.

West, C. E., and Redgrave, T. G.: Reservations on the use of polyunsaturated fats in human nutrition. *Amer. Lab. (Jan.)*:23, 1975.

Whyte, H. M., and Havenstein, N.: A perspective view of dieting to lower the blood cholesterol. *Amer. J. Clin. Nutr. 29*:784, 1976.

Wilson, D. E., Schreibman, P. H., Brewster, A. C., and Arky, R. A.: The enhancement of lipemia by ethanol in man. *J. Lab. Clin. Med. 75*:264, 1970.

Wilson, W. S., Hulley, S. B., Burrows, M. I., and Nichaman, M. Z.: Serial lipid and lipoprotein responses to the American Heart Association fat-controlled diet. *Amer. J. Med. 51*:491, 1971.

Yanigihara, H.: Health development in Japan. *J.A.M.A. 235*:314, 1976.

Zelis, R., Mason, D. T., and Spann, J. F., Jr.: The hyperlipoproteinemias. A simplified classification and approach to therapy. *Calif. Med. 112*:32, 1970.

Zelis, R., and Salel, A. F.: Type 4 hyperlipoproteinemia: one theory of atherogenesis. *Chest 64*:486, 1973.

Plate 1   Skin turgor reflects the thickness of the skin and its underlying tissues. Prolonged malnutrition causes thinning of the skin itself and loss of both fat and collagen from subcutaneous tissues. Often there is evidence of bruising and bleeding. Loss of turgor develops gradually as people grow older, but malnutrition exaggerates and accelerates the process.

Plate 2   Increased vascularity of the bulbar conjunctivae can result from a variety of causes including trauma, allergy, infection or malnutrition. Although riboflavin deficiency causes a very severe degree of conjunctival hyperemia, other deficiencies may produce similar changes.

Plate 3   Magenta colored tongue. Severe malnutrition is usually accompanied by an abnormal color of the tongue. This is not changed by giving any number of vitamins, but will revert to normal within a few days, once positive caloric and nitrogen balance have been established.

Plate 4   A corneal arcus occurring in a person less than 60 years of age is an indication for lipid studies. In homozygous Type II hyperlipoproteinemia, an arcus may appear before age 20. Courtesy Elaine Feldman and *Resident and Staff Physician.*

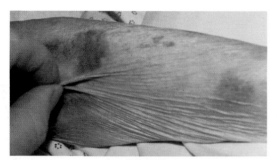

PLATE 1

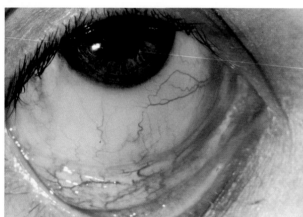

PLATE 2

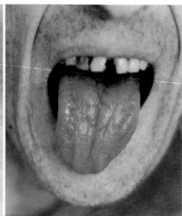

PLATE 3

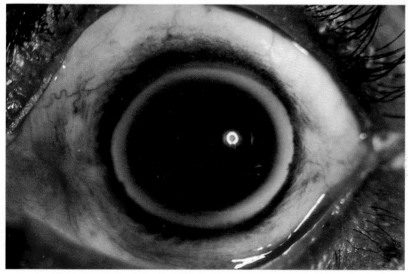

PLATE 4

5

NUTRITION AND THE NERVOUS SYSTEM

Robert E. Hodges, M.D.

In the chapters on Reproduction and on Hematopoiesis, evidence is presented to show the essentiality of specific nutrients for new cell formation. In this chapter, which deals with the nervous system, emphasis will be placed on the vital role of the nutrients in *preserving* functions of this highly specialized organ system.

Both the central nervous system and the peripheral nerves are continuously dependent upon a high degree of homeostasis. This includes not only an abundant supply of oxygen but also a readily available source of energy with all of the vitamins and minerals that participate in its many enzyme systems and metabolic functions.

Some nutrients, such as glucose, are so rapidly metabolized by the brain that coma and convulsions can be induced in a short time by giving enough insulin to lower plasma glucose levels, a form of therapy formerly used in treating patients with schizophrenia. Infusion of glucose intravenously promptly corrects both the hypoglycemia and the convulsive disorder.

But most deficiencies develop slowly: for vitamin B_{12}, there may be a delay of several years before a dietary deficiency becomes clinically apparent. And secondary deficiencies that result from drug-nutrient interactions may have an even longer latent period. As an example, the deficiency of vitamin D that results from prolonged use of anticonvulsant medications may not become apparent for many years (Rødbro and Christiansen, 1975).

Nutritional factors play many other roles in the normal and abnormal physiology of the nervous system. Current interest has been particularly keen in a variety of situations in which nutrition is

136

thought to influence the nervous system. Perhaps the greatest degree of interest has been generated by reports that maternal nutrition may have an impact on development and maturation of the fetal brain. The implications of this concept are enormous, especially for the developing nations. But this theory remains to be proved.

Another area of interest and controversy is the concept that various food additives may have a toxic effect on children and may even contribute to the so-called "hyperkinetic" syndrome. And another widely held view is that many common complaints may arise from "hypoglycemia", with or without fasting.

In addition, nutritionists and psychiatrists are perplexed by conflicting reports about the alleged benefits of "megavitamin" therapy of mental disorders. This dilemma has not been resolved by use of the term "orthomolecular psychiatry", even though some highly respected people endorse this concept.

Metabolic and endocrine disorders such as diabetic coma, uremia, or myxedema have long been known to have profound effects on the functions of the brain. Recent trends in medical practice have underscored the importance of these and other syndromes, especially in patients who must be fed by total parenteral nutrition. Development of non-ketotic hyperosmolar coma or of hypophosphatemia requires prompt diagnosis and appropriate therapy to avoid a fatal outcome.

Although epidemiologists have long suggested that dietary sodium chloride may play a role in hypertension and stroke, few predicted that the *type* of dietary fat was of great importance. Both of these factors are under active investigation and may prove to be important in prevention and management of cerebrovascular diseases.

A message that has been delivered (and ignored) countless times is that poverty and ignorance contribute to malnutrition. But now there is a growing sense of conviction that many people, especially children, who were unfortunate enough to be born in one of the *developing* countries may not have the energy and ability needed to perform at a high intellectual level. As a result, these people may not receive adequate education and training to raise them out of the ranks of the unskilled laborer.

NUTRITIONAL NEEDS OF THE BRAIN

The nervous system, and especially the brain, is highly susceptible to functional derangement from a variety of nutritional deficits. At present, a great deal of interest centers on the potential damage that may occur to the brain of a fetus whose mother is malnourished. Certainly in experimental animals the basic principles have been established: maternal malnutrition, when severe, leads to intrauterine or neonatal death. Less severe malnutrition early in pregnancy can cause malformations, stunted growth, and eventually, impaired performance. During periods of rapid growth the nervous system is extraordinarily susceptible to malnutrition. Fortunately, the effects of malnutrition are not always permanent. The outcome depends upon the stage of development of the brain, the severity and duration of deficiency, and the type of deficiency.

Feeding experiments in subhuman animals may give misleading results because of the disparity between fetal/maternal weight ratios of various species and humans. For example, a sow gives birth to a litter of pigs whose total weight is a substantial percentage of her own weight, but a woman weighing 65 kg characteristically gives birth to a baby weighing about 3.25 kg, or about 5 per cent of her weight. Thus, the nutritional drain on a woman is usually less than that on a mother of some lower species. In an effort to compensate for this defect, several investigators have studied the effects of malnutrition on the offspring of various subhuman primates that usually have a single baby. Elias and Samonds (1977) found that both diet and environmental stimuli were important in behavioral development of Cebus monkeys. On the other hand, Cheek and others (1976) fed diets containing varying amounts of protein and energy to pregnant Rhesus monkeys and found that the fetal brains were remarkably well protected. Barnes (1976) reviewed the effects of environmental deprivation and of malnutrition on intellectual development of the child and remarked, "The interaction between poor nutritional status and poor environmental stimulation must be a prominent factor in devising strategies to combat the intellectual retardation common to those living in poverty." Studies by Graves (1976) are in accord with this concept. Undernourished children between the ages of seven and eighteen months were found to have less vigor and less emotional attachment to their mothers, even though they had closer physical contact.

In adults, the consequences of malnutrition are generally slow to develop and less severe than they are in children. It is fortunate that deficiency syndromes usually remain latent when there is also severe caloric restriction. Thus, during periods of famine, the populace may become emaciated and apathetic but they probably will not develop such syndromes as scurvy, pellagra, and beriberi, which might be fatal within a short time. During World War II, many citizens of Western Europe survived for several years without adequate food supplies, presumably because undernutrition caused them to reduce their metabolic activity to a minimum.

This provides an important lesson in the management of patients who, because of chronic illness, depression, or poverty, have become severely starved and malnourished. If one feeds them too rapidly or if one starts parenteral feedings at too high a level, they may develop acute deficiency syndromes and die. The keynote must be *gradual* restoration of food.

In the case of most adults in the United States, nutritional deficiencies are rare *unless* the individual is addicted to alcohol. When this occurs there is double jeopardy because: (1) many alcoholic patients either cannot or will not eat regular meals, and so may consume a diet deficient in one or more essential nutrients; and (2) alcohol supplies an abundant number of calories (7 kcal/gm), thus depriving the patient of the protection from deficiency syndromes otherwise afforded by semistarvation. Little wonder, then, that alcoholic patients are far more apt than most to have deficiency diseases.

Glucose

As noted previously, glucose is the primary source of energy for the nervous system. Sudden reduction in the concentration of glucose in the brain results in serious disruption of function. In patients who have been starved for several weeks, hypoglycemia develops gradually and the brain acquires an ability to metabolize fatty acids and ketone bodies as sources of energy. Brozek and colleagues (1948), who studied human starvation both in wartime prison camps and under experimental conditions, observed the onset of weakness, hypothermia, bradycardia, fatigue, and apathy in their subjects. Although these subjects had some degree of hypoglycemia, it probably was not the primary cause of their hunger or their apathy, which presumably resulted from multiple deficiencies.

Amino Acids and Neurotransmitters

Most tissues of the body have a requirement for amino acids that is proportional to the rate of cellular regeneration. But the brain, and presumably the spinal cord as well, uses certain amino acids as substrates from which several neurotransmitters are formed. The fascinating topic of behavioral pharmacology, dealing as it does with receptors, transmitters, depressants, and hallucinogens (Goldfarb, 1976), is beyond the scope of this chapter. But a few of the neurotransmitters, such as norepinephrine, serotonin, acetylcholine, and histamine, have been well known for years (Goldfarb and Wilk, 1976). And there is preliminary evidence that the distribution and functions of these neurotransmitters may have some relationship to the recognized manifestations of several neurologic and psychiatric disorders (Omenn,

1976). Studies of factors that regulate serotonin synthesis in the brain indicate that there is a high-affinity-uptake of tryptophan in patients with certain neuroses that are termed "serotonergic." Administration of lithium results in a net increase in tryptophan concentration in certain portions of the brain (Mandell and Knapp, 1977). To some extent diet controls the synthesis of monoamine neurotransmitters in the brain. For example, Wurtman and Fernstrom (1975) observed that after administering tryptophan and injecting insulin there was an increase in brain tryptophan. A similar result followed a meal of carbohydrates. But a meal of protein lowered the concentration of both tryptophan and serotonin in the brain. Although there is no consensus regarding the effects of the various neurotransmitters on mental illness, there is agreement that most of the antipsychotic drugs exert their action by augmenting or suppressing specific neurotransmitters.

The Vitamins

Undoubtedly the vitamins are essential for development and maintenance of the nervous system, but deficiencies of only a few have been associated with characteristic dysfunctions of the brain itself.

Pyridoxine Deficiency: Vitamin B_6 is the generic name that refers to three closely related substances — pyridoxal, pyridoxamine, and pyridoxine — but the term pyridoxine is also used generically. The effect of this vitamin upon the nervous system was well established by animal studies that demonstrated the occurrence of a convulsive disorder when the diet contained none of this vitamin. Because convulsions in humans can be controlled by giving phenobarbital, this medication was given in large doses to dogs that had become pyridoxine deficient as a result of dosing with the vitamin antagonist, desoxypyridoxine. The result was complete control of their convulsions. But when these animals were given repleting doses of pyridoxine they promptly became oversedated by the phenobarbital. This experiment clearly demonstrated the interactions that can occur between nutrients and drugs, especially when one is studying functions of the central nervous system.

These studies of convulsions in experimental animals later proved to be life saving. Coursin (1954) had become interested in electroencephalograms (EEGs) in infants with convulsions, and requested practitioners in his area to refer such patients to him. Within a short span of time he had an unprecedented number of referrals of infants who had convulsions but who were otherwise entirely healthy. He quickly suspected a common factor and discovered that they had all been fed the same brand of commercial infant formula. Communication with the manufacturer disclosed that several packages of their product had in recent months become moldy, so they had modified their technique of sterilization. In so doing, they had unwittingly destroyed a portion of the pyridoxine in the infant formula. Administration of pyridoxine to these infants quickly cured their convulsions and no residual damage could be detected. Of course physicians promptly tried giving large doses of vitamin B_6 to infants and adults with a variety of convulsive disorders but the results were negative. It is possible to detect early signs of pyridoxine deficiency by means of electroencephalography. Similar EEG abnormalities have been observed as a result of deficiencies of thiamin, riboflavin, niacin, folic acid, and biotin (Anonymous Review, 1975a).

Another phenomenon relating to pyridoxine was discovered serendipitously when Lepkovsky and Nielson (1942) were studying pyridoxine deficiency in rats and, because of limited funds, employed inexpensive cages made from galvanized iron hardware cloth. Newspapers were placed beneath the cages because wood shavings were more expensive. It was noted that the urine from rats in the pyridoxine-deficient group reacted with the zinc-coated iron cages and stained the newspapers green. The substance responsible for this was actually yellow before it reacted with zinc. This was found to be a derivative of tryptophan, xanthurenic acid. Feeding large amounts of tryptophan resulted in excretion of large amounts of xanthurenic acid in the urine of vitamin B_6–deficient animals, but not in normal controls. This tryptophan-load test has become a standard method for evaluating the adequacy of pyridoxine nutrition in humans. Subjects who are deficient in vitamin B_6 will excrete abnormal amounts of xanthurenic acid in their urine following an oral load of 5 gm L-tryptophan.

Needless to say, this test was performed in a wide variety of patients. This resulted in another surprise when it was found that tryptophan-load testing of healthy pregnant women resulted in excretion of excessively large amounts of xanthurenic acid in their urine. Administration of 50 mg doses of pyridoxine prior to tryptophan loading prevented the abnormality. Does this mean that pregnant women need more pyridoxine than they usually consume? The question remains unanswered.

Shortly after the introduction of the oral contraceptive steroids (OCS) an effort was made to evaluate those few individuals who complained of nervousness, irritability and headache while taking "the pill". Tryptophan-load tests confirmed the suspicion that women taking OCS behave metabolically like pregnant women; they excrete excessive amounts of xanthurenic acid in their urine. And oral administration of 50 mg of pyridoxine prior to tryptophan loading prevents xanthurenuria. Some of these women reported that their symptoms of nervousness, irritability, and headache disappeared when they took additional pyridoxine. Studies of this type are continuing, but it does appear that vitamin B_6 requirements may be increased by either pregnancy or OCS.

Thiamin Deficiency: Thiamin deficiency has become rare in the United States since the advent of the enrichment and fortification programs initiated in the 1940's. Commercially manufactured bread and flour sold in retail markets contains added thiamin, niacin, and riboflavin as well as iron. Why, then, should we discuss thiamin deficiency? Because it still occurs in patients who are addicted to alcohol and who eat very little food. Often this results from lack of funds to purchase *both* food and alcoholic beverage, and most alcoholic patients will choose their bottle. Another factor relates to the energy-related requirements for thiamin; the greater the total amount of food energy consumed, the greater the need for thiamin (Figure 5–1). This is unequivocal in the case of carbohydrate energy and also applies to ethanol, whereas fat calories actually reduce the need for thiamin. The familiar Wernicke-Korsakoff's syndrome occurs al-

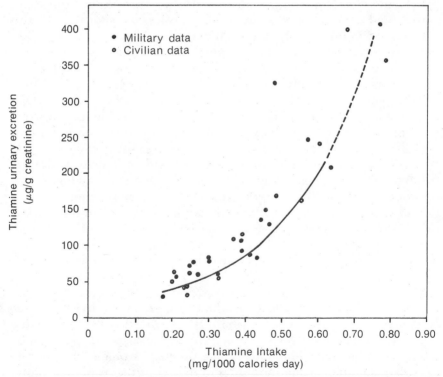

Figure 5–1 In subjects fed a mixed diet thiamine excretion increases when intake exceeds a certain level per 1,000 kilocalories. As energy intake rises, so does total requirement, but requirement per 1,000 kilocalories remains constant.

most exclusively in persons who not only drink large amounts of alcohol but also eat an inadequate diet. Usually this syndrome is divided into its two components: Wernicke's disease and Korsakoff's psychosis. The illness begins with diplopia and an unsteady gait — scarcely surprising in the case of an alcoholic patient. But the symptoms do not disappear after an appropriate period of abstinence. Instead they progress to include weakness and lethargy. Eventually, the ailing patient is transported to a hospital where examination discloses the classical signs of Wernicke's disease: impaired ocular motility, ataxia, especially in the lower extremities, and impaired mentation. Often there is also evidence of peripheral neuropathy. Even if a patient is hospitalized and given the customary treatment — abstinence from alcohol, injections of thiamin, and regular meals — not only may the signs of alcohol withdrawal develop, such as tremor, agitation, delusions and hallucinations, but the salient features of Korsakoff's psychosis may become manifest within a few days. This is characterized by a very short memory span coupled with awareness that mental function is defective. As a result, the patient tries to "cover up" and resorts to confabulation and fabrication. This patient may have difficulty performing even simple tasks relating to personal hygiene and be totally unable to recall events of the very recent past.

Whether this syndrome results solely from deficiencies of thiamin and other essential nutrients or partially from the toxic effects of alcohol is not known. Pathologically, there are characteristic lesions in the mamillary bodies and in the midbrain which can explain the ataxia and the extraocular motor dysfunction. Unfortunately, the prognosis is poor, perhaps because few patients can be successfully withdrawn from alcohol. But hemorrhagic lesions in the brain result in scarring which almost certainly contributes to persistence of ataxia and mental aberrations.

Thiamin deficiency can also result in a form of peripheral neuropathy or "dry beriberi." Various accounts of this syndrome give differing descriptions of the disorder but there is general agreement on several points. In times of war, when traditional food sources may become unavailable, thiamin deficiency generally is the first syndrome to appear. Human studies suggest that the body's reserves of thiamin are sufficient to last only about two weeks. If people continue to be physically active, in contrast to imprisoned groups, there is a likelihood that caloric expenditures will be greater than food intake. Peripheral neuropathy is first manifested by weakness of the lower extremities, and specifically by quadriceps weakness. If a subject is asked to perform a deep knee bend he or she will be unable to rise without assistance. This is the beginning of "dry beriberi" in contrast to the "wet beriberi" resulting from myocardial failure with marked edema. In wet beriberi, the patient becomes incapacitated by cardiac failure and physically unable to expend much energy — hence, theoretically, at least, his thiamin requirements are less. A diagnosis of "dry beriberi" is established on the basis of a low intake of thiamin with a good intake of calories, a history of progressive fatigue, chiefly of leg muscles, and physical findings indicating loss of deep tendon reflexes with some sensory impairment. Thiamin deficiency has been found to develop whenever the total intake of thiamin falls much below 0.3 mg/1000 non-fat kcal. The finding of low levels of transketolase in the blood confirms the diagnosis. This procedure is not generally available in most hospitals in the United States because the need for it is relatively infrequent. There is some disagreement as to whether thiamin is also needed for metabolism of ethanol, but its role in decarboxylation of alpha keto acids and in the hexose monophosphate shunt suggests that metabolically it is involved chiefly with carbohydrates.

Therapy of thiamin deficiency consists of three important measures: (1) administration of thiamin both orally and parenterally, 100 mg t.i.d. orally and 50 mg subcutaneously daily for one week, accompanied by (2) provision of an adequate diet supplemented with multiple vitamins and (3) *complete abstinence* from alcohol (because most patients are heavy users of alcoholic beverages).

Niacin Deficiency: Deficiency of nicotinic acid (pellagra) has a long history in the United States. In the South, black slaves were fed a diet in which ground corn supplied the major portion of calories. The disease was seasonal, becoming most severe during late summer when physical work was at its height, and when people were exposed to bright sunlight: this was a combination of inflammation, desquamation, and pigmentation. Mental confusion, hallucinations, and acute psychoses were present in severe cases. Diarrhea was profuse and prolonged. Coma and death were not uncommon. But pellagra did not disappear with the end of slavery — indeed it persisted until Goldberger fathomed its mysteries in the 1930's.

Presently, pellagra is rare in the United States, partly because few people depend chiefly upon corn for their sustenance and partly because farinaceous foods are fortified with niacin. But it still occurs in an occasional patient who either has a severely limited diet because of alcoholism or who has some form of intestinal malabsorption. Foods that contain liberal amounts of niacin (the term now used to include nicotinic acid and nicotinamide) include proteins of animal origin (meat, milk, and eggs) as well as proteins of vegetable origin (nuts and legumes) and cereal products that have been fortified with niacin, thiamin, and riboflavin.

Part of the mystery of pellagra was solved when Krehl and others (1945) discovered that tryptophan could be converted to nicotinic acid. Since corn (maize) is low in *both* niacin and tryptophan, it is easy to understand why pellagra was common in those who used it as a staple food. In general, the conversion of tryptophan to niacin is thought to require about 60 mg of the amino acid to provide about 1 mg of niacin equivalent. Average diets in the United States contain about 16 to 33 niacin equivalents, whereas the recommended allowance is 14 to 20 mg of niacin/day. The greatest needs occur in young men who consume the most protein; hence the most niacin.

Clinically, pellagra produces not only the characteristic actinic dermatitis and mental aberrations but also severe inflammation of mucous membranes including the tongue, buccal and gingival mucosa, and the esophagus. But it may also cause inflammation of mucous membranes, resulting in urethritis, vaginitis, and proctitis, often accompanied by diarrhea.

The diagnosis of pellagra rests upon a history of faulty diet or intestinal malabsorption coupled with clinical findings of mucocutaneous lesions and mental derangement. The familiar "four D's" are appropriate: dermatitis, dementia, diarrhea, and death. Laboratory tests that aid in the diagnosis are not widely available even in modern hospital laboratories. Measurement of the rate of urinary excretion of 2-pyridone and of N-methyl nicotinamide appears to be the most promising method of evaluating niacin status.

Niacin functions as a component of diphosphopyridine nucleotide (DPN) and triphosphopyridine nucleotide (TPN) or nicotinamide adenine dinucleotide (NAD-NADH).

Treatment of pellagra consists of giving a proper diet plus supplements of niacin. Oral doses of 50 mg t.i.d. for 5 days should be adequate unless anorexia, nausea, vomiting, or diarrhea occurs. In this event, parenteral administration of a mixture of water-soluble vitamins should be given with a dose that provides approximately 50 mg of niacin/day for 5 days. By the end of this time the patient should be able to consume a normal diet and the cutaneous and mucosal lesions should be visibly improved.

But even more dramatic is the improvement in mental function. Indeed this is the phenomenon that led some psychiatrists to try giving large doses of niacin to patients with schizophrenia or other psychiatric illness. This subject is discussed in the chapter dealing with food fads and megavitamin therapy.

Pantothenic Acid Deficiency: Pantothenic acid is, as its name implies, "present everywhere". It is virtually impossible to eat a diet composed of regular foods without ingesting 5–15 mg daily. During World War II, a group of Americans imprisoned in a Japanese prison camp developed a neurologic disorder characterized as "the burning foot" syndrome. The skin of the feet was exquisitely sensitive to light touch. When these men were liberated some of them were given, one at a time, injections of each of the water-soluble vitamins in an effort to determine what accounted for the burning foot syndrome. There were no specific mental or emotional symptoms that could be ascribed to this deficiency. When pantothenic acid was given, all symptoms subsided. Later, in studies of men fed a diet deficient in pantothenic acid and also given a vitamin antagonist, omega-methyl-pantothenic acid, Hodges and colleagues (1959) observed a syndrome that included paresthesias of the feet and legs. These symptoms disappeared within a few days after pantothenic acid was restored to their diet.

Vitamin B_{12} Deficiency: Deficiency of vitamin B_{12}, for any one of several reasons, resulted in a gradually developing anemia, usually accompanied by the neurologic signs and symptoms of a spinal cord lesion formerly known as subacute combined lateral sclerosis and now termed combined systems disease. Both the hematologic and the neurologic characteristics of this disease have been presented in some detail in the chapter on Hematology. Treatment with vitamin B_{12} is also described. Reynolds (1976) has presented evidence that suggests that neurologic and hematologic metabolic mechanisms may be similar.

But the cerebral manifestations of pernicious anemia are often ignored, or ascribed to the severe anemia which undoubtedly causes some degree of tissue hypoxia. Among the many symptoms reported, loss of recent memory and change in personality are relatively common. Some patients clearly have impairment of consciousness and may also neglect their personal cleanliness. Others complain of lack of taste and begin to eat less. The prompt response of these patients to therapeutic vitamin B_{12} is most convincing, long before any change occurs in hematologic values.

Folic Acid Deficiency: Deficiency of folic acid may result in vague neurologic symptoms and cause mental changes that are often ascribed to "senile dementia". This has no specific characteristics, but develops gradually as a blunting of memory and thought processes. Occasionally, it develops in patients who have been taking anticonvulsant medications such as phenytoin for prolonged periods of time. In such patients the level of folates in serum may be greater than the level in cerebrospinal fluid. This suggests blood-brain barrier problems or an abnormal rate of removal of folates from the brain. Folate derivatives are known to be neuroexcitatory, whereas the folate antagonist, methotrexate, is an antiepileptic drug. Serum folate levels have been reported to be low in 10 to 33 per cent of patients on admission to psychiatric hospitals. But only a few of these patients have a folate-responsive psychosis (Anonymous Editorial, 1976a).

A common cause of poor absorption or faulty utilization of folates is an excessive intake of alcohol. This results not only from inhibition of the bowel mucosal enzyme that removes glutamate groups from the pteroic acid molecule, but also from interference with utilization of folates even when given parenterally.

Ascorbic Acid Deficiency: Until recently, most nutritionists assumed that neurologic symptoms were not a part of the scorbutic syndrome resulting from lack of ascorbic acid. A review of ancient accounts of scurvy, however, coupled with clinical studies of experimental scurvy, discloses both mental and peripheral neurological abnormalities. Historical accounts described patients with scurvy as having lassitude and reluctance to move about. Recent studies defined a "neurotic triad" characterized by depression, hysteria and hypochondriasis in men who developed scurvy as a result of consuming a diet deficient in vitamin C (Kinsman and Hood, 1971). Peripheral nerve involvement has been found to result from hemorrhage into a nerve sheath. Recovery was slow but complete. Ascorbic acid also plays a role in the synthesis of epinephrine and in the maintenance of vascular tone. Failure of this mechanism can explain postural dizziness or even syncope in scorbutic patients, but in general such symptoms are rather mild. Perhaps the relative mildness of cerebral changes is a result of a natural protective phenomenon that regulates the concentration of vitamins in such a way as to provide an "ultrastable" environment. Spector (1977) observed that vitamin C levels in cerebrospinal fluid remained constant except at very low or very high plasma levels. Presumably the blood-brain barrier may have been responsible.

Vitamin E Deficiency: Despite many claims made by authors of popular paperback books, vitamin E does not appear to play a major role in the function of the adult nervous system. It does help to maintain the integrity of cell membranes, perhaps as a result of its ability to prevent peroxidation of unsaturated fatty acids, but this has not been translated into a disease or syndrome. Experiments with chick embryos indicate that lack of vitamin E, during and subsequent to the time when the neural crest is developing, can result in encephalomalacia. Excessive intakes of vitamin E have not been shown to prevent or cure any disease.

Vitamin A Deficiency: Although this vitamin is known for its ability to preserve night vision and to protect epithelial structures, very little has been learned about other functions relating to the nervous system. Studies of vitamin A–deficient calves demonstrated increased cerebrospinal fluid (CSF) pressure in the *deficient* animals. Excessive doses of vitamin A also have been shown to elevate CSF pressure in humans, sometimes to the point of producing headache and papilledema of the retinal discs. Studies by Hodges and Canham (1971) of vitamin A deficiency in otherwise healthy men confirmed the elevation of CSF pressure with deficiency and demonstrated marked loss of vestibular function, presumably as a result of loss of cilia from the semicircular canals. Loss of dark adaptation was accompanied by marked impairment of both taste and smell. All of these abnormalities responded promptly and completely to therapy with vitamin A.

A daily dose of 5000 IU of vitamin A or 1000 RE* will rapidly reverse all evidence of vitamin A deficiency. In the event of inability to absorb fatty substances from the digestive tract, one should give 1000 RE of vitamin A parenterally each day.

Essential Fatty Acid Deficiency: The essential fatty acids — linoleic acid and arachidonic acid — have been thought to play a role in the normal metabolism of the brain. But recent studies by Sanders and others (1977) suggest that in pregnancy, the mother can desaturate and elongate short chain polyunsaturates to produce long chain polyunsaturates. Nonetheless, it is wise to consider the essential fatty acids to be analogous to a vitamin, especially in pregnancy.

The Minerals

Derangements of fluid and electrolyte balance will cause mental symptoms, disorientation, and even coma. Deficiencies of calcium or magnesium can lead to hyperirritability of the nervous system and excess of either can have a depressant effect. Little is known about the effects of trace minerals on the functions of the brain, even though copper and zinc are known to participate in numerous enzyme systems.

In the rare familial disorder known as Wilson's disease or hepatolenticular degeneration there is a defect in the copper transport protein, ceruloplasmin, in the plasma. Perhaps as a result, copper is deposited in certain portions of the brain and in the liver. These unfortunate people can be benefited temporarily by restricting the amount of copper in their diet and by giving chelating substances such as penicillamine, which increases urinary excretion of copper. For many years investigators have argued about the mechanism responsible for deposition of excessive amounts of copper in the brain and liver. A recent report (Anonymous Review, 1975b) indicates that administration of toxic amounts of copper to rats causes storage of this metal in their liver and brain. But this mechanism is difficult to accept because patients with Wilson's disease have abnormally low concentrations of copper in their plasma, while the experimental animals presumably had excessive concentrations.

Deficiency of zinc, like lack of vitamin A, can cause loss of taste and smell. And also like vitamin A, this deficiency may lead to reduced food intake and consequently to dwarfism. Catalanotto and Lacy (1977) observed that zinc-deficient rats will eat greater-than-normal amounts of salt, perhaps as a result of impaired taste.

---

*Retinol Equivalents (RE) have replaced International Units (IU).
1 RE = 1 μg Retinol = 3.33 IU Retinol = 6 μg β-carotene = 10 IU β-carotene

FUNCTIONS OF THE BRAIN

Infant and Child Behavior

Reference has already been made to the concept that both maternal nutrition and neonatal nutrition may have an effect on subsequent behavior and performance of children and, later, of adults. Certainly childhood malnutrition of the type called protein-energy-malnutrition (PEM) has an obvious effect. At one extreme children are literally starved as a result of inadequate food: calories, protein, fats, and accessory food factors. This is termed marasmus and children suffering from it are likely to be irritable, restless, and understandably miserable. At the other extreme of PCM, children who were breast fed until they were a year or more of age find themselves abruptly displaced by the arrival of a new sibling. Often these children are given food containing chiefly carbohydrates and as a result they develop hypoalbuminemia, edema, and ascites. Often there are pigmentary changes in their skin and hair. This syndrome, known as kwashiorkor, has a different effect on behavior than marasmus. These children are listless, apathetic, dull, and less aggressive than marasmic children. Teotia and Teotia (1975) studied serotonin metabolism in children with kwashiorkor and found that those with steatorrhea had increased levels of serotonin in their serum and increased urinary excretion of 5-hydroxyindole acetic acid. After these children were refed and had recovered from kwashiorkor, their serotonin metabolism returned to normal.

The Hyperkinetic Child

As most mothers and every elementary school teacher knows, some children seem to be inherently difficult. A certain child may be inattentive, disobedient, disruptive, and unteachable. Recently claims have been made that certain food additives — chiefly preservatives and artificial colorings and flavorings — may cause this condition which is called "the hyperkinetic child syndrome". Few authorities can agree on a definition of this condition; some claim that these children actually have minimal brain damage from unknown causes. But Dr. Benjamin Feingold has advised parents of hyperkinetic children to avoid all foods that contain food additives, especially those that are related to aspirin. Since a great many food additives are phenolic derivatives, the families of these children are hard pressed to find foods that are at the same time nutritious, palatable, and free of any type of food additive. This topic was recently reviewed (Anonymous Review, 1976) in the light of "a Scientific Status Summary by the Institute of Food Technologists' Expert Panel on Food Safety and Nutrition, and the Committee on Public Information". Among the points emphasized were the following: (1) There are no fixed criteria for diagnosis; (2) When Feingold's recommendations are followed, more than diet is changed. Often the child becomes the center of interest at home or at school; (3) Thus, suggestibility may be a factor; (4) Methods of making observations have been more subjective than objective; (5) The chemical basis of this syndrome has not been defined; (6) Results of dietary change are similar to those of other approaches; and (7) The results of a controlled study suggest that additional studies should be performed. In the meantime, family physicians and pediatricians will have to deal with many questions from parents who have read or heard of the Feingold theory of hyperkinesis. They need facts on which to base their recommendations, and those facts are not yet available.

Diet and Stroke

As mentioned in the chapter on cardiovascular disorders, dietary salt has been shown to have an effect on blood pressure, both epidemiologically and in experimental animals. Similarly, there is strong epidemiologic evidence to link cerebral vascular disease with hypertension.

Undoubtedly cerebral vascular occlusion results most often from atheromatous changes that eventually lead to atherothrombotic brain infarction (ABF). For decades physicians have recognized the "little strokes" that now are called transient ischemic attacks (TIA). Studies by Dougherty and colleagues (1977), and others, have shown that blood platelets are aggregated or clumped in more than half of patients with a completed stroke (ABF) and in about one-third of patients with TIA. These findings were very significantly different from those of matched patients with other neurologic disorders. And they certainly support the view that platelet aggregation is likely to be abnormal in patients with acute cerebral ischemia. The obvious questions are, how can one decrease the propensity of platelets to clump or aggregate, and if this is possible, will it prevent strokes or lessen the amount of damage they cause? At present, we have fragments of information suggesting that diets containing much saturated fat and cholesterol favor platelet aggregation, whereas diets low in saturated fat and cholesterol may have an opposite effect. Vergroesen (1977) described several functions of linoleic acid in the diet including a platelet antiaggregation effect. While there is support for inclusion of moderate amounts of polyunsaturated fats in the diet (10 per cent of total calories has been suggested) to help lower plasma levels of cholesterol, there is not enough information to justify a specific quantitative recommendation for the optimal amount of linoleic acid in the diet. As an essential fatty acid, the suggested intake is 1 to 2 per cent of total kcal, or up to 7 gm for a person consuming 3000 kcal/day. But this is considerably lower than the amount of total polyunsaturates recommended as a preventive measure.

The Neurotransmitters

As the knowledge of the chemistry and pharmacology of the brain grows in depth and scope, there is increasing evidence that dietary factors also influence the inner workings of this amazing organ. And even more exciting are the apparent links between some of the neurotransmitters and mental illnesses. Horrobin (1977) has studied metabolism of prostaglandins in patients with schizophrenia and has found that some of the antischizophrenic drugs produce a rise in the production of prolactin, which in turn stimulates formation of prostaglandins. He noted that schizophrenic-like symptoms occur as a side reaction to drugs that are prostaglandin antagonists. A report by Growdon and others (1977) lends more support to the concept that deficiency of some of the neurotransmitters may be a characteristic of certain mental diseases. They noted that levels of serotonin and of acetylcholine can be enhanced by feeding tryptophan and choline, respectively. Along a similar line, Chouinard and others (1977) observed that while feeding tryptophan to depressed patients might have some antidepressant effects, the magnitude was weak at best. Since tryptophan is destroyed by a pyrrolase in the liver, and since nicotinamide can inhibit the effect of tryptophan pyrrolase, these authors gave both tryptophan and nicotinamide to 11 depressed patients and after 4 weeks observed significant improvement. Similarly, Fernstrom and Lytle (1976) attempted to link "corn malnutrition" with brain concentrations of serotonin and with behavior. They suggested that malnutrition can have a profound effect on behavior. This is scarcely a new idea: the dementia of pellagra has long been known to corn-eating populations.

Almost every disease for which there is no known cause becomes the target for widespread speculation. Although this practice occasionally results in a significant discovery, it also produces many disappointments. Recently several reports have suggested that wheat gluten is a pathogenic factor in schizophrenia. Singh and Kay (1976) fed a diet devoid of both gluten and milk to patients with schizophrenia and observed apparent improvement. When gluten was added to their diet they worsened. Nonetheless, the authors stressed that the cause of schizophrenia has not yet been established (Anonymous Editorial, 1976b).

Migraine and Epilepsy

For many years authorities have argued the pros and cons of a relationship between the vascular headaches and idiopathic epilepsy. Both are familial and tend to be exacerbated during periods of stress. Both are thought to be related to certain neurotransmitters or to vasoactive substances. But there are many differences as well. Dietary factors tend to be much greater in the opinion of patients with migraine than patients with epilepsy. Starvation-ketosis was employed many years ago as treatment of epilepsy but it may initiate a migrainous attack. And consumption of alcohol is more likely to bring on an epileptic seizure than it is to cause a vascular headache. It seems that the differences are greater than the similarities, at least with relation to diet. Friedman (1971) editorially reviewed the metabolic abnormalities of migraine from the standpoint of both diet and the neurotransmitters. He noted that the three principal suspects are serotonin, the catecholamines (chiefly norepinephrine), and certain polypeptides (chiefly bradykinin). He concluded that although some migrainous patients are "food sensitive", especially to foods containing tyramines, most of them are not. Indeed, neither tyramines nor absence of food (hypoglycemia) causes headache in *most* migrainous patients. Martin and others (1975) reported the results of a survey of 240 patients with migraine. They were asked to answer a questionnaire regarding the foods they avoided. Many patients avoided several foods but chocolate (73 per cent) and dairy products (cheese) (48 per cent) headed the list. Actually, many patients are not at all certain whether these or other foods have an effect on the frequency or severity of their headaches.

With the onset of a migrainous headache, plasma levels of serotonin may fall (Gilroy and Meyer, 1975), but patients who regularly awaken with early morning headache were found by Hsu and colleagues (1977) to have elevated levels of catecholamines in their plasma three hours before awakening.

Certain drugs, as well as diets, may have an effect on vascular headaches. Van Den Noort (1977) observed that oral contraceptive steroids, nitrates, and amphetamines, in addition to dietary tyramines, may precipitate headaches. Mechanisms whereby drugs or foods cause headaches still are poorly understood. Harper and others (1977) studied cerebral spinal fluid in migrainous patients and observed that various circulating vasoactive substances cause a fall in cerebral spinal fluid (CSF) pressure. A similar fall in CSF pressure occurs with the onset of migrainous prodromata. These workers postulate that the blood-brain barrier may become disrupted, thus allowing monoamines and perhaps prostaglandins to enter the brain more freely. This interesting concept deserves more scrutiny.

TOXIC AND METABOLIC DISORDERS OF THE NERVOUS SYSTEM

The Inherited Aminoacidurias

At least 25 forms of primary aminoaciduria have been recognized in children. Most of them are characterized by mental retardation and some by convulsive disorders. The best known is phenylketonuria, which is managed by feeding a diet that provides only enough phenylalanine to meet the child's requirements but not enough to overload his or her limited capacity to metabolize it. Many children with the syndrome of phenylketonuria (PKU) have made apparently satisfactory mental progress while eating this diet. The remaining forms of primary aminoaciduria carry a much poorer prognosis although investigations provide some hope for the future.

Vitamin Deficiencies

Deficiencies of several vitamins have already been discussed in relation to nutritional needs of the brain. Two of the most important vitamins in terms of proper functioning of the nervous system are folic acid and vitamin B_{12}. In addition to the mental blunting that occurs with lack of either one, and the spinal cord damage that characterizes lack of vitamin B_{12}, there is evidence for a metabolic derangement of nervous tissue resulting from lack of vitamin B_{12}. Neurological changes were observed in fruit bats fed a diet devoid of vitamin B_{12} for a period of 200 days. They had ataxia, difficulty climbing and flying, and histologic evidence of demyelination of the spinal cord (Anonymous Review, 1975c). Somewhat similar abnormalities developed in five patients who were vegetarians and who developed malabsorption. They had low serum levels of vitamin B_{12}, neurologic abnormalities, and megaloblastosis, all of which responded to injections of vitamin B_{12} (Dastur et al., 1975). Deficiency of vitamin B_{12} also develops in some patients who undergo maintenance dialysis for chronic renal failure. Rostrand (1976) found that the mean plasma levels of vitamin B_{12} were 312 pg/ml in 60 dialysis patients compared with 793 for a similar group of non-dialyzed patients with chronic renal failure. Nineteen of the 60 had levels below 200 pg/ml and 51 of the 60 had decreased nerve conduction velocities.

The widely held concept that it is hazardous to give folic acid to patients who are deficient in vitamin B_{12} was mentioned earlier in this chapter. Indeed, a few investigators have reported improvement of neuropathy following administration of folates either alone or with vitamin B_{12}. Manzoor and Runcie (1976) successfully treated ten patients with folates alone. These patients had either mental confusion or evidence of spinal cord lesions or both. Their responses to folates were prompt and convincing. Melsom and colleagues (1977) studied a man who had undergone a subtotal gastrectomy 23 years previously and who had developed muscular weakness and dementia. He was found to have normal levels of vitamin B_{12} and hemoglobin, but his serum folate level was low and he had an abnormal Schilling test. Administration of vitamin B_{12} and folic acid resulted in prompt improvement of his mental disorder and slower recovery from his neuropathy. These authors suggest that measurement of plasma levels of only vitamin B_{12} may not give an accurate evaluation of a patient's status.

Hyperosmolar Coma

The introduction of total parenteral nutrition (TPN) into the therapeutic resources of physicians has brought to light at least two syndromes that were seldom encountered previously. These are nonketotic hyperosmolar coma and the hypophosphatemic syndrome. Hyperosmolar coma is most apt to occur in an elderly patient who has mild to moderate diabetes mellitus of the adult-onset type. These patients often have some renal changes that result in elevation of the renal threshold for glucose. When such a patient is fed parenterally, it is most important to obtain frequent determinations of blood glucose levels. Urinary glucose excretion may not provide an accurate evaluation of the patient's status. When blood levels of glucose rise to 600 mg/dl or higher, there is often a marked degree of glycosuria that causes an osmotic diuresis with its inevitable loss of water and electrolytes, especially sodium. Unless the situation is accurately diagnosed and promptly treated, the patient soon becomes hypotensive and obtunded. Once coma has developed the outlook is grave; about 30 per cent of these patients die. The diagnosis is based on finding clinical evidence of dehydration, hypotension, and mental changes. Evaluation of body weight and intake-output data provides presumptive evidence of the syndrome, and finding very high levels of blood glucose confirms the diagnosis. Treatment consists of rehydration and supportive measures. Infusion of 0.9 per cent saline solution should begin at once. A patient may need 8 to 10 liters in the first 24 hours, but rising blood pressure and secretion of urine will provide evidence of satisfactory rehydration. As soon as possible, the patient should be allowed to drink fluids. If this is not possible, additional fluids, 0.45 per cent saline, should be given intravenously. Generally, the blood glucose level will fall rapidly as a result of rehydration but it may be necessary to give small, frequent doses of regular insulin. If resumption of eating can be tolerated there is no need to give potassium in the parenteral infusions; otherwise, patients will require 40 to 120 mEq per day to compensate for losses.

Hypophosphatemia

The second metabolic defect that may be precipitated by parenteral nutrition is the hypophosphatemic syndrome. This represents an exaggeration of a normal phenomenon — the lowering of serum levels of phosphate following a carbohydrate meal, since phosphorylation is an essential part of the oxidative degradation of glucose. Corredor and others (1969) reported that the physiologic hypophosphatemia that ordinarily accompanies an oral glucose tolerance test was accentuated in obese patients by a fast of 10–14 days. And in that same year, Lichtman and others (1969) reported that erythrocyte adenosine triphosphate became depleted in a uremic patient who developed hypophosphatemia as a result of a diet low in protein plus administration of aluminum hydroxide antacid medication. But the significance of these isolated publications could not be appreciated at that time. Soon this syndrome of hypophosphatemia was to assume much greater importance when clinicians began to observe its occurrence in patients receiving total parenteral nutrition (TPN). Ruberg and colleagues (1971) observed that hypophosphatemia occurred in some patients receiving TPN, but it did not result from excessive urinary losses of phosphates; indeed, urinary excretion of phosphorus was diminished. These authors suggested that addition of phosphates to the infusion fluid would prevent the syndrome. Silvis and Paragas (1971) studied hypophosphatemia in animals and solved several of its perplexing problems. They observed that starved dogs could not tolerate massive infusions of glucose or amino acids or both, whereas normal dogs could. Serum levels of inorganic phosphorus (Pi) fell very low in the starved dogs, all of which died. But normal animals receiving the same infusions had little change in their Pi levels and all survived. Furthermore, infusion of phosphates into hypophosphatemic dogs did not prevent death, even though their serum levels of Pi returned to normal. The authors concluded that the hypophosphatemic syndrome could be avoided by limiting the initial infusion of nutrients to the point where the patients did not gain weight for one week. If serum levels of Pi began to fall, slowing of the infusion rate would correct this. They also suggested that phosphates should be added to the parenteral nutrition formula. Travis and others (1971) studied alterations of erythrocyte glycolytic intermediates and of oxygen transport as a consequence of hypophosphatemia occurring in patients who were fed parenterally. Five of eight patients treated with TPN had a fall in serum levels of Pi to less than 1.0 mg/dl (normal = 3.0–4.5). All of the phosphorylated glycolytic intermediates were reduced in red blood cells. Presumably as a result of low concentrations of 2,3-diphosphoglycerate, there was a marked shift to the left of the erythrocyte oxygen-carrying capacity. This, of course, would mean that hemoglobin could trap oxygen more easily than normal, but that it could not release it at the tissue level. This obviously creates a very serious situation. Lichtman and others (1971) also observed that hypophosphatemia produced lower levels of red cell 2,3-diphosphoglycerate and adenosine triphosphate. They also described an increased affinity of hemoglobin for oxygen, which in turn produced a reduction in tissue oxygen. Silvis and Paragas (1972) observed the hypophosphatemic syndrome in three starved patients who had received infusions of parenteral nutrition fluids. Two complained of paresthesias, had convulsions, and became comatose. One died. A third patient recovered uneventfully. These authors recognized the significance of a preceding period of starvation, the abrupt initiation of high caloric parenteral feeding, the prompt fall in serum Pi, and the onset of neurologic symptoms within 4–7 days. They emphasized the importance of slow initial infusion rates, prompt reduction of flow rates if the serum level of Pi falls, and the need for phosphates in parenteral nutrition fluids. They also noted that the hypophosphatemic syndrome was not related to the syndrome of non-ketotic hyperosmolar coma.

Alcohol

The patient who abuses himself or herself with alcohol has a number of health problems; yet almost no branch of medicine wants to claim this patient. The alcoholic might well belong under the care of the psychiatrist or the internist (more specifically the hepatologist or the gastroenterologist) or, sometimes, the surgeon. And, since nutritional problems constitute a major part of the alcoholic patient's ills, he or she may properly come under the care of a nutritionist.

Few patients are more in need of professional help or more discouraging to treat than those with chronic alcoholism. In fact, it is difficult even to *define* alcoholism, let alone cure it. But as a point of departure, it can be defined as the chronic or episodic use of quantities of alcohol that are harmful, either to the patient or to persons associated with the patient. Habitual intake of more than 20 per cent of total calories as ethanol is likely to be harmful after a period of months or years.

Nutritionally, alcohol is a food without virtue: it supplies 7 kcal of energy per gram but most alcoholic beverages contain few if any other nutrients. The average serving of alcohol supplies about 80 kcal as ethanol. Alcohol can and often does interfere with utilization of dietary folates. It may, even in the presence of an excellent diet, cause hepatic damage. And frequently the person who becomes addicted to alcohol develops dietary habits that are grossly inadequate. Beer drinkers are often obese and hyperlipidemic, while those who choose other forms of alcoholic beverages are less apt to become obese and some are even emaciated. Advanced liver disease accompanied by multiple nutritional deficiencies justifies the description of the chronic alcoholic patient as a "nutritional derelict". The list of nutrients that are most commonly deficient in the diet of the alcoholic patient includes thiamin, folates, ascorbic acid, and niacin, as well as iron and zinc.

We have already discussed Wernicke-Korsakoff's syndrome, peripheral neuropathy, and dry beriberi as manifestations of thiamin deficiency. Folates, which are abundant in fresh fruits and vegetables, liver, and eggs, are often lacking in the diet of alcoholic patients. Furthermore, failure to deconjugate these large molecules results in failure to absorb folic acid. Deficiency not only affects hematopoiesis and synthesis of cells throughout the body but also may result in impairment of absorptive functions of the bowel. Thus, secondary malabsorption syndromes can occur.

Ascorbic acid deficiency also occurs in alcoholic patients. It results entirely from inadequate intake. A minimal intake of 10 mg/d will prevent scurvy, yet many individuals fail to eat even this small amount. Those who eat one potato each day or several servings of potato chips may avoid scurvy, and a salad or a piece of fresh fruit will suffice. But the alcoholic person seldom eats more than a bowl of soup and a hamburger sandwich, neither of which is apt to contain enough ascorbic acid.

Deficiency of niacin occurs in those individuals who do not eat even a hamburger or a handful of peanuts. These are the patients who develop frank pellagra, which may be unnoticed on the hospital wards. The patient with wasted muscles, sagging skin, and staring eyes attracts little attention from busy nurses and medical staff. Neither does pigmented scaling dermatitis in areas exposed to sunlight command attention when the patient in the next bed is vomiting blood. But the pellagrous alcoholic patient needs attention as promptly as the patient with upper gastrointestinal bleeding and may die of his or her illness just as quickly. Prompt and appropriate therapy may result in gratifying improvement. A good rule is to perform a "nutritional" history and physical examination on every alcoholic patient. Special tests should be performed to determine the presence or absence of specific deficiencies (blood transketolase, serum ascorbic acid, retinol, carotene, folate and vitamin B_{12} levels, serum iron, and total binding capacity (TIBC). Specific deficiencies should be treated promptly; then the patient should receive each day a single multivitamin capsule by mouth in addition to his or her diet.

Hepatic Encephalopathy

Although there are some exceptions, the majority of patients who develop hepatic encephalopathy have used excessive amounts of alcohol for many years. This dread complication of liver failure is difficult to manage and the mortality rate is high, but new information may improve the prognosis.

So many alcoholic patients have multiple reasons for apparent confusion — disorientation, agitation, memory loss, slurred speech, and ataxia — that it may be difficult to separate acute withdrawal from sedative medications, trauma, vitamin deficiencies, or impending hepatic coma. If, however, the patient's state of mentation is deteriorating instead of improving, and if fluid and electrolyte imbalances are at least controlled, then impending hepatic coma must be considered. Daily examination of the patient may demonstrate asterixis or flapping tremor, and if the patient's handwriting deteriorates, then definitive therapy should be considered.

In our present state of ignorance we have little to offer other than saline catharsis or enemas to lessen bacterial breakdown of nitrogenous products, administration of neomycin orally and removal of protein from the diet, and provision of adequate carbohydrate calories. But recent progress suggests that a better understanding of hepatic coma has evolved and that more effective therapy may soon be available. Some suggest that the problem of hepatic coma revolves around tryptophan and its rate of entry into the brain (Daniel et al., 1975). Normally tryptophan competes with the branched-chain amino acids — leucine, isoleucine and valine — for entry into the brain. These same amino acids are metabolized chiefly by peripheral tissues, especially skeletal muscle. Insulin hastens their entry into muscle cells. To set the stage, Munro calls attention to the failure of a cirrhotic liver to extract normal amounts of pancreatic insulin from the portal blood. As a result, the peripheral circulation contains more insulin than normal. This in turn causes the concentrations of the branched-chain amino acids in the peripheral circulation to fall. As a result, tryptophan can more easily enter the brain where it is metabolized into serotonin and other neurotrophic amines. Johnson and others (1977) suggest that degradation of insulin is impaired. Fischer, who studied dogs with portocaval shunts, observed that hepatic coma could be induced readily by feeding an abundance of protein. If, however, he gave a special amino acid mixture parenterally he could salvage these animals (Soeters and Fischer, 1976). This special preparation contains additional amounts of the branched-chain amino acids and less-than-average amounts of the aromatic amino acids and methionine. Recently, a similar amino acid preparation has become available for oral administration. This new understanding of the mechanisms involved in hepatic coma may result in effective therapy within the near future.

Parkinsonism

The recent discovery that L-dopa could benefit patients with parkinsonism was only slightly dimmed by the observation that this drug was also an antivitamin that caused some degree of pyridoxine deficiency. But the enzyme that converts L-dopa to Dopamine is a vitamin B_6–dependent decarboxylase that becomes more active when large amounts of the vitamin are given. As a consequence, vitamin B_6 cannot be given to patients who are treated with L-dopa without impairing the effectiveness of this drug. And since amino acids compete with L-dopa for absorption from the digestive tract, patients taking this drug should eat a diet that contains only enough protein to meet requirements, and should not take their medication with meals.

The Chinese Restaurant Syndrome

This exotic-sounding syndrome was first described by Schaumburg and Byck (1968). Schaumburg experienced severe distress in his neck, face, and chest shortly after eating a bowl of chinese soup. After investigation, he discovered that he and others reacted to monosodium glutamate added to the soup as a flavor enhancer. Since that original report, some have confirmed and others have denied the existence of this strange syndrome.

Reif-Lehrer (1976) not only confirmed Schaumburg's findings, he also suggested that the Chinese restaurant syndrome (CRS) may represent a benign inborn error of metabolism. He found that 25 per cent of persons consuming Chinese restaurant food reported adverse reactions compatible with the CRS. In the light of the known neuroexcitatory acitvity of monosodium glutamate, he postulated that some form of inborn error might be present. The same author (1977) investigated the prevalence of the CRS in a group of 197 employees of a biomedical research institute and subsequently a group of 1286 members of a medical school faculty. The results confirm that appreciable numbers (about 30 per cent) of people react to monosodium glutamate. There seems to be no evidence of permanent damage, although some patients have become quite alarmed by the symptoms.

MEGAVITAMIN THERAPY OF MENTAL ILLNESS

Recent publication of a popular book has heightened the interest of the general population in the possibility that most forms of mental disease may be benefited by large doses of one or several vitamins. In each instance the vitamin selected had at least *some* relation to the functions of the central nervous system. Wolman (1976) has reviewed the theories and the evidence for and against this form of therapy. This topic is discussed in more detail in Chapter 13, Food Fads and Megavitamin Therapy. Another form of megavitamin therapy has recently been shown to be deleterious. Ch'ien and colleagues (1975) observed eight epileptic patients who had been treated for a year or longer with Dilantin. Six were observed to have low levels of folates in their serum and were given very large doses of folic acid (75 mg) intravenously in a period of 30 minutes. Because of recent claims that folates can counteract the anticonvulsant action of Dilantin, the investigators studied electroencephalographic (EEG) tracings in these subjects but found no changes. One subject was then given 150 mg of folic acid intravenously and he had EEG changes as a result. Another patient developed EEG changes within 3 minutes after administration of 7.2 mg of folic acid. A third patient had convulsive seizures following rapid infusions of folic acid. This experiment seems to confirm the clinical impression that folic acid in large doses can interfere with the anticonvulsant action of Dilantin and, presumably, other anticonvulsant drugs.

REFERENCES

Anonymous Editorial: Folic acid and the nervous system. *Lancet* 2:836, 1976a.
Anonymous Editorial: Gluten and schizophrenia. *Lancet* 1:844, 1976b.
Anonymous Review: Central nervous system changes in deficiency of vitamin B_6 and other B-complex vitamins. *Nutr. Reviews* 33:21, 1975a.
Anonymous Review: Copper toxicity, rats, and Wilson's disease. *Nutr. Reviews* 33:51, 1975b.
Anonymous Review: Neurological damage in vitamin B_{12}-depleted bats. *Nutr. Reviews* 33:217, 1975c.
Anonymous Review [Special Report]: Diet and hyperactivity: Any connection? (A scientific status summary by the Institute of Food Technologist's Expert Panel on Food Safety and Nutrition, and the Committee on Public Information.) *Nutr. Reviews* 34:151, 1976.
Barnes, R. H.: Dual role of environmental deprivation and malnutrition in retarding intellectual development. *Amer. J. Clin. Nutr.* 29:912, 1976.

Brozek, J., Chapman, C. B., and Keys, A.: Drastic food restriction. Effect on cardiovascular dynamics in normotensive and hypertensive conditions. *J.A.M.A.* 137:1569, 1948.

Catalanotto, F. A., and Lacy, P.: Effects of a zinc-deficient diet upon fluid intake in the rat. *J. Nutrition* 107:436, 1977.

Cheek, D. B., Holt, A. B., London, W. T., Ellenberg, J. H., Hill, D. E., and Sever, J. L.: Nutritional studies on the pregnant Rhesus monkey — The effect of protein-calorie or protein deprivation on growth of the fetal brain. *Amer. J. Clin. Nutr.* 29:1149, 1976.

Ch'ien, L. T., Krumdieck, C. L., Scott, C. W., Jr., and Butterworth, C. E., Jr.: Harmful effect of megadoses of vitamins: Electroencephalogram abnormalities and seizures induced by intravenous folate in drug-treated epileptics. *Amer. J. Clin. Nutr.* 28:51, 1975.

Chouinard, G., Young, S. N., Annable, L., and Sourkes, T. L.: Tryptophan-nicotinamide combination in depression (Letter to the Editor). *Lancet* 1:249, 1977.

Corredor, D. G., Sabeh, G., Mendelsohn, L. V., Wasserman, R. E., Sunder, J. H., and Danowski, T. S.: Enhanced postglucose hypophosphatemia during starvation therapy of obesity. *Metabolism* 18:754, 1969.

Coursin, D. B.: Convulsive seizures in infants with pyridoxine-deficient diet. *J.A.M.A.* 154:406, 1954.

Daniel, P. M., Love, E. R., Moorhouse, S. R., and Pratt, O. E.: Amino acids, insulin, and hepatic coma. *Lancet* 2:179, 1975.

Dastur, D. K., Santhaderi, N., Quadros, E. V., Gagrat, B. M., Wadia, N. H., Desai, M. M., Singhal, B. S., and Bharucha, E. P.: Interrelationships between the B-vitamins in B_{12}-deficiency neuromyelopathy. A possible malabsorption-malnutrition syndrome. *Amer. J. Clin. Nutr.* 28:1255, 1975.

Dougherty, J. H., Jr., Levy, D. E., and Weksler, B. B.: Platelet activation in acute cerebral ischaemia. *Lancet* 1:821, 1977.

Elias, M. F., and Samonds, K. W.: Protein and calorie malnutrition in infant Cebus monkeys: Growth and behavioral development during deprivation and rehabilitation. *Amer. J. Clin. Nutr.* 30:355, 1977.

Fernstrom, J. D., and Lytle, L. D.: Corn malnutrition, brain serotonin, and behavior. *Nutr. Reviews* 34:257, 1976.

Friedman, A. P.: Metabolic abnormalities in migraine (Editorial). *Ann. Intern. Med.* 75:801, 1971.

Gilroy, J., and Meyer, J. S.: Headache, migraine, epilepsy, and syncope. In *Medical Neurology*, Second edition. Macmillan Publishing Company, New York, 1975, pp. 301–363.

Goldfarb, J.: Introduction to Pharmacology. In *Behavioral Pharmacology*, Stanley D. Glick and Joseph Goldfarb (eds.). C. V. Mosby Company, St. Louis, 1976, pp. 58–84.

Goldfarb, J., and Wilk, S.: Neuroanatomy, neurophysiology and neurochemistry. In *Behavioral Pharmacology*, Stanley D. Glick and Joseph Goldfarb (eds.). C. V. Mosby Company, St. Louis, 1976, pp. 14–57.

Graves, P. L.: Nutrition, infant behavior, and maternal characteristics: A pilot study in West Bengal, India. *Amer. J. Clin. Nutr.* 29:305, 1976.

Growdon, J. H., Cohen, E. L., and Wurtman, R. J.: Treatment of brain disease with dietary precursors of neurotransmitters. *Ann. Intern. Med.* 86:337, 1977.

Harper, A. M., MacKenzie, E. T., McCulloch, J., and Pickard, J. B.: Migraine and the blood-brain barrier. *Lancet* 1:1034, 1977.

Hodges, R. E., Bean, W. B., Ohlson, M. A., and Bleiler, R.: Human pantothenic acid deficiency produced by omego-methyl pantothenic acid. *J. Clin. Invest.* 38:1421, 1959.

Hodges, R. E., and Canham, J. E.: Vitamin deficiencies. Studies of experimental vitamin C deficiency and experimental vitamin A deficiency in man. *Proceedings of the Workshop on Problems of Assessment and Alleviation of Malnutrition in the United States; 13–14 January, 1970*, Nashville, Tennessee, pp. 115–128, 1971.

Horrobin, D. F.: Schizophrenia as a prostaglandin deficiency disease. *Lancet* 1:936, 1977.

Hsu, L. K. G., Crisp, A. H., Kalucy, R. S., Koval, J., Chen, C. N., Carruthers, M., and

Zilkha, K. J.: Early morning migraine. Nocturnal plasma levels of catecholamines, tryptophan, glucose, and free fatty acids and sleep encephalographs. *Lancet 1*:447, 1977.

Johnston, D. G., Alberti, K. G. M. M., Faber, O. K., Binder, C., and Wright, R.: Hyperinsulinism of hepatic cirrhosis: Diminished degradation or hypersecretion? *Lancet 1*:10, 1977.

Kinsman, R. A., and Hood, J.: Some behavioral effects of ascorbic acid deficiency. *Amer. J. Clin. Nutr. 24*:455, 1971.

Krehl, W. A., Tepley, L. J., Satma, P. S., and Elvehjem, C. A.: Growth retarding effect of corn in nicotinic acid-low rations and its counteraction by tryptophane. *Sci. 101*:489, 1975.

Lepkovsky, S., and Nielson, E.: A green pigment-producing compound in urine of pyridoxine-deficient rats. *J. Biol. Chem. 144*:135, 1942.

Lichtman, M. A., Miller, D. R., and Freeman, R. B.: Erythrocyte adenosine triphosphate depletion during hypophosphatemia in a uremic subject. *New England J. Med. 280*:240, 1969.

Lichtman, M. A., Miller, D. R., Cohen, J., and Waterhouse, C.: Reduced red cell glycolysis, 2,3-diphosphoglycerate and adenosine triphosphate concentration, and increased hemoglobin-oxygen affinity caused by hypophosphatemia. *Ann. Intern. Med. 74*:562, 1971.

Mandell, A. J., and Knapp, S.: Regulation of serotonin biosynthesis in brain: Role of the high affinity uptake of tryptophan into serotonergic neurones. *Fed. Proc. 36*:2142, 1977.

Manzoor, M., and Runcie, J.: Folate responsive neuropathy: Report of 10 cases. *Brit. Med. J. 1*:1176, 1976.

Martin, D. W., Jr., Watts, H. D., and Smith, L. H., Jr.: Migraine. *West. J. Surg. 123*:211, 1975.

Melsom, H., Kornstad, S., and Abildgaard, U.: Reversible neuropathy of vitamin-B_{12} deficiency with normal haemoglobin and serum-vitamin B_{12} (Letter to the Editor). *Lancet 1*:803, 1977.

Omenn, G. S.: Neurochemistry and behavior in man. *West. J. Med. 125*:434, 1976.

Reif-Lehrer, L.: Possible significance of adverse reactions to glutamate in humans. *Fed. Proc. 35*:2205, 1976.

Reif-Lehrer, L.: A questionnaire study of the prevalence of Chinese Restaurant Syndrome. *Fed. Proc. 36*:1617, 1977.

Reynolds, E. H.: The neurology of vitamin B_{12} deficiency. Metabolic mechanisms. *Lancet 2*:832, 1976.

Rødbro, P, and Christiansen, C.: Prophylactic vitamin D supplement to epileptic children on anticonvulsant drugs (Letter to the Editor). *New England J. Med. 293*:306, 1975.

Rostrand, S. G.: Vitamin B_{12} levels and nerve conduction velocities in patients undergoing maintenance hemodialysis. *Amer. J. Clin. Nutr. 29*:691, 1976.

Ruberg, R. L., Allen, T. R., Goodman, M. J., Long, J. M., and Dudrick, S. J.: Hypophosphatemia with hypophosphaturia in hyperalimentation. *Surg. Forum 22*:87, 1971.

Sanders, T. A. B., Ellis, F. R., and Dickerson, J. W. T.: Polyunsaturated fatty acids and the brain. *Lancet 1*:751, 1977.

Schaumburg, H. H., and Byck, R.: SIN CIB-SYN: Accent on glutamate (Letter to the Editor). *New England J. Med. 279*:105, 1968.

Silvis, S. E., and Paragas, P. V., Jr.: Fatal hyperalimentation syndrome. Animal studies. *J. Lab. Clin. Med. 78*:918, 1971.

Silvis, S. E., and Paragas, P. V., Jr.: Paresthesias, weakness, seizures, and hypophosphatemia in patients receiving hyperalimentation. *Gastroenterology 62*:513, 1972.

Singh, M. M., and Kay, S. R.: Wheat gluten as a pathogenic factor in schizophrenia. *Science 191*:401, 1976.

Soeters, P. B., and Fischer, J. E.: Insulin, glucagon, amino acid imbalance, and hepatic encephalopathy. *Lancet 2*:880, 1976.

Spector, R.: Vitamin homeostasis in the central nervous system. *New England J. Med. 296*:1393, 1977.

Teotia, M., and Teotia, S. P. S.: Serotonin metabolism in children with kwashiorkor. *Amer. J. Clin. Nutr. 28*:1284, 1975.

Travis, S. F., Sugerman, H. J., Ruberg, R. L., Dudrick, S. T., Delivoria-Papadopoulos, M., Miller, L. D., and Oski, F. A.: Alterations of red cell glycolytic intermediates and oxygen transport as a consequence of hypophosphatemia in patients receiving intravenous hyperalimentation. *New England J. Med. 285*:763, 1971.

Van Den Noort, S.: Drugs and diet as causes of vascular headaches. *Audio-Digest Ophthalmology.* Extracted and published in *West. J. Med. 126*:459, 1977.

Vergroesen, A. J.: Physiological effects of dietary linoleic acid. *Nutr. Reviews 35*:1, 1977.

Wolman, W.: Megavitamin claims not proved. Questions and *Answers. J.A.M.A. 236*:2224, 1976.

Wurtman, R. J., and Fernstrom, J. D.: Control of brain monoamine synthesis by diet and plasma amino acids. *Amer. J. Clin. Nutr. 28*:638, 1975.

6

NUTRITION AND THE MUSCULOSKELETAL SYSTEM

Robert E. Hodges, M.D.

THE BONES AND TEETH

The bones, teeth, and muscles are considered together because they are physically dependent upon each other. And they share another common feature: they represent the major storage mechanism for important nutrients—calcium and phosphorus in the skeleton, and protein in the muscles.

Development and Growth

Development of the skeleton is well established in the fetus, but growth and ossification will continue for about two decades after birth. The bones and teeth contain 99 per cent of the calcium in the body. This calcium is in dynamic equilibrium with the calcium present in plasma and in cells. During the developmental period, an infant or child must consume adequate amounts of energy as well as all of the essential nutrients—protein, vitamins, and minerals—that support growth. Fortunately, children can and do achieve reasonably normal development of their bones and teeth despite a wide range of diets varying from excellent to poor. Thurm and others (1976) described the effects of feeding inadequate diets to monkeys for 20 weeks. Deficiency of either protein or calcium retarded the rate of bone growth and caused "late-forming" epiphy-

164

ses. Similar abnormalities have been reported among children in South Africa whose intake of calcium was low. Walker (1972) found that this diet had an adverse effect on bone composition and dimensions, dental caries, rickets, osteomalacia, and osteoporosis. Furthermore, the physiologic processes of growth, pregnancy, and lactation were prejudiced. Lutwak, with his colleagues (1974), has shown that the calcium and phosphorus in the diet have a measurable effect upon the skeleton, and he suggests that lifelong neglect of this consideration leads to progressive demineralization of bones.

Deficiency Syndromes

Deficiency of Vitamin D. Certain specific deficiencies can impair growth and development, sometimes permanently. Deficiency of vitamin D, although uncommon now because of fortification of milk supplies, still occurs occasionally in this country, and commonly in children of the developing countries. Rickets results in permanent deformities of the legs of children who have reached the "toddler" age (Figure 6–1); and pelvic deformities in girls may later result in serious reproductive problems. Rickets usually results from ignorance on the part of parents or, rarely, from a defect of the digestive tract that impairs absorption of fat-soluble vitamins. Exposure of an infant or child to sunlight for less than an hour daily will produce enough vitamin D, from activation of 7-dehydrocholesterol

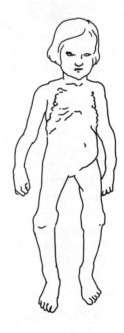

Figure 6–1 Rickets causes softening of bones, which become disjointed as a result of muscle pull and bearing weight. This results in the classical "rachitic rosary" and bowed legs of childhood and in adults. The forearms also are bowed and the pelvic deformities result in faulty posture that contributes to a "pot-belly."

in the skin, to prevent rickets. Some authorities feel that actinic exposure is more important than dietary sources of vitamin D.

Edward Mellanby's classical investigations of rickets (1919) called attention to the apparent lack of resistance to infections that accompanied the bony deformities of this disease, which was so common in the cities of Great Britain early in the 20th century. Surely the smoke and fog must have contributed to the prevalence of rickets by obscuring the sun. Mellanby recognized that vegetable oils, unlike fish liver oils, could not prevent or cure this disease. Many investigators have since made valuable contributions to our understanding of vitamin D and the diseases it prevents. Kodicek (1956) described his early efforts at studying the absorption and metabolism of ^{14}C-labeled vitamin D. He showed that bile salts do not facilitate absorption of vitamin D, while lecithin does. Steendijk (1968) observed that the aminoaciduria that accompanies vitamin D–deficient rickets in children may result from the effects of parathyroid hormone on renal tubular transport of amino acids. The marked hypocalcemia of early rickets was found to disappear as the rickets became more severe. This stimulation of parathyroid glands to release more hormone resulted from the initial hypocalcemia. Steendijk (1971) went on to review the major forms of metabolic bone disease in children, defined as "all generalized skeletal diseases in which the mass, structure, growth, composition, or metabolism of bone are deranged." Lack of appropriate therapy for many children with metabolic diseases of bone is primarily a result of ignorance of the normal physiology of bone and of calcium metabolism.

A fact often ignored is the difference between vitamin D deficiency in actively growing children and similar deficiency in adults. The child who is rapidly growing is far more vulnerable to rickets than the adult or even the undernourished child whose growth has been stunted by inadequate amounts of food. Lapatsanis and others (1976) described two types of nutritional rickets in infants: one as a result of vitamin D deficiency, and the other, a lack of phosphorus. Both types are responsive to vitamin D, and in both there is a close correlation between the concentration of inorganic phosphorus in serum and the appearance of bones by x-ray. Although the serum calcium concentration is often low, these authors could find no correlation between calcium levels and x-ray findings. In an infant, the usual radiologic abnormalities are widening, cupping, fraying, and demineralization in metaphyseal areas, periosteal new bone formation and demineralization along the shafts, and a shaggy, irregular appearance in the cortex of long bones. In older children who have begun to stand or walk, the long bones of the lower extremities become bowed. Other characteristics include enlargement of the costochondral junctions to produce the classic "rachitic rosary" and hypocalcemia, sometimes so severe as to cause convulsions (Schneider et al., 1976). Treatment of rickets consists of giving vitamin D, first in large doses, then smaller therapeutic doses, and when healing is complete, in maintenance amounts. Now that 1,25-dihydroxycholecalciferol is recognized as the active form of vitamin D, we can expect new definitions of appropriate therapy.

The chain of events leading to identification of the active form of vitamin D included meticulous animal studies, years of clinical experience, and development of sophisticated technology. Chemical synthesis of ^{14}C-cholecalciferol, development of new chromatographic systems, and advances in high resolution mass spectroscopy each contributed to the recognition of vitamin D as a substance with multiple functions, somehow linked with those of parathyroid hormone and calcitonin (Kodicek, 1974). As the structure of the several metabolites of vitamin D was evolving, the biological activity of some was found to be great, and that of others, insignificant (Proscal et al., 1976). In brief, the substance known as cholecalciferol (CC) or vitamin D_3 is biologically active but only after a period of time varying from one to several days. Hydroxylation of this compound on the 25-carbon yields 25-hydroxycholecalciferol (25-HCC) which is more active and more rapidly effective than the parent compound. Later studies disclosed that a second hydroxylation is accomplished in the kidney, this time on the first carbon. The final product, 1,25-dihydroxycholecalciferol (1,25-DHCC) is very potent and works more rapidly than any of its analogues, but there is still some delay. This results from the fact that 1,25-DHCC stimulates synthesis of a calcium-binding protein which becomes attached to the epithelial surface of the small bowel, where it facilitates absorption of calcium and phosphorus. 1,25-dihydroxycholecalciferol also has a calcium-mobilizing effect on bone. Certain errors of metabolism result in failure to hydroxylate cholecalciferol in a normal fashion. Another factor that inhibits formation of 1,25-DHCC is the effect of anticonvulsant drugs on the liver (Christiansen et al., 1973). Both of these problems can be bypassed by giving 1,25-DHCC itself, but synthesis of this compound is difficult and costly. A synthetic analog of 1,25-DHCC is 1-alpha-hydroxycholecalciferol (1-α-HCC), which is active either orally or parenterally and seems to function in a maner similar to that of the natural compound. It may even have an advantage over 1,25-DHCC in that it does not require the presence of parathyroid hormone, whereas the natural compound does (DeLuca and Neer, 1976).

Deficiency of Calcium. For several decades, authorities have argued over the optimal amount of calcium in the human diet. Americans who routinely consume about 800 to 1000 mg of calcium daily seem to have about the same amount of bone demineralization and of dental caries as people of other countries where the intake of calcium is only half as great. Hegsted (1967) expressed the opinion that osteoporosis has not been shown to be related to calcium intake. An expert Committee of the FAO/WHO* (World Health Organization, 1962) stated that "No clear-cut disease due to calcium deficiency has ever been described in the human male. Deficiency disease can be produced experimentally in animals, but it is not possible to apply figures derived from such experiments to human nutrition." Results of two studies in a total of 36 men suggested that their calcium requirements averaged between 400 and 450 mg daily. Since women generally have a smaller skeleton than men, they probably need less calcium in their diets unless they are pregnant or lactating. The amount of calcium used by the fetus is about 30 gm and lactation for six months accounts for another 50 gm. Lack of calcium can probably contribute to osteomalacia in women whose diets are lacking in vitamin D, yet no clear-cut calcium deficiency disease has been described in women. And similarly no frank ill effects resulting from calcium deficiency in children have been described (World Health Organization, 1962). Walker (1972) supported this view by calling attention to some rather convincing data. Most "Western" people ingest an average of about 500 to 1000 mg of calcium daily, at least half of which is derived from milk and milk products. By contrast, the South African Bantu generally consumes 175 to 475 mg/day. Walker observed that in these and other populations ingesting about half as much calcium as Western people, the prevalence of dental caries, rickets, osteomalacia, and osteoporosis is low, provided the people live in open spaces where exposure to sunlight is ample. But in major cities throughout the world, habitation therein results in less exposure to sunlight and greater prevalence of diseases that result from lack of vitamin D. Walker acknowledges that calcium is a very important dietary essential but the *amount* required is still to be established.

These views are not shared by Lutwak and colleagues (1974), who contend that chronic dietary deficiency of calcium or excess of phosphate or both may lead to secondary hyperparathyroidism, which results in resorption of trabecular bone. Osteoporosis of the jaw leading to periodontal disease may be an early manifestation of osteoporosis in other patients. Lutwak (1974) pointed out that a slight negative calcium balance, if sustained for a long time, can cause enough mineral loss to be recognized radiographically as osteoporosis. In the hypothetical case of a woman 50 years of age who weighs 65 kg, at age 20 she might have had about 1200 gm of calcium in her skeleton. If her daily intake of calcium has averaged 400 mg (a

---

*Food and Agriculture Organization/World Health Organization

common finding in women who do not consume milk or milk products), and if she has absorbed 45 per cent of this, her effective intake would be 180 mg daily. Her losses of calcium (urine, feces, and integument) would average 270 mg each day. Thus, she has been in a negative balance of 90 mg daily, which over a span of 30 years could total more than 900 gm or three-fourths of her entire skeletal calcium by age 50.

Nancy Raper (1977) recently reviewed the dietary interrelations of calcium and phosphorus. Although 99 per cent of the total body calcium is deposited in bony tissue (including teeth) only 80 per cent of the total phosphorus is so bound. Accordingly, soft tissues, especially skeletal muscle, contain far more phosphorus than calcium. Several investigators have proposed that an excess of dietary phosphorus in relation to calcium may contribute to the prevalence of osteoporosis. In fact, the American diet *is* heavily slanted toward a high intake of phosphorus, which is matched by calcium only if an individual consumes generous amounts of milk and milk products. Table 6–1 shows the Ca:P ratio of a number of common foods. The calcium content of bread and of tortillas was formerly enhanced by stone grinding with limestone implements. But modern technology has removed this source of "contamination" of cereals and grains. Green leaves contain oxalates that inhibit calcium absorption.

TABLE 6–1   CALCIUM TO PHOSPHORUS RATIO OF SOME COMMON FOODS*

FOOD	CA:P
Corn on the cob	0.03
Baked ham, lean	0.04
Halibut, fresh	0.06
Chicken breast	0.07
Beef chuck, lean	0.10
Peanuts	0.19
Split pea soup	0.19
Egg, whole	0.26
Tomato juice	0.36
Whole-wheat bread	0.44
Raisin pie	0.45
Almonds	0.46
Salmon, canned (with bones)	0.8
Sardines, canned (with bones)	0.9
Cheese, American	0.9
White bread, enriched	0.9
Whole milk	1.3
Collard greens (leaves)	3.6

*The optimal ratio of calcium-to-phosphorus is about 1:1 or 1.0. The average American diet has an excess of phosphorus, largely as a result of the large amount of meat consumed. Soft drinks (not listed) may also contribute large amounts of phosphorus.

Walker and Linkswiler (1972) made an important contribution to our understanding of calcium metabolism by comparing the effects of low, average, and high intakes of protein on the retention of dietary calcium. Calcium retention was best with a low-protein diet and poorest with a high-protein intake. The mechanism is not known, but the major loss of calcium was urinary. Perhaps the high phosphorus content of meat contributed to this effect.

Studies of factors that impair calcium absorption or utilization are urgently needed. Bell and colleagues (1977) observed the physiologic responses of adults to diets rich in phosphorus. This caused intestinal distress with soft or liquid stools, elevation of serum phosphorus levels, and a decrease in serum calcium levels. Their urinary excretion of hydroxyproline was increased, suggesting that bone matrix might be wasted. Indeed, Lutwak has proposed that the excessive intake of phosphates by Americans may increase their need for dietary calcium to help prevent osteoporosis. It seems sensible for several reasons to reduce our consumption of meats and to maintain a good intake of milk, preferably skim.

Other factors that impair absorption of calcium from the digestive tract include oxalates, fats, and phytates. Under normal circumstances, part of the calcium in food combines with oxalates in the lumen of the bowel to form a highly insoluble salt that is excreted in the feces. A certain amount of calcium forms other insoluble compounds in the bowel (such as calcium stearate and calcium palmitate). In patients with malabsorption and steatorrhea, the excess fats in the lumen of the bowel compete with oxalates for the available calcium. The result is less absorption of calcium and more absorption of oxalate, which in turn is excreted in the urine. Certain foods, especially deep-green leafy vegetables, contain large quantities of oxalates that interfere with absorption of calcium. As a result, foods like spinach, beet greens, and mustard greens are of little value as a dietary source of calcium even though they may be listed as excellent sources. Similarly, much of the calcium contained in whole grains may not be available for absorption because the phytic acid in these foods can form insoluble compounds — especially if unleavened bread is made. Fortunately the leavening process, which depends on growth of yeast, releases phytase that degrades phytic acid (inositol hexaphosphate), thus avoiding interference with calcium absorption. Many Indians and Pakistanis eat *chapatis* made from unleavened whole-wheat flour that contains much phytic acid (Wills et al., 1972). These same people have pigmented skin that may not be highly efficient in synthesizing cholecalciferol when exposed to sunlight. Whatever the cause, nutritional rickets is not uncommon in immigrants from India and Pakistan to Great Britain.

Scurvy. Infantile scurvy can resemble rickets in a superficial way. The peak age of onset is about 9 months, and it occurs in children whose formula has not been supplemented with a source of ascorbic acid. Breast-fed infants seldom develop scurvy even when the mother's intake of vitamin C is low. This has led to speculation that the human breast may be capable of synthesizing some vitamin C. The child with scurvy is pale and fretful, and lies in the "pithed-frog" position with the knees drawn up and hips externally rotated. Any attempt to move this child precipitates crying because movement is painful. There may be swelling and tenderness of the knees and ankles as a result of subperiosteal hemorrhage and epiphyseal displacement. Often the child is febrile because of some intercurrent infection that may in itself have triggered the onset of scurvy. There may be a few petechial hemorrhages, particularly on the lower extremities. X-ray of the knees and ankles will often show dislocation of the epiphysis and calcification of subperiosteal hemorrhages with generalized demineralization of the shafts of long bones. Scurvy must be treated promptly with appropriate amounts of ascorbic acid, preferably by mouth if tolerated. A dose of 50 mg three times daily will produce prompt relief of symptoms, but complete healing may require several weeks. Parents of these children must be taught how to provide proper nutrition in the future.

Metabolic and Nutritional Factors

The Teeth. Although Americans have the highest standard of living in the world, based on per capita income, national food supply, and availability of health care, their dental health leaves much to be desired. The usual childhood index of Decayed-Missing-Filled (DMF) teeth is high compared with children of developing countries. The usual reasons proposed include American dietary levels of calcium and phosphorus (which are high by world standards), neglect of dental hygiene (most Americans own a toothbrush, whether they use it or not), and ingestion of sweets including candy and soft drinks (which Americans love).

Dental health does depend in part on dietary practices, but it also depends upon the amount of fluoride in drinking water. Newbrun (1975) reports that dental caries is the most prevalent disease of childhood. By age 5 or 6 years the average child has five decayed teeth and by age 15 this has risen to 11 decayed teeth. Fluoridation of community water supplies to an optimal concentration of about 1 part per million or 1 mg/L has been shown to lower the caries score by 50 to 70 per cent. The aim of any fluoridation project is to provide optimal protection against caries with minimal toxicity. Authorities agree that maximal caries prevention occurs with intakes averaging 1 mg daily (1 mg/L), whereas dental fluorosis or mottling begins to appear at levels of 0.6 mg/L. Most people are willing to accept the small (10 per cent) risk of mottled teeth in exchange for an average 50 to 70 per cent reduction in dental caries. Furthermore fluorides have been associated with a lowered incidence of osteoporosis in older people. Accordingly, Lee (1975) advocates fluoridation at such a level as to provide total fluoride ingestion of 0.5 to 1.0 mg/day for children and 1.0 to 1.5 mg/day for older children. But Lee cautions against fluoridation of water supplies without careful evaluation of *total* sources of this mineral. For example, atmospheric pollution may increase the fluoride content of broad-leaved plants such as cabbage and lettuce. Contamination of pasture land with fluoride may increase the amount of this mineral in milk. And foods processed or manufactured in another part of the country may contain surprising amounts of fluorides. Nonetheless, the desirability of insuring an adequate intake of fluorides seems to be firmly established.

Since the beginning of this century the consumption of sugar in the United States has increased enormously, but in the past 25 years there has been little change. Based on disappearance data, the total consumption of sugar has been about 100 to 120 lb. per person per year or between 25 and 30 per cent of total calories. Less than 30 per cent of this is packaged for home use. Most sugar is used industrially in the manufacture of soft drinks, bakery products, confections, ice cream, syrups, jellies, and jams. Sucrose is the most abundant food additive because it has a great many desirable characteristics as a preservative, an enhancer of flavor, and a hydrophylic softener.

Many claims have been made, without convincing evidence, that an excessive intake of sugar contributes to the prevalence of atherosclerosis, myocardial infarction, and maturity-onset diabetes mellitus. Most epidemiologists discredit these claims. But the evidence for an association between dietary intake of sugar and dental caries is irrefutable (Newbrun, 1973). It makes no difference whether this sugar grew naturally in fruits and vegetables or whether it was added in processing. Some believe that glucose and fructose are virtually equivalent to sucrose in terms of cariogenicity. But Newbrun believes that cleavage of the sucrose molecule releases energy that can be used by a caries-producing group of bacteria (streptococcus mutans), and that this leads to a lower pH in the dental plaque, favoring erosion of enamel. There seems to be no doubt that cariogenicity of sugars depends in large measure on the length of time they are in contact with the teeth. Therefore, the sugar consumed with a meal should have less effect on teeth than that same amount of sugar eaten as candy over a longer span of time. Consumption of sweetened soft drinks can lead to prolonged contact of sugar with the teeth; and sticky sweets such as caramels are more deleterious than those that can be quickly washed away by saliva. The practice of brushing teeth after meals and of drinking fluoridated water can reduce the prevalence of dental caries very substantially.

But what should physicians advise their patients about sugar and other sweets? The author believes that a common-sense approach is best. Encourage them to eat a wide variety of foods, including some that contain sugar. But in the interest of restricting calories (for those whose weight is above normal), the routine consumption of candies, soft drinks, and sugary desserts should be curtailed substantially. By doing so, the patient may reduce not only his or her caloric intake, but also some of the risk of dental caries.

Other dietary factors that influence dental health are those that influence dental plaque formation and those that affect periodontal disease (Lutwak and Nizel, 1973). A diet containing little protein and much sugar is most favorable to plaque formation. There is evidence that chewing foods that are firm or fibrous removes some plaque by mechanical abrasion; but brushing the teeth after meals probably is more effective. Periodontal disease, especially that resulting from osteoporosis, occurs most commonly after age 35 and may reflect lack of vitamin D, inadequate calcium intake, or (according to Lutwak) an excess of phosphorus in the diet. It is worth noting that milk is an excellent source of calcium and of vitamin D (as a result of fortification) and it contains appropriate amounts of phosphorus. By contrast, soft drinks contain sugar, and many contain substantial quantities of phosphates added for flavor.

Osteoporosis and Osteomalacia. Osteoporosis, as described in the preceding pages, is literally "loss of bone", a condition in which the ratio of minerals to matrix remains unchanged. But osteomalacia, or "softening of bones", is characterized by demineralization of the matrix. As a result, the ratio of minerals to matrix is reduced. But is is difficult, from a nutritional viewpoint, to draw a sharp line between the two processes, because either can result from lack of vitamin D, calcium, and phosphorus. Successful treatment of the osteoporosis of aging with 1-α-HCC, 2 μg, plus 1000 mg of calcium has been described by Lund and colleagues (1975). No doubt further experience with this synthetic compound will establish its proper role in management of a number of diseases of bone.

In Great Britain there is an "unacceptable prevalence" of rickets among immigrant school children and of osteomalacia among adults of Asiatic origin, especially those from India and Pakistan (Stamp et al., 1976). Their diet of coarse, whole-grain, unleavened bread is deficient in vitamin D, and probably in calcium as well.

Other forms of bone disease occur but are not as prevalent. Reddy and Sivakumar (1974) reported two cases of rickets that did not respond to massive doses of vitamin D. Because both patients had low serum levels of magnesium, they were given 20 mEq of magnesium as $MgCl_2$ daily and both made rapid recoveries. Obviously, any patients with presumed vitamin D–resistant rickets should have measurements of the amounts of magnesium in their serum.

Mention has been made of the effect of anticonvulsant drugs on vitamin D metabolism. Hahn and others (1972) surveyed 48 patients who were taking phenobarbital and phenytoin for control of epilepsy. They found hypocalcemia in 19 per cent and low levels of 25-HCC in 33 per cent of patients. The authors suggest that adult epileptic patients who are receiving chronic combined anticonvulsant therapy should also be given supplemental vitamin D. Since these patients either fail to hydroxylate cholecalciferol or actually destroy it, it would be of interest to observe the effect of 1-α-HCC on their calcium metabolism.

A variety of names have been applied to certain metabolic defects that result in rickets. The essential features of these conditions are deformed long bones, short stature, low serum phosphorus levels, and failure to respond to normal doses of vitamin D. In about two-thirds of cases there is evidence of familial hypophosphatemia. Some patients have aminoaciduria, glycosuria, or other renal defects. Conventional treatment consists of giving massive doses of vitamin D with (Glorieux et al., 1972) or without (Wenner, 1977) supplemental phosphate. There are some reported trials of 1,25-DHCC in which the response has been prompt and convincing. This would seem to indicate that the defect consists of inability to hydroxylate cholecalciferol either at the 25th carbon or the 1st carbon or both (Fraser et al., 1973). Once again, it will be of great interest to see what effects 1-α-HCC may have in patients with this syndrome.

Patients with advanced stages of chronic renal failure often become hypocalcemic and their parathyroid glands respond with an excessive output of parathyroid hormone. This results in demineralization of bone. In all likelihood, this is a consequence of the inability of the kidneys to hydroxylate 25-HCC on the 1st carbon. Administration of 1,25-DHCC will help to correct the calcium defect but phosphorus accumulation results from renal failure. Preliminary trials of 1-α-HCC have reportedly given encouraging results.

Gout. The ancient "disease of kings" has a continuing fascination because optimal management combines diet and the use of drugs like allopurinol that inhibit formation of uric acid. The traditional dietary advice has been to avoid organ meats (liver, kidney, pancreas), seafoods (especially sardines, caviar, and anchovies), and gravies that might be rich in nucleic acids. Most physicians have come to minimize the importance of diet in management of gout. But recent studies (Clifford et al., 1976; Clifford and Story, 1976) indicate that diet can and does play an important role in regulating uric acid levels. Clifford and his group first studied the effects of seven different purines, fed one at a time, to normal subjects, to hyperuricemic subjects without gout, and to patients with gout. Hypoxanthine had the greatest effect on uric acid levels in the serum of gouty patients; but adenine and xanthine were intermediate in their effects. Clifford and Story then measured the purine content of a variety of foods and observed their metabolic effects in rats. These animals were fed those purines found most commonly in certain groups of foods. These groups and the purines that were most abundant are, in descending order:

Organ meats: xanthine, hypoxanthine, guanine, adenine
Fresh seafoods: xanthine, guanine, adenine, hypoxanthine
Canned seafoods: xanthine, guanine, adenine, hypoxanthine
Dried legumes: adenine, guanine, xanthine, hypoxanthine

Although traditional advice has been to avoid all organ meats, sardines, and anchovies, Clifford's work suggests that this advice is not strictly accurate. Among the organ meats, liver has high levels of xanthine and hypoxanthine and should be restricted. There seems to be little reason to restrict sardines and anchovies. On the other hand, lentils have the highest concentration of adenine of all the foods studied. Presumably, lentil soup (which is often prescribed for a gouty patient) is not a good choice.

Obviously much more work remains to be done but two facts are obvious: certain foods can elevate serum levels of uric acid markedly, and traditional dietary advice to gouty patients is faulty.

THE MUSCLES

Reservoirs of Protein and Calcium

The skeletal muscles constitute by far the largest protein reservoir in the human body. Yet it is important to realize that the body does not have any "protein stores". Every molecule of protein serves a useful purpose as contractile tissue, as a supporting structure, as an enzyme or hormone or carrier protein, or as something else. Despite this, in emergencies, the body will destroy protein to obtain glucose and ketones for energy and to supply essential amino acids for repair. This protein breakdown may be lifesaving, but it is also debilitating. It has been thought to be mediated through the so-called catabolic hormones: catecholamines, adrenal cortical steroids, and glucagon. An alternate view is that the normal rate of protein breakdown continues while *synthesis* stops.

In infants and children, the problem is more urgent than in adults because their muscle mass is relatively smaller and they have a growth requirement. Thus, an acute illness can cause more rapid weight loss and greater protein depletion on a percentage basis.

The protein resources of an adult man can be grossly estimated as shown in Table 6–2. One might speculate that the body would have certain "orders of priority" in utilizing its vital tissues. And to some extent this appears to be true, although accurate data are difficult to find. O'Keefe has presented data that change our concept of nitrogen equilibrium. He found, in patients undergoing surgical operations, that the rate of protein breakdown remained quite constant at about 300 gm daily. But the rate of *synthesis* fell, thus resulting in the familiar negative nitrogen balance of a catabolic state. If synthesis is slowed or halted, then one would expect those proteins that normally have the shortest half-life to be depleted first. And this could explain the very rapid depletion of certain plasma proteins, especially albumin. Table 6–3 lists the apparent "Orders of Priority" as tentatively derived from a variety of sources. Fortunately, the central nervous system is spared.

Munro has depicted the protein metabolism of a 70 kg man in a very useful diagram (Figure 6–2). Normal intake of protein may vary from about 32 to 90 gm daily, yet the rates of protein breakdown and synthesis remain unaffected. Excessive intake of protein affects only the amount of urinary nitrogen excreted. Normally, the rates of protein breakdown and synthesis are equal at about 300 gm daily. And the pool of free amino acids in circulation is only about 70 gm at any given time. Yet this small quantity (2.5 per cent of total body proteins) can and does permit maintenance and repair of the entire 12,000 to 14,000 gm of protein tissue.

Both the skeletal muscle mass and the bony skeleton play active roles in regulating amino acid metabolism and mineral metabolism respectively. The patient who has sustained massive injuries, such as the trauma of an automobile accident or a thermal burn involving 50 per cent of more of the skin surface, will have a sudden and severe loss of nitrogen. Assuming that protein catabolism continues at the rate of 300 gm daily, and that synthesis falls to zero, the rate of weight loss might approximate 1500 gm daily (since most protein-containing tissues average about 20 per cent protein, 70 per cent water and 10 per cent fat). Furthermore, the acutely injured patient will lose additional weight as a result of depletion of

TABLE 6–2 ESTIMATES OF PROTEIN RESOURCES OF A 70 Kg MAN*

Skeletal muscle mass	4200 grams
Skin and subcutaneous tissue	3500 grams
Formed elements of the blood including hemoglobin	1500 grams
Digestive tract	1000 grams
Liver	400 grams
Nervous system	350 grams
Bone matrix	350 grams
Plasma proteins	250 grams
Heart and vessels	150 grams
Spleen, lymph nodes, pancreas	150 grams
Kidneys and adrenals	100 grams
Lungs	50 grams
Total	12000 grams

*The soft tissues of the body of a 70 kg man contain about 12 to 14 kg of protein. Much of this will be depleted by a prolonged period of catabolic illness, especially if starvation is superimposed.

glycogen stores, lipolysis of fat stores, and loss of fluids. Thus, a critically injured patient may lose more than 2 kg of weight daily for the first few days. The presence or absence of good protein "reserves" may make the difference between recovery and death. Fortunately, the recent advent of improved methods for giving nutrients parenterally has improved the chances for survival of all patients, but those who were in the best nutritional state prior to illness or injury will have the best chance of recovery.

TABLE 6–3 APPARENT ORDERS OF PRIORITY
OF TISSUE CATABOLISM*

1. Plasma proteins (albumin)
2. Formed elements of the blood (leukocytes, erythrocytes)
3. Organ tissues
    lymphatic structures
    digestive tract
    liver
    heart and vessels
4. Skeletal muscle
5. Bone matrix, skin, subcutaneous tissues
6. Central nervous system (spared)

*In patients who are severely catabolic, the levels of albumin and hemoglobin decline promptly and remain low until anabolism is firmly re-established. Measurements of the diameter and skin-fold thickness of the upper arm give evidence of rapid shrinkage of skeletal muscle and thinning of subcutaneous tissues. The above "orders of priority" are gross approximations and may be changed as new evidence becomes available. It seems likely that the half-life of each protein determines its rate of depletion when protein synthesis is impaired. Thus, proteins with a very short half-life, such as retinol-binding protein or transferrin, may be depleted quickly, while structural proteins persist much longer.

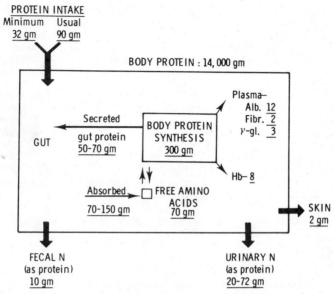

Figure 6–2 *Protein metabolism.* (Courtesy of Dr. Hamish Munro.) Although the protein intake of healthy adults may vary from about 30 to 90 gm daily, the rates of protein synthesis and of breakdown remain constant at about 300 gm daily. Urinary losses of nitrogen parallel dietary intakes.

Returning to calcium metabolism, the rate of dissolution and deposition in a young adult probably approximates 700 mg daily or about 0.06 per cent of the 1200 gm present in the skeleton, and the rate of turnover is thought to decrease with advancing age. One of the mysteries of calcium metabolism is the marked dissolution of bone that results from loss of weight bearing, either as a result of injury or as a result of confinement to bed. Indeed, the extreme loss of calcium experienced by the astronauts during space flight was a matter of considerable concern. In chronically ill or severely injured patients, the skeleton may lose calcium at a rapid rate. We do not have sufficient knowledge of the mechanisms involved to permit us to offer suitable advice on the best way to prevent or correct this problem. Early mobilization is effective if it is not contraindicated by other factors.

Protein Allowances

The perennial question of how much protein should be fed to children and adults in health and in disease is still being debated. The World Health Organization advocates 0.5 gm of protein per kg of body weight for normal adults. Infants and children require much more — about three times this amount. In the United States, adults are given 0.8 mg/kg and children proportionately more. Many surgeons have studied this problem and generally suggest much larger amounts. They regard an injured patient as having the protein needs of an infant in terms of synthesis of protein and formation of new cells.

In the field of athletic performance, an old and erroneous idea persists: heavy muscular work increases caloric needs but it does *not* increase protein requirement, once physical conditioning has been achieved. Consolazio and others (1975) fed two levels of protein to young men during a period of intensive physical training. One group received the customary and ample allowance provided by the armed forces: 1.4 gm/kg. The second group was given twice this amount. Those consuming the larger amount of protein gained more weight and retained more nitrogen than the control subjects. They also lost more nitrogen in their urine and sweat. For a time, the high-protein group had lower hemoglobin values than the controls. The muscle mass of the high-protein group was increased but their physiological work performance did not change. The essentially unchanged blood hemoglobin and serum protein levels indicate that the control group was consuming adequate amounts of protein to maintain protein equilibrium under conditions of fairly heavy physical activity (3700 kcal/d).

Nutritional Myopathies

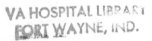

Although deficiency of vitamin E may result in nutritional myopathy in some species of animals, none of the spontaneously occurring myopathies of mankind responds to therapy with vitamins or other nutrients. There are, however, certain specific deficiencies that do result in muscular dysfunction. Perhaps the best known is the tetany that occurs in patients who become deficient in calcium or magnesium. Ravid and Robson (1976) described a peculiar form of myopathy involving chiefly the proximal muscles of patients who become hypophosphatemic as a result of medical therapy. The most common cause is administration of large and frequent doses of aluminum hydroxide gel as an antacid. This causes fecal loss of phosphates and eventual depletion of circulating levels of inorganic phosphorus. Another cause of hypophosphatemia is parenteral nutrition, a topic that will be covered in Chapter 15 (Feeding Patients). Another little-known cause of skeletal muscle dysfunction is iron deficiency. Hematologists have long recognized that severely anemic, iron-deficient patients often complain of weakness, but this has been ascribed to the anemia. Recent studies (Anonymous Review, 1977) demonstrated that in iron-deficient rats there was a decrease in the rate of mitochondrial phosphorylation of α-glycerophosphate. This was accompanied by a shortened running time. Control animals were made anemic without becoming iron-deficient, and it was found that their running time was not a function of hemoglobin level but was affected by iron nutrition. Another form of myopathy results from carnitine deficiency. This rare syndrome (Editorial, 1973) is accompanied by muscular weakness and mitochondrial changes of the skeletal muscle fibers. But the most common cause of muscle weakness is depletion of glycogen, either as a result of starvation, strenuous and prolonged exercise, or a metabolic disorder such as poorly controlled insulin-dependent diabetes mellitus.

ATHLETIC MEDICINE

Since both the skeleton and the skeletal muscles are major participants in athletic performance, it seems appropriate to introduce this topic in the chapter on the skeletomuscular system. This subject often perplexes the practicing physician. In addition to the sound physiologic principles of physical conditioning, the physician may find that high school or college coaching staffs are greatly concerned about the roles of diet and vitamins and special drinks in the performance of their athletes. The most *common myths* are:

1. *Heavy physical exertion requires a heavy intake of protein.* This is false. Once an athlete has achieved optimal muscle mass he or she does not need extra protein as fuel. The muscles metabolize both glucose and fatty acids. An excess of protein necessitates deamination of amino acids, the residues of which can be metabolized as glucose or fatty acids, but the amino groups must be converted to urea and excreted. This results in unnecessarily large losses of water because of the high solute load the kidneys must excrete.

2. *Megavitamins can help* an athlete achieve greater strength and endurance. This idea is false. In every carefully controlled study of athletic performance as influenced by excessive doses of vitamins, there has been no evidence of benefit from large amounts of vitamin C or vitamin E or multiple B-complex vitamins. This applies both before and after conditioning of athletes.

3. *The anabolic steroid hormones are effective in producing larger muscles and in achieving maximal performance.* This topic is open to debate. There is no doubt that such androgenic steroids as testosterone do have an anabolic effect on muscle metabolism. This is the reason men are more muscular than women. For centuries, farmers have castrated chickens, cattle, sheep, and hogs to eliminate androgenic hormones and thereby produce meat that is more tender. Apparently, most Olympic athletes who need maximal muscular strength (weight lifters, shot-putters, wrestlers) have used the

anabolic steroids during training, but recent evaluations (Hervey et al., 1976) question their value. Several problems are associated with their use. Do they have an additive effect in men who already have adequate amounts of androgens? Are they justified in women who experience the obvious side effects of hirsutism, deepening of the voice and hypertrophy of the clitoris? Should the anabolic steroids be permitted in high school and collegiate sports in view of their potential damage to hepatic function? In the opinion of the author, anabolic steroids should be banned, not only because of potential toxicity but because they represent a form of pharmacologic manipulation that could be extended to other agents such as caffeine, amphetamines, and even "blood doping" (the practice of transfusing an athlete with his or her own blood that had been withdrawn a few weeks before an athletic event).

4. *"Quick energy" foods* such as honey or glucose *should be eaten before athletic events* to improve performance. For events of short duration, this idea is illogical. The body has ample stores of glycogen to provide energy for muscle contraction. In endurance sports where sustained physical activity is maintained for many hours, carbohydrate foods may have a significant effect (Felig and Wahren, 1975; Bergström and Hultman, 1972).

5. *Abstain from all liquids* when preparing for an athletic event where weight limits must be met (wrestling, boxing). Some athletes try to "sweat off" the extra pounds if necessary (Paul, 1966). This is a deplorable practice, and should be rigidly prohibited. Young athletes may weaken themselves to such an extent as to have serious consequences, even death, when they attempt to compete after dehydrating themselves.

6. *Salt tablets* and extra water should be taken before every strenuous workout (Greenleaf, 1967). An athlete will lose excessive amounts of salt during the early phases of training but as he or she becomes conditioned, the rate of salt lost in perspiration declines. The salt consumed with meals is generally adequate. Thirst is the best guide to water regulation. The use of commercial drinks, containing not only salt and water but also other minerals along with glucose, lactic acid, and so on, is unnecessary but probably harmless.

7. Every athlete should *eat* a steak dinner *two hours before* a major athletic event (Asprey et al., 1968). This is arbitrary and impractical for many athletes. There is no special advantage to steak, and each individual is apt to have different tastes. Some will be too tense to eat at all and they should not be forced to do so. Some may relish a substantial meal. Others may want only liquids. The best advice is to give each athlete a choice.

Many coaches rely upon a certain food or drink to provide a psychological advantage to team members. This is not objectionable so long as the substance is harmless and does not lead to unphysiologic practices. The physician who chooses to work with a high school or college athletic department will find much gratification in providing sound advice based upon fact rather than fiction. Athletes seem to need their "rabbit's foot" as a symbol of good fortune, but they also need good nutrition in terms of both quality and timing.

The best nutritional advice for athletes was given by Mayer and Bullen (1960), who said: "The optimum diet for an athlete in training is not essentially different from that of any normal individual: however, certain modifications may seem advisable from the particular circumstances under which the athlete is to perform. To meet the standards of nutritional adequacy, the diet should comply with the needs of the individual in terms of growth, maintenance, and superimposed activity requirements."

REFERENCES

Anonymous Review: A specific skeletal muscle dysfunction in iron deficiency. *Nutr. Reviews* 35:76, 1977.

Asprey, G. M., Alley, L. E., and Tuttle, W. W.: Effect of eating at various times on subsequent performances in the one-mile free style swim. *The Research Quarterly* 39:231, 1968.

Bell, R. R., Draper, H. H., Tzeng, D. Y. M., Shin, H. K., and Schmidt, G. R.: Physiological responses of human adults to foods containing phosphate additives. *J. Nutrition* 107:42, 1977.

Bergström, J., and Hultman, E.: Nutrition for maximal sports performance. *J.A.M.A.* 221:999, 1972.

Christiansen, C., Rødbro, P., and Lund, M.: Incidence of anticonvulsant osteomalacia and effect of vitamin D: Controlled therapeutic trial. *Brit. Med. J.* 4:695, 1973.

Clifford, A. J., Riumallo, J. A., Young, V. R., and Scrimshaw, N. S.: Effect of oral purines on serum and urine uric acid of normal, hyperuricemic, and gouty humans. *J. Nutrition* 106:428, 1976.

Clifford, A. J., and Story, D. L.: Levels of purines in foods and their metabolic effects in rats. *J. Nutrition* 106:435, 1976.

Consolazio, C. F., Johnson, H. L., Nelson, R. A., Dramise, J. G., and Skala, J. H.: Protein metabolism during intensive physical training in the young adult. *Amer. J. Clin. Nutr.* 28:29, 1975.

DeLuca, H. F., and Neer, R. M. (Reviewers of): Recent developments in vitamin D. *Dairy Council Digest* 47:13, 1976.

Editorial: Carnitine deficiency myopathy. *J.A.M.A.* 225:165, 1973.

Felig, P., and Wahren, J.: Fuel homeostasis in exercise. *New England J. Med.* 293:1078, 1975.

Fraser, D., Kooh, S. W., Kind, H. P., Holick, M. F., Tanaka, Y., and DeLuca, H. F.: Pathogenesis of hereditary vitamin-D-dependent rickets. *New England J. Med.* 289:817, 1973.

Glorieux, F. H., Scriver, C. R., Reade, T. M., Goldman, H., and Roseborough, A.: Use of phosphate and vitamin D to prevent dwarfism and rickets in x-linked hypophosphatemia. *New England J. Med.* 287:481, 1972.

Greenleaf, J. E.: Exercise and water-electrolyte balance. In *Nutrition and Physical Activity*, Gunnar Blix (ed.). Almquist & Wiksells, Upsalla, 1967, pp. 47–58.

Hahn, T. J., Hendin, B. A., Scharp, C. R., and Huddad, J. G., Jr.: Effect of chronic anticonvulsant therapy on serum 25-hydroxycalciferol levels in adults. *New England J. Med.* 287:900, 1972.

Hegsted, D. M.: Nutrition, bone, and calcified tissue. *J. Amer. Dietet. Assoc.* 50:105, 1967.

Hervey, G. R., Hutchinson, I., Knibbs, A. V., Burkinshaw, L., Jones, P. R. M., Norgan, N. G., and Levell, M. J.: "Anabolic" effects of methandienone in men undergoing athletic training. *Lancet* 2:699, 1976.

Kodicek, E.: Metabolic studies on vitamin D. In *Bone Structure and Metabolism*, G. E. W. Wolstenholme and Celia M. O'Connor (eds.). Little, Brown and Company, Boston, 1956, pp. 161–174.

Kodicek, E.: The story of vitamin D from vitamin to hormone. *Lancet* 1:325, 1974.

Lapatsanis, P., Makaronis, G., Vretos, C., and Doxiadis, S.: Two types of nutritional rickets in infants. *Amer. J. Clin. Nutr.* 29:1222, 1976.

Lee, J. R.: Optimal fluoridation. *West. J. Med.* 122:431, 1975.

Lund, B., Hjorth, L., Kjaer, I., Reimann, I., Friis, T., Andersen, R. B., and Sørensen, O. H.: Treatment of osteoporosis of aging with 1α-hydroxycholecalciferol. *Lancet* 2:1168, 1975.

Lutwak, L., Singer, F. R., and Urist, M. R.: Current concepts of bone metabolism. *Ann. Intern. Med.* 80:630, 1975.

Lutwak, L.: Continuing need for dietary calcium throughout life. *Geriatrics* 29:171, 1974.

Lutwak, L., and Nizel, A. E. (reviewers): The impact of food and nutrition on oral health. *Dairy Council Digest* 44:13, 1973.

Mayer, J., and Bullen, B.: Nutrition and athletic performance. *Physiol. Reviews* 40:369, 1960.

Mellanby, E.: An experimental investigation on rickets. *Lancet* 1:407, 1919 reprinted in *Nutr. Reviews* 34:338, 1976.

Newbrun, E.: Sugar, sugar substitutes, and noncaloric sweetening agents. *Int. Dent. J.* 23:328, 1973.

Newbrun, E.: Water fluoridation and dietary fluoride ingestion. *West. J. Med.* 122:437, 1975.

Paul, W. D.: Crash diets and wrestling. *J. Iowa Med. Soc.*, 56:835, 1966.

Proscal, D. A., Okamura, W. H., and Normal, A. W.: Vitamin D, its metabolites and analogs: A review of the structural requirements for biological activity. *Amer. J. Clin. Nutr.* 29:1271, 1976.

Raper, N. R.: Calcium and phosphorus — dietary concerns. *Nutrition Program News*, U.S. Department of Agriculture, Washington, D.C., pp. 1–8, January–April 1977.

Ravid, M., and Robson, M.: Proximal myopathy caused by iatrogenic phosphate depletion. *J.A.M.A.* 236:1380, 1976.

Reddy, V., and Sivakumar, B.: Magnesium-dependent vitamin-D-resistant rickets. *Lancet* 1:963, 1974.

Schneider, J. A., Weller, M., Gersh, E. S., Trauner, D., and Nyhan, W. L.: Rickets. *West. J. Med.* 125:203, 1976.

Stamp, T. C. B., Exton-Smith, A. N., and Richens, A.: Classical rickets and osteomalacia in Britain (Letter to the Editor). *Lancet* 2:308, 1976.

Steendijk, R.: Vitamin D and the pathogenesis of rickets and osteomalacia. *Folia Med. Neerl.* 11:178, 1968.

Steendijk, R.: Metabolic bone disease in children. *Clin. Orthop.* 77:247, 1971.

Thurm, D. A., Samonds, K. W., and Hegsted, D. M.: The effects of a 20-week nutritional insult on the skeletal development of Cebus albifrons during the 1st year of life. *Amer. J. Clin. Nutr.* 29:621, 1976.

Walker, A. R. P.: The human requirement of calcium. Should low intakes be supplemented? *Amer. J. Clin. Nutr.* 25:518, 1972.

Walker, R. M., and Linkswiler, H. M.: Calcium retention in the adult human male as affected by protein intake. *J. Nutrition* 102:1297, 1972.

Wenner, S. M.: Vitamin D metabolism and vitamin D resistant rickets. *Orthop. Review* 6:75, 1977.

Wills, M. R., Day, R. C., Phillips, J. B., and Bateman, E. C.: Phytic acid and nutritional rickets in immigrants. *Lancet* 1:771, 1972.

World Health Organization: Calcium requirements report of an FAO/WHO Expert Group. *Technical Report Series no. 230*, pp. 22–24, Geneva, 1962.

7

NUTRITION AND THE
ENDOCRINE SYSTEM

Robert E. Hodges, M.D.

Among the many endocrine disorders that may be influenced by nutrients, only one, diabetes mellitus, is of major importance to the practicing physician. Accordingly, most of this chapter is devoted to diabetes.

An even more common problem, that of energy metabolism, is not really a direct result of endocrine malfunctioning, even though most lay persons and many physicians assume that any patient who is overweight "must have a glandular problem." Actually this concept is largely incorrect, and as recounted in Chapter 15, obese patients very seldom have a primary endocrine disorder.

HORMONES AND OBESITY

It would be wrong to assume that hormonal factors do *not* influence food intake, body composition, and fat deposition. For uncounted centuries, castrating male animals raised for their meat has been a part of animal husbandry, because the absence of testicles results in production of meat that is more tender. In recent decades, farmers have used estrogens to enhance the quality of poultry, beef, and other meats. Estrogens cause more fat to be deposited between muscle fibers — a quality known as "marbling." Perhaps the most striking effects of increasing estrogen production become apparent when a girl reaches menarche and has increased deposition of fat in her breasts and buttocks. The "normal" triceps skin-fold thickness of a

184

young adult woman is about 26 mm, but that of a young adult man is only about 16 mm. Another example of an endocrine effect is the well-known tendency for women to acquire unwanted fat with each pregnancy. One might assume that estrogens cause fatness, but paradoxically some women acquire added fat *after* menopause. Another manifestation of the effects of hormones on adiposity can be seen every day on our city streets. Women, when they become obese, tend to deposit more fat in their buttocks and thighs, while men tend to deposit fat in the upper half of their torso. Both men and women develop enlarged abdomens. There are notable exceptions to these rules, but they apply most of the time. The unfortunate fact is that, according to the World Almanac (1978) statistics, both men and women gain an average of 18 to 20 pounds between their early 20s and their mid 50s. Whether this results from decreasing physical activity, increasing ability to purchase more attractive foods, or declining endocrine function is still debated.

But from the practical standpoint, obesity, as it is seen in a physician's office or in a clinic, is not an endocrine abnormality and will not respond to endocrine manipulation. Furthermore, the author considers the practice of obtaining an "endocrine profile" of every obese patient unnecessary and wasteful. To be sure, the occasional patient will give a history that suggests a need for specific endocrine studies. And the physical examination might disclose an abnormality, such as goiter or hirsutism, that warrants endocrine tests. But routine endocrine testing fortifies the patient's fond hope that the problem is really "glandular," and lessens the likelihood that other forms of management will be successful.

An interesting phenomenon demonstrates the reverse effect: nutritional status can alter endocrine functions. Women who become massively obese — two or more times normal body weight — often develop amenorrhea. And young women with anorexia nervosa who have lost 40 to 50 per cent of their body weight almost always have amenorrhea. Less is known about men who are massively obese or severely emaciated, but impotence was reported to be almost universal in starved inmates of German prison camps during World War II.

THYROID FUNCTIONS

Although hypothyroidism is rarely a factor in the causation of obesity, an overactive thyroid gland can cause thyrotoxicosis and marked weight loss. This weight loss can be prevented by vigorous dietary means, but the underlying endocrinopathy is not corrected by diet.

In several parts of the world the soil has become severely depleted of iodides, presumably as a result of thousands of years of leaching by rainwater. Foods grown on these soils are understandably low in iodine. Until this century, the result was endemic cretinism; whole villages were sometimes affected. These unfortunate people had dwarfed stature, large goiters, and stupid expressions. Indeed their mentality *was* severely impaired. Eventually public health authorities identified the problem and introduced iodized salt. Fortification of table salt with appropriate amounts of potassium iodide has been shown to prevent cretinism in the present generation, but of course nothing can repair the mental damage done by lack of iodine during the developing months of pregnancy and neonatal life.

In the United States, a "goiter belt" was identified early in this century, presumably as a result of iodine-deficient soil. Iodization of table salt was effective in reducing the prevalence of goiter, as predicted by Taylor (1960). But today, some authorities (Vought, 1972) believe that iodized salt should no longer be used because the average American diet contains an abundance of iodine from other sources. These include organic iodides in bread as well as inorganic iodides that are widely available in seafoods and fruits and vegetables imported from coastal regions where the soil is rich in iodides. In addition, meats, dairy products, and eggs are produced by cattle, sheep, hogs, and chickens fed rations containing ample amounts of iodine and other trace minerals. The net result is an increased dietary source of iodine, but the magnitude and distribution are largely unknown. The daily intake of iodine should be about 100 to 300 μg for adults but intakes up to 1000 μg daily are considered safe (Recommended Dietary Allowances, 1974).

THE ADRENALS

The classical description by Harvey Cushing of the appearance of patients afflicted with pituitary tumors secreting adrenal corticotrophic hormone is well known. Among other characteristics, there is a peculiar form of truncal obesity with a puffy face, a "buffalo" hump at the junction of the neck with the thorax, and purple striae on the abdomen as a result of rapid expansion of girth. We now recognize an iatrogenic form of Cushing's syndrome in patients who receive large doses of adrenal corticoids for therapy of some illness. This form of obesity is so unlike the common forms of obesity as to suggest that the adrenals are not likely to be involved in the etiology of ordinary obesity. Yet many obese women do have an unusual degree of hirsutism. And studies of adrenal function have shown modest elevations of plasma and urinary levels of adrenocortical steroids in obese subjects. The significance of these findings is not clear but adrenal dysfunction does not play an important role in the etiology of exogenous obesity; it results from an excess of food.

DIABETES MELLITUS

Incidence and Types

Diabetes is one of the most common endocrine abnormalities in the American population. Estimates vary from 5 to 10 per cent, depending upon whether the investigator is describing overt diabetes or one of the less completely developed forms such as "latent" diabetes, "suspected" diabetes, and "pre" diabetes. This discussion will deal primarily with adult patients.

More than 80 per cent of adult diabetic patients are overweight at the time their disorder is diagnosed. It is convenient to divide patients with diabetes into two major categories: the milder adult-onset (non-insulin-dependent) type which is more common and the juvenile-onset (insulin-dependent) type. Virtually all of the adult-onset patients are obese, and a great many have hyperlipidemia, especially of the types characterized by elevated triglycerides. By contrast, the juvenile-onset type (which generally develops before age 30) typically begins with rapid loss of weight. Many of these patients would die without insulin.

Characteristics

Diabetes has been characterized by West (1976) as being a disorder in which deficiency of insulin, either relative or absolute, results in certain symptoms, signs, and laboratory findings. These include polyuria, polydipsia, and weight loss in those individuals with moderate or marked hyperglycemia. In older people, a mild form of diabetes may be present for months or years with few, if any, symptoms.

Diabetic patients with either mild or severe forms of the disease are prone to develop degenerative changes in arteries and in nerves. Patients with severe, insulin-dependent diabetes may develop extreme hyperglycemia, ketoacidosis, and dehydration with electrolyte depletion which may be fatal. Nutritional problems in these patients include muscle wasting and hyperlipidemia. By contrast, patients with mild diabetes generally remain obese and often hyperlipidemic, and although degenerative changes occur, they may develop at a more gradual pace.

Early Methods of Treatment

It is of interest to examine standard medical texts from the 19th century (Von Noorden, 1895) and to note that physicians of that time had a remarkable understanding of diabetes. They recognized the same two major types (but used different names) and employed similar forms of diet therapy. Of course, insulin and the oral hypoglycemic drugs were yet to be discovered. Physicians of the last century sharply restricted the total caloric allowance of obese diabetics and confidently predicted that these subjects, if successful in losing weight, had a good chance of living a near-normal life for many years. On the other hand, diabetic patients who became ketotic and acidotic and who lost weight rapidly had to be fed frequently from early in the morning to late at night. Their diet consisted of meats, eggs, fats, vegetables, and alcoholic beverages (Tables 7–1, 7–2, 7–3). It may surprise today's medical profession to learn that many (though not most) of these diabetic patients improved enough to enjoy a few more years of life. But serious infections with their accompanying ketosis and coma were a constant threat.

TABLES 7–1, 7–2, 7–3

Diets prescribed for patients with juvenile-onset diabetes in 1895, 1950, and 1975 are compared. In the pre-insulin era, weight loss was a serious problem, so an abundance of food was encouraged; even alcoholic beverages. Obviously, this diet was ketogenic, but it allowed many patients to survive for a time. Like the diets of later years, this restricted simple sugars severely and spaced meals throughout the day. Actually, we seldom provide six feedings daily for our patients but the comparison is obvious.

The major differences between these diets are:

	1895	1950	1975
Total Calories	2900	2000	2000 (or less)
Fat Calories	57%	40%	35% (or less)
Carbohydrate Calories	0	40%	50% (mostly complex CHO)
Alcohol Calories	19%	None	None
Protein, G/Kg (normal body weight)	2.0	1.4	1.1
Cholesterol Mg/D	>1300	~700	<300

The author views this as a beneficial trend.

TABLE 7–1 A SAMPLE BILL OF FARE, 2500 CALORIES
(VON NOORDEN, 1895)

		ALBUMIN gm	FAT gm	ALCOHOL gm	CALORIC VALUES
8:00 o'clock first breakfast	100·gm ham	25	36		497
	1 cup tea				
	1 glass cognac			8.5	
10:30 o'clock second breakfast	2 eggs	14	11		234
	fried in 10 gm butter		8		
12:30 o'clock luncheon	150 gm cold roast meat	57	8		912
	Mayonnaise made w/yolk of 1 egg and 1 spoonful of oil	3	18		
	Raw cucumber, w/5 gm vinegar, 1 spoonful of oil, salt and pepper		15		
	15 gm Gorgonzola cheese	4	5		
	Half-bottle of Moselle			25	
	1 cup of coffee with 1 tablespoon of cream		5		
5:00 o'clock tea	1 cup of tea				144
	1 boiled egg	7	6		
	1 glass cognac			8.5	
7:30 o'clock dinner	1 cup of bouillon w/15 gm marrow		14		1074
	80 gm boiled salmon	18	11		
	1/3–1/2 lb asparagus w/20 gm butter		16		
	30 gm smoked ox tongue	8	6		
	100 gm capon	17	12		
	Salad w/5 gm vinegar and 1 spoonful of oil		15		
	Half-bottle of burgundy			30	
10:00 o'clock nightcap	1 glass cognac w/seltzer water			8.5	59
	Total	150	185	80	2900

TABLE 7-2 A SAMPLE BILL OF FARE, 2000 CALORIES (1950s)

2000 calories: 20% protein = 100 gm protein (400 calories)
40% fat = 90 gm fat (~800 calories)
40% carbohydrate = 200 gm carbohydrate (800 calories)

SERVINGS		PROTEIN	FAT	CARBOHYDRATE
whole milk	2	16	20	24
vegetable	1	2	7	
fruit	5			50
bread	8	16		120
meat	9	63	45	
fat	5		25	
		97	90	201

8:00 o'clock
  first breakfast

  coffee or tea
  3/4 cup corn flakes
  1 glass whole milk
  1/2 cup orange juice
  30 gm ham

10:30 o'clock
  second breakfast

  1 hard boiled egg
  1 slice toast
  1 teaspoon butter (5 gm)
  tea

12:30 o'clock
  luncheon

  1 glass whole milk
  3 oz roast beef
  2 slices bread   }Sandwich
  1 tablespoon Mayonnaise (5 gm)
  1 banana
  coffee
  1 tablespoon cream

5:00 o'clock
  tea

  tea
  2 squares graham cracker

7:30 o'clock
  dinner

  broth
  4 oz salmon (120 gm)
  1/2 cup peas
  1/2 cup rice
  1 dinner roll
  1 teaspoon butter (5 gm)
  Salad w/5 gm vinegar and 5 gm oil (1 tsp) and salt,
      pepper
  1/2 cup water packed fruit cocktail

10:00 o'clock
  nightcap

  1/2 cup grapefruit juice
  5 vanilla wafers

TABLE 7–3 A SAMPLE BILL OF FARE, 2000 CALORIES (1970s)

2000 calories: 15% protein = 75 gm protein (300 calories)
35% fat = 80 gm fat (~700 calories)
50% carbohydrate = 250 gm carbohydrate (1000 calories)

SERVINGS		PROTEIN	FAT	CARBOHYDRATE
skim milk	2	16		24
vegetable	1	2		7
fruit	6			60
bread	10	20		150
meat	6	42	30	
fat	10		50	
		80	80	241

8:00 o'clock
first breakfast

coffee or tea
3/4 cup corn flakes
1 glass skim milk
1/2 cup orange juice

10:30 o'clock
second breakfast

1/2 cup water-packed applesauce
2 slices toast
2 teaspoons margarine (10 gm)
tea

12:30 o'clock
luncheon

1 glass skim milk
3 oz roast beef ⎫
2 slices bread ⎬ Sandwich
2 teaspoons Mayonnaise ⎭
1 banana
Salad w/10 gm vinegar and 10 gm oil (2 tsp) and salt,
   pepper
coffee

5:00 o'clock
tea

tea
2 squares graham cracker

7:30 o'clock
dinner

broth
3 oz salmon (90 gm)
1/2 cup peas
1/2 cup corn
1/2 cup rice
1 dinner roll
2 teaspoons margarine (10 gm)
Salad w/10 gm vinegar and 10 gm oil (2 tsp) and salt,
   pepper
1/2 cup water-packed fruit cocktail

10:00 o'clock
nightcap

1/2 cup grapefruit juice
5 vanilla wafers

Advent of Insulin

With the advent of insulin in 1922 came a new era for the juvenile-onset diabetic (though not for the adult-onset diabetic). Not only could ketoacidosis and extreme hyperglycemia be controlled, but insulin-dependent diabetic patients could be fed *some* carbohydrates without dangerous consequences. Gradually, in the half-century that has passed since the introduction of insulin, physicians and dietitians have cautiously increased the carbohydrate content of diets fed to patients with both forms of diabetes. This has been done without apparent ill effects on either diabetic control or insulin requirement. Meanwhile, the life span of insulin-dependent diabetics has lengthened considerably. The life span of an average male infant born in the U.S. is now about 70 years, but that of a diabetic child is estimated to be at least 20 years less. Very few adult diabetics have the likelihood of dying from ketoacidosis or electrolyte imbalance or acute infections. Most of them die from cardiovascular disorders, particularly coronary heart disease and renal disease.

This applies not only to insulin-dependent diabetic patients, but also to the seemingly more fortunate adult-onset diabetic patients. These people are usually obese when their diabetes starts, and most of them stay obese. In some ways, the advent of oral hypoglycemic drugs may have been an unfortunate event for them; otherwise, they might have dieted more conscientiously and controlled their diabetes in this fashion. By taking the oral hypoglycemic medications, either sulfonylurea derivatives or the biguanides, they can control their hyperglycemia and glycosuria *while they continue to overeat.* Indeed, when the first oral hypoglycemic agent became available one of my professors complained ". . . and now they can eat all they want, and stay fat." The much publicized University Group Diabetes Program (UGDP) called attention to the apparent *increase* in deaths from cardiac disease among patients taking oral hypoglycemic drugs, and their judgment appears to have been substantiated by subsequent experience. Very recently, phenformin was removed from the market. The important point is this: *Diet is the primary form of therapy for all diabetic patients — but what diet?*

Diabetologists, like most other physicians, have differing opinions about the best dietary management of their patients. Despite these differences, however, there are areas of general agreement that should be stressed. These are:

1. A diabetic patient — man, woman, or child — is a person and should be treated as such. The emotional trauma of referring to him or her as a "diabetic," rather than as a person, can do incalculable harm by generating feelings of rebellion and negativism.

2. All people — normal or diabetic — have similar nutritional requirements for vitamins, minerals, proteins, and energy. These must be met by their diets.

3. The proper amount of food energy must be supplied daily — neither too much nor too little. But here a *distinction should be made* between adult-onset diabetic patients, who are obese, and juvenile-onset diabetic patients, who are usually lean and sometimes emaciated. In the case of obese diabetic patients, the important point is to *reduce total energy* intake by appropriate methods. The amount and type of carbohydrates and the timing of meals are of less importance.

4. For the insulin-dependent diabetic patient, meals must be spaced so as to provide a reasonably *constant source of energy.* The pattern may have to be altered to comply with the form, dose, and frequency of insulin given.

5. The diet may have to be adjusted to meet the everyday stresses of life. A patient who develops an acute upper respiratory infection may need more insulin or less food than usual, whereas the same patient, when engaging in unusually strenuous physical activity, will need more food or less insulin to compensate. An intelligent, well-informed patient can handle these problems with little difficulty but some, such as elderly patients and children, may need special assistance at times.

6. In the opinion of the author, every effort should be made to prevent the common complications of diabetes. The commonest cause of death in adult diabetic patients is coronary heart disease. Almost half will die of this disease. And women, who generally have a statistical advantage over men, lose their inherent advantage when they develop diabetes and become as susceptible to coronary disease as diabetic men. The overall incidence of coronary heart disease in men examined postmortem was 10 per cent for non-diabetics and 19.5 per cent for diabetics. For women the figures were 5.8 per cent for non-diabetics and 17.4 per cent for diabetics — a threefold rise (Clawson and Bell, 1949).

Epidemiologic studies of coronary heart disease have repeatedly shown that certain "risk factors" are statistically related to death rates from this disorder. Among the most significant are elevated levels of cholesterol in plasma, elevated blood pressure, and cigarette smoking. For the past decade, the American Heart Association has recommended that the American public attempt to reduce its risk of coronary heart disease by making certain changes in its way of life. These changes include dietary modifications designed to lower plasma cholesterol and triglycerides. In brief, this involves (1) adjustment of food intake to achieve and maintain normal body weight; (2) reduction of total fat in the diet from about 42 per cent to 30–35 per cent of calories; (3) reduction of saturated fat (chiefly animal fats and hydrogenated fats) to about 10 per cent of calories; (4) maintaining the level of polyunsaturated fats in the diet at 10 per cent of calories; (5) reduction of dietary cholesterol from 600 to 700 mg to less than 300 mg/d; and (6) reducing use of simple sugars and alcohol to a minimum. In the view of the author, the same recommendations can and should be made for diabetic patients.

In 1965, Stone published the results of a study in which he fed a modified diet to diabetic patients, and compared their diabetic control, their insulin needs, and their plasma lipids with those of a control group of diabetic patients fed the traditional American Diabetes Association diet. The results were highly favorable in terms of lipid responses. Furthermore, the level of diabetic control was not impaired and the requirement for insulin remained the same.

This result was, of course, to be anticipated. Diabetologists in China and Japan have always fed their patients the same basic diet consumed by their non-diabetic countrymen. This diet is, by American standards, very low in fat (10 to 12 per cent of calories) and quite high in carbohydrates (70 to 75 per cent of calories). At the same time, the intake of cholesterol is very low: 100 to 200 mg/day.

A study of the complications that occur in Japanese diabetic patients is very informative. Cardiovascular diseases in the late 1950's to the early 1960's were half as common in the Orient as they were in American diabetic patients and the death rate from coronary heart disease was only 6 per cent compared with 53 per cent in the U.S. These data suggest that some degree of modification of the traditional diet for diabetic patients is in order (Shigeta et al., 1970); and indeed, many diabetologists are doing this.

Others remark that the diet–cholesterol–heart disease theory remains unproven and that, besides, diabetic children have been found to have thickened basement membranes in their arterioles at the time diabetes is first diagnosed. In either event, coronary heart disease results from atherosclerosis, not from thickening of the basement membrane, and there is reason to hope that a modified diet may slow the rate of development of vascular disease in all people — diabetics and non-diabetics alike. Studies currently in progress will help to elucidate this problem; meanwhile, to the author, it seems logical to reduce plasma lipid levels in diabetic as well as in non-diabetic patients, and to suggest that all patients attempt to minimize their risk of developing coronary heart disease by avoiding cigarette smoking, controlling hypertension when it exists, and maintaining a high level of physical activity.

Complications of Diabetes

Aside from the greater-than-average incidence of atherosclerotic heart disease and peripheral vascular disease, diabetic patients have a number of other complications. Prominent among these are disorders of the smaller arteries and arterioles, and degenerative changes of peripheral nerves. The most devastating results of "small vessel disease" include retinopathy with loss of vision, and nephropathy which often proves to be fatal. The most common form of neurological involvement is "diabetic neuropathy" which may affect either the peripheral or the autonomic nerves or both. Campbell and others (1976) studied nerve conduction in the peroneal nerves of seven diabetic patients during ketoacidosis, and again after diabetic control had been achieved. They found that the function of the peripheral nerves was quite susceptible to the acute metabolic damage of ketoacidosis; but more often, there is little or no relationship between the level of diabetic control and the functional status of the nervous system of diabetic patients.

Importance of Diabetic Control

Many physicians, the author included, were taught that the best interests of a diabetic patient were served by providing good diabetic control. This was defined as avoidance of both ketoacidosis and hypoglycemia and maintenance of near-normal levels of glucose in samples of blood drawn fasting, at midmorning and midafternoon. Many physicians believed that this type of control of insulin-dependent diabetic patients would minimize the likelihood of vascular and neurologic complications in future decades.

But other physicians, who were equally conscientious and equally able, felt that more permissive control was preferable. Their insulin-dependent diabetic patients were taught to eat well-balanced meals at regular intervals, but that they need not weigh their food. They were advised to eat generous amounts of protein and to avoid excesses of concentrated sweets, but otherwise lived a relatively normal life. They tested their urine occasionally for acetone, but were not encouraged to worry about glycosuria unless it became so marked as to cause polyuria, thirst, and weight loss. In such patients, a blood sugar level of 200 to 300 mg/dl was no cause for alarm, but any suggestion of hypoglycemia was to be corrected promptly by eating food. Indeed some evidence *has* been assembled to suggest that "tight" control of diabetic patients leads to frequent periods of hypoglycemia and that these, in turn, produce central nervous system changes.

On the other hand, those diabetologists who have insisted on good diabetic control now have at least some evidence to support their position. Jarrett and Keen (1976) in a review of several epidemiologic studies of patients with adult-onset diabetes, concluded that "the risk of specific diabetic complications becomes important only in people with capillary whole blood sugar concentrations exceeding 200 mg/dl two hours after a 50 gm oral glucose load" (given after an overnight fast).

Recently diabetologists have become interested in a derivative of hemoglobin A (HbA) termed HbA_{1C}. Normally this comprises 3 to 6 per cent of the total hemoglobin in healthy persons, but in patients with juvenile-onset diabetes mellitus this rises to 6 to 12 per cent. The structure of HbA_{1C} is the same as HbA except for the addition of a glucose molecule to the terminal valine molecule of the beta chain. Studies in mice have shown that the glucose molecule can be added at any time after HbA has been synthesized. Furthermore, the amount of HbA_{1C} formed is linearly correlated with the area under the curve of a glucose tolerance test. Koenig and others (1976) studied the levels of HbA_{1C} in five patients who were hospitalized because their diabetes was out of control. Before control, their average fasting blood sugar was 343 mg/dl and during optimal control it fell to an average of 84 mg/dl. At the same time the concentration of HbA_{1C} fell from an average of 9.8 per cent to an average of 5.8 per cent. These authors suggest that periodic measurement of HbA_{1C} provides a useful way of documenting the degree of control of glucose metabolism, as well as a means for relating diabetic control to development of complications.

Cahill and others (1976) reviewed the evidence for and against the theory that good diabetic control may decrease or delay diabetic nephropathy and retinopathy. An abundance of retrospective evidence seems to support those who advocate tight control, but one cannot accept such evidence as proof. Good prospective studies are not available in sufficient numbers to answer the question of whether close control is worthwhile. Certainly the University Group Diabetes Project proved that none of the five types of treatment used (placebo, tolbutamide, insulin in variable doses, insulin in a standard dose, and later, phenformin) prevented death, which is the ultimate complication (Goldner et al., 1971).

Yet, as Cahill and colleagues point out, recent studies in diabetic animals have demonstrated that reduction of hyperglycemia, by a variety of means, prevents or minimizes formation of diabetic-like lesions in eyes, kidneys, and nerves. Biopsies of kidneys and muscles suggest that microvascular lesions do not develop until diabetes has existed for a few years, thus excluding an independent inherited phenomenon. These researchers conclude that ". . . optimal regulation of glucose levels should be achieved in the treatment of diabetics, particularly in young and middle-aged persons, who are at greatest risk of the microvascular complications." They go on to say that "current means of therapy are only partly effective at best . . ." and ". . . high priority must be assigned to the development of more physiologic delivery systems. . . ." "Finally, good diabetic management necessitates education and training of both patients and health professionals. . . ." The American Diabetes Association accepts as policy the concept that the microvascular complications of diabetes are decreased by reduction of blood glucose concentrations.

More credence is given to this theory by a recent report by Gabbay (1977), in which measurements were made of HbA_{1a}, A_{1b}, and A_{1c}. All three of these glycosylated forms were found to be elevated in diabetic patients. Gabbay and his group suggest that this test "is probably an index of diabetic control over time," and may provide a valuable clue to the development of diabetic complications.

On the other hand, a number of diabetologists remain skeptical of these enthusiastic views. Siperstein and colleagues (1977) state that "when subjected to critical analysis, . . . the various clinical studies attempting to demonstrate a beneficial effect of rigid glucose control have been, at best, inconclusive." They go on to state, "Though the arguments advanced are notable, we are not convinced that the findings in animals can be directly applied to diabetes in man, and we question the conclusions of the clinical studies quoted." They caution against strict acceptance of the American Diabetes Association statement recommending that physicians strive "to achieve levels of blood glucose as close to those in the non-diabetic state as feasible," especially in juvenile diabetes. Instead, they recommend the best possible control of blood glucose in the diabetic patient, but never at the severe price of hypoglycemic attacks.

But the controversy over microvascular lesions in diabetic patients is only part of the picture. There is at least as much disagreement about the role of diabetes in the metabolism of fats and cholesterol and in the mechanisms whereby diabetes increases the risk of premature death or disability from atherosclerotic disease, including the coronary, cerebral, and peripheral arteries. We have already discussed the differences in the clinical patterns of these diseases among Japanese and American populations. Bennion and Grundy (1977) have compared the cholesterol metabolism of diabetic Pima Indians with that of the same subjects after their diabetes had been treated with insulin. Their food intake was greater when their diabetes was untreated and this may have influenced lipid metabolism. Plasma levels of cholesterol were higher in the untreated state and at the same time the cholesterol balance was more strongly positive. Both fecal bile excretion and total bile acid pool were larger in untreated patients. The presumption was that hyperglycemia led to an excessive rate of synthesis of cholesterol. In the one patient serum cholesterol was fractionated into lipoprotein components: this cholesterol was largely low density lipoprotein cholesterol.

The amount of protein that should be included in a diabetic patient's diet is also subject to debate. Some advocate large amounts, because the surplus provides a steady supply of glucose as a result of gluconeogenesis. Others oppose the use of excessive amounts of protein because many foods rich in protein also contain large amounts of fats and cholesterol. This is especially true of most forms of animal protein. Felig and others (1977) studied the effects of dietary protein on amino acid metabolism in diabetic patients. Compared with normal subjects, diabetic patients responded to a protein meal by converting more protein to glucose, by increasing levels of branched chain amino acids in arterial blood, and by developing higher serum levels of glucose. This suggests that excesses of protein are not advisable.

Summary of Optimal Management of Diabetes

As mentioned above, dietary treatment of diabetes mellitus is *the most important aspect* of medical management. Yet it often is the most neglected because too few physicians understand the basic principles. The objectives of dietary management are different for the two types of diabetes.

In the more common adult-onset form of diabetes mellitus the prime objective is correction of obesity by reducing total energy intake and increasing exercise. Secondary objectives are to reduce insulin resistance, reduce hyperglycemia, reduce hyperlipidemia, and if possible, delay or reduce the severity of diabetic complications, including microvascular disease, neuropathy, and atherosclerosis.

Patients with juvenile-onset diabetes mellitus have much different requirements. These patients are usually lean or even emaciated and they usually require exogenous insulin. In an effort to provide adequate amounts of energy and to avoid extremes of hyper- or hypoglycemia, it is necessary to give small meals at regular intervals. Often, it is desirable to provide snacks between meals and at bedtime to avoid hypoglycemic episodes. These patients must be instructed in many aspects of their diet, including caloric values, food exchange lists, and appropriate methods for adjusting to late meals, unusual exercise, or intercurrent illnesses.

In both types of diabetes it is sensible to attempt to apply the same principles that aid in reducing blood lipids in non-diabetic persons. These are: avoidance or correction of obesity, reduction of total dietary fats to about 30 to 35 per cent of calories, reduction of saturated fats to about 10 per cent of calories and inclusion of polyunsaturated fats at a level of about 10 per cent of calories. Although there is still some dispute about the amount of cholesterol that should be allowed in the diet, the author believes that this figure should be less than 300 mg/day. The use of simple sugars and of alcohol by diabetics should be limited, chiefly because of the propensity of these individuals to develop hypertriglyceridemia when they consume substantial amounts of either.

Recent controversy over the potential harm that could result from ingestion of such artificial sweeteners as the cyclamates and saccharine has led several legislators to make emotional appeals to the Food and Drug Administration to rescind the prohibition. Their argument is that patients with diabetes mellitus will suffer serious injury if they cannot use artificial sweeteners. This logic is difficult to follow, for there is no "dietary requirement" for sweets. Indeed, many people might be healthier if they ate no sweets, because they might find it easier to curtail their excessive intake of food.

But the total amount of carbohydrates advocated for most diabetic patients has been increased substantially (West, 1977). This enables the physician to limit his or her patients' intake of saturated fats and cholesterol and yet provide an attractive and balanced diet. Newer diabetic diets may contain 25 to 35 per cent of calories from fats, 12 to 24 per cent from protein, and about half (35 to 60 per cent) from carbohydrates. This would include 30 to 45 per cent of calories from starches and other polysaccharides and only 5 to 15 per cent from sugars and dextrins derived almost exclusively from sugars in fruits, vegetables, and milk.

The author agrees with those critics who say "you have no proof" that diets can retard the development of microvascular disease, degenerative changes, or atherosclerosis. But I do believe that these are worthy goals and that we shall never attain them unless we try. The diets proposed are, in my opinion, safe and sensible. Time will provide the final answer, but meanwhile I believe that good diabetic control, avoidance of both ketoacidosis and hypoglycemia, and reduction of hyperlipidemia are worthwhile clinical objectives.

REFERENCES

Bennion, L. J., and Grundy, S. M.: Effects of diabetes mellitus on cholesterol metabolism in man. *New England J. Med.* 296:1365, 1977.

Cahill, G. F., Jr., Etzwiler, D. D., and Freinkel, N.: "Control" and diabetes. *New England J. Med.* 294:1004, 1976.

Campbell, I. W., Fraser, D. M., Ewing, D. J., Baldwa, V. S., Harrower, A. B. D., Murray,

A., Neilson, J. M. M., and Clarke, B. F.: Peripheral and autonomic nerve function in diabetic ketoacidosis. *Lancet* 2:167, 1976.

Clawson, B. J., and Bell, E. T.: Incidence of fatal coronary disease in nondiabetic and diabetic persons. *Arch. Pathol.* 48:105, 1949.

Felig, P., Wahren, J., Sherwin, R., and Palaiologos, G.: Amino acid and protein metabolism in diabetes mellitus. *Arch. Intern. Med.* 137:507, 1977.

Gabbay, K. H.: Blood test may start new era in diabetes therapy evaluation. *J.A.M.A.* 237:847, 1977.

Goldner, M. G., Kantterud, G. L., and Prout, T. E.: Effects of hypoglycemic agents on vascular complications in patients with adult-onset diabetes. *J.A.M.A.* 218:1400, 1971.

Jarrett, R. J., and Keen, H.: Hyperglycemia and diabetes mellitus. *Lancet* 2:1009, 1976.

Koenig, R. J., Peterson, C. M., Jones, R. L., Saudek, C., Lehrman, M., and Cerami, A.: Correlation of glucose regulation and hemoglobin A_{1C} in diabetes mellitus. *New England J. Med.* 295:417, 1976.

Recommended Dietary Allowances. Eighth revised edition. Iodine. Washington, D. C., Food and Nutrition Board, National Research Council — National Academy of Sciences, 1974, pp. 96–97.

Shigeta, Y., Oji, N., Shichiri, M., and Hoshi, M.: Pathogenesis and clinical characteristics of obese diabetics in Japan. In *Diabetes Mellitus in Asia, Proceedings of a Symposium, Kobe, Japan, 24 May, 1970.* S. Tsuji, and M. Wada (eds.). Amsterdam, Excerpta, 1971, p. 159.

Siperstein, M. D., Foster, D. W., Knowles, H. C., Jr., Levine, R., Madison, L. L., and Roth, J.: Control of blood glucose and diabetic vascular disease. *New England J. Med.* 296:1060, 1977.

Stone, D. B.: A rational approach to diet and diabetes. *J. Amer. Dietet. Assoc.* 46:30, 1965.

Taylor, S.: Genesis of the thyroid nodule. *Brit. Med. Bull.* 16:102, 1960.

The World Almanac and Book of Facts. New York, Newspaper Enterprise Association, Inc., 1978, p. 956.

Von Noorden, C.: Diabetes Mellitus in Twentieth Century Practice of Modern Medical Science. New York, William Wood & Company, 1895.

Vought, R. L.: Upward trend in iodide consumption in the United States. In *Trace Substances in Environmental Health, V., Proceedings of University of Missouri's 5th Annual Conference on Trace Substances in Environmental Health.* Delbert D. Hemphill (ed.). Columbus, Mo., Curators of the University of Missouri, 1971, pp. 303–312.

West, K. M.: Prevention and therapy of diabetes mellitus. In *Present Knowledge in Nutrition.* D. M. Hegsted, C. O. Chichester, W. J. Darby, K. W. McNutt, R. M. Stalvey, and E. H. Stotz (ed. comm.). New York, The Nutrition Foundation, Inc., 1976, pp. 356–364.

West, K.: Diabetes mellitus. In *Nutritional Support of Medical Practice.* H. A. Schneider, C. E. Anderson, and D. B. Coursin (eds.). Hagerstown, Md., Harper & Row, 1977, pp. 278–296.

8

NUTRITION AND HEMATOPOIESIS

Robert E. Hodges, M.D.

In the field of hematology, one can see clear evidence of the vital role that nutrients play in the synthesis, function, and maintenance of the body's tissues — in this instance, the blood-forming tissues. Here is proof that certain specific nutrients are needed for synthesis of hemoglobin, others for maturation of blood cells, and still others for proper functioning and life-span of the erythrocyte.

Both curiosity and resourcefulness were necessary for elucidation of some of the intricate interrelationships between nutrients and disease: witness the complexities of pernicious anemia, intrinsic factor, and Vitamin B_{12}. Yet despite all the brilliant work that has brought the science and art of hematology to its present esteemed position, there is one serious flaw: epidemiologic surveys repeatedly show that many people, both within and outside the industrialized nations, continue to have a substantial incidence of the nutritional anemias (Ten State Nutrition Survey, 1972); (Anonymous, 1972). This often results from poverty, ignorance, and indifference but it also results from another factor: those same essential nutrients that were studied so diligently in laboratories are not commonly consumed as chemicals. They are eaten as food. And food of many kinds and descriptions contains not only essential nutrients but often substances that can interfere with or even inactivate the essential nutrients.

Here the nutritionist can be of help, for people need information about which choices they should make from familiar foods. They may readily understand the difference between meat and bread, but they also know that, because of poverty, they can't afford to make drastic changes. Wise and experienced nutritionists can offer advice that is at the same time acceptable, effective, and compatible with their way of life.

DEFICIENCIES OF ESSENTIAL NUTRIENTS

Iron Deficiency and Surplus

Although deficiency of iron is by far the most common cause of nutritional anemia, lack of several other nutrients may result in hematopoietic disorders. Typically, surveys of population groups show a higher incidence of anemia among the poor, and especially among children and women who are in their reproductive years. One such survey of 334 urban children, ages 1 to 16 years, disclosed an incidence of anemia of 23 per cent accompanied by low serum iron levels, but more than twice this number of people had low iron values (Margo et al., 1977). None of the cases of anemia could be ascribed to deficiency of folates or vitamin B_{12}.

By far the commonest nutritional deficiency in the United States, and presumably in the rest of the world, is lack of adequate iron. It occurs in every age group: infancy, childhood, adolescence, the childbearing years, middle age, and old age. Although it accounts for few deaths, iron deficiency contributes to the impairment of health and substandard performance of millions of persons throughout the world. Gardner and others (1977) recently reported studies of the work performance of 75 women who worked on a tea estate in Sri Lanka, Ceylon. Their hemoglobin values ranged from 6.1 to 15.9 g/100 ml and their work performance correlated significantly with their hemoglobin level. These authors found that there was a 20 per cent decrement in work performance in subjects with hemoglobin concentrations between 11.0 and 11.9 g/100 ml when compared to subjects with hemoglobin concentrations of greater than 13 g/100 ml. Accordingly, Gardner and colleagues made a strong plea for correction and prevention of iron deficiency, not only because of decreased work performance but also on a basis of economics and health.

Recommended Dietary Allowances and Fortification. But this view is not shared by everyone. Indeed, Crosby (1975) is critical of the Food and Drug Administration for proposing an increase in the amount of iron to be added to all enriched bread and flour; of the Department of Health, Education, and Welfare for stating that 95 per cent of American women and children eat iron-deficient diets; and of the Food and Nutrition Board of the National Academy of Sciences for recommending a high level of iron fortification of foods derived from grain.

On the other hand, many established authorities are deeply concerned about the problem of iron deficiency in the United States as well as the rest of the world. Finch and Monsen (1972) estimate that there are 25 million women in the United States who are deficient in storage iron and about 5 million of these probably have iron-deficiency anemia. Those who have supported the Food and Drug Administration's proposal to increase the amount of iron added to our food supply include The Council on Foods and Nutrition of the American Medical Association (1972), Arnold Schaefer (1972), The Food and Nutrition Board of the National Academy of Sciences — National Research Council (1973), and the late Grace Goldsmith (1973).

The major concerns of those who oppose higher levels of iron fortification of foods are:

1. Iron deficiency anemia is not a serious condition except in infants and in pregnant women.

2. The available data are not sufficient to support the proposal for higher levels of iron fortification.

3. Fortification of farinaceous foods is an added risk to people with unrecognized hemochromatosis.

4. There is a need for long-term studies to assess the effectiveness of iron fortification and the effects on iron stores of the body.

Those who favor iron fortification at higher levels argue that fortification of flour and bread is safe at the proposed level (estimated average intake would approximate 18 mg per day for adult women and 30 mg for men). They cite two studies of the Ethiopian population, the ICNND Survey (1959) and the studies by Hofvander (1968), which showed intakes of about 300 mg of iron daily by many of these people. Yet there was no evidence of iron storage disease in the individuals studied. The previous studies of hemosiderosis among the Bantu, who make beer by fermenting grain in large iron kettles, are not comparable (Charlton et al., 1973). Many of these people had diets that were deficient in ascorbic acid and all of them consumed rather large amounts of alcohol. Both of these factors are believed to affect deposition of iron in the liver.

Iron deficiency, like many other deficiency syndromes, is insidious in its onset and difficult to diagnose until it reaches an advanced stage (Figure 8–1). In its mildest, or pre-latent, form the only detectable abnormality is depletion of storage iron in the bone marrow as manifested by reduced microscopic staining with Prussian blue. "Early" iron deficiency occurs when the iron stores are virtually exhausted and the plasma iron level is decreased. At the same time the transferrin (and, of course, the total iron-binding capacity) rises. Still, the patient will be only mildly or moderately anemic, and at this stage the erythrocytes are usually normocytic and normochromic.

NUTRITIONAL STATUS	DIET INTAKE	TOTAL RESERVES	PLASMA LEVELS	BIOCHEMICAL OR PHYSIOLOGICAL	TISSUE INTEGRITY
OPTIMAL NUTRITION	N	N	N	N	N
SUBOPTIMAL NUTRITION	$\rightarrow$	N±	N	N	N
SLIGHT DEFICIENCY	↓	$\rightarrow$	N±	N	N
MODERATE DEFICIENCY	O	↓	$\rightarrow$	N±	N±
MARKED DEFICIENCY	O	O	↓	$\rightarrow$	$\rightarrow$
ADVANCED DEFICIENCY	O	O	O	↓	↓
SEVERE DEFICIENCY	O	O	O	O	O
DEATH	O	O			

N = Normal
N± = Less than normal
→ = Decidedly low values
↓ = Deficient
O = Prolonged deficiency

Figure 8–1 Various hypothetical stages in the development of nutritional deficiency syndromes are schematically depicted. With less than adequate intakes of nutrients, the factor of time becomes important; and with total absence of a nutrient, the rate at which a deficiency develops varies inversely with the ability of the body to store that nutrient. For example, thiamin deficiency may develop in a few weeks, but vitamin B_{12} deficiency may not occur for several years, despite a diet devoid of this nutrient. In almost every instance, physical abnormalities represent a far advanced stage of deficiency.

TABLE 8-1

Hemoglobin Fe	1500–3000 mg
Storage Fe	1000–1500 mg
Other tissue Fe	100– 300 mg
TOTAL	2600–4800 mg

With more advanced deficiency, all measures of iron status indicate a severe deficiency: there is no stainable iron in bone marrow, plasma iron levels are low, transferrin levels are elevated, per cent iron saturation is low, anemia is pronounced, and the erythrocyte indices show microcytosis and hypochromia (Wintrobe et al., 1974).

The total amount of iron in adults is usually said to average about 4 grams or slightly less (35 mg/kg for women, 50 mg/kg for men). This iron is distributed throughout the body as shown in Table 8-1.

In order to maintain these stores of iron, dietary intake multiplied by amount absorbed must equal losses. If intake ranges from 12.0 to 15.0 mg daily and absorption varies from 5 to 10 per cent, then total iron absorbed would range from 0.6 to 1.5 mg daily. Average losses of iron vary from 0.5 to 1.5 mg daily, but some women lose about 2.5 mg daily as a result of menstrual losses.

Based upon the above, the estimated dietary iron needs of various people are:

Infants	10 mg daily
Children	10–15 mg daily
Adolescents (male and female)	18 mg daily
Pregnant or Lactating Women	Supplements of 30–60 mg/d.
Women of Reproductive Age	18 mg daily
Men	10 mg daily

The National Research Council recognizes that women cannot get 18 mg of iron daily from the average mixed diet (the average diet contains about 6 mg of iron/1000 Kcal). Accordingly, supplemental iron should be given, especially during pregnancy (Committee on Dietary Allowances, 1974).

At least part of the inadequacy of the American diet can be attributed to our excessive concern over cleanliness. Our vegetables and fruits are thoroughly washed and peeled. Food is cooked in stainless steel, porcelainized or Teflon-coated pans, and our water supply passes through plastic or copper pipes. Much of the former opportunity for contamination of our food with iron and other essential minerals has been lost. Moore (1965), White (1968), and Butterworth (1972) have called attention to the beneficial effects of cooking in old-fashioned black-iron pots and pans. Indeed, the author's wife does so and finds them easy to use and highly acceptable for many foods. The few exceptions include vegetables and fruits, which may become discolored. Also, boiling acid foods will erode the seasoned surface of ironware.

Metabolism of Iron. In recent years, studies with ^{59}Fe have helped to elucidate the intricate mechanisms that regulate iron absorption. Helbock and Saltman (1967) demonstrated not only a gradient-dependent mechanism but also an active membrane-bound facilitating carrier. This serosal-to-mucosal transport system is inhibited by iron deficiency anemia. Thus the amount of iron in the body is regulated by control of absorption as well as by dietary intake. Most iron absorption takes place in the jejunum. Although it is commonly believed that iron must be reduced to its ferrous state before it can be absorbed, Saltman's group has shown that chelated or complexed forms of ferric iron are absorbed even better than ferrous sulfate (Spiro and Saltman, 1969; Bates et al., 1972; Bates et al., 1973; Christopher et al., 1974; Carmichael et al., 1975; Saltman et al., 1976). The problem is to make iron salts that are soluble so they can cross the mucosal barrier. Indeed, the recent popularity of taking large amounts of ascorbic acid provided Cook and Monsen (1977) with an opportunity to study the effects of vitamin C on iron absorption. Studies performed by Moore (1955) had shown that large amounts of orange juice, consumed with breakfast, enhanced the availability of iron in eggs. Cook and Monsen confirmed Moore's observations and found that this effect of ascorbic acid was dose-related at least between the ranges of 25 and 1000 mg. Furthermore, this was a sustained effect that could result in greater-than-average long-term absorption of iron. They estimated that ingestion of ascorbic acid could increase iron absorption as much as ninefold, provided that it is consumed with meals. Taking vitamin C in large doses three times daily increases average absorption of iron about threefold, whereas taking it once each morning results in doubling of iron absorption.

But other substances can interfere with iron absorption — these include some of the antibiotics (tetracyclines) (Greenberger, 1973) and presumably other medications, as well as substances naturally occurring in food, such as phosphates, oxalates, phytates, and indigestible fiber (Jacobs, 1973; Jenkins et al., 1975). Even milk may interfere with iron absorption (Moore, 1965), unless the iron is chelated.

Studies of nutrient absorption always are difficult to interpret. The rate and efficiency of absorption of a single nutrient, such as iron, may be altered by incorporation of that nutrient into a single food such as cereal, milk, meat, and so on (Monsen and Cook, 1976), and the problem becomes even more complex when absorption of a nutrient is studied in subjects consuming an entire meal. Several investigators

TABLE 8-2 FOOD SOURCES OF IRON AROUND THE WORLD*

	CEREAL-GRAIN	VEGETABLE-FRUIT	ANIMAL PROTEIN
Far East	50%+	10%	15%
Near East	50%+	10%	15%
Africa	40%	25%	10%
Latin America	35%	10%	20%-
Europe	30%	10-20%	35%
U.S.A.	30%	10%	35%

*Modified from FAO/WHO Report No. 452 (1970).

have observed that iron is less well absorbed when it is fed as part of a full meal (Cook and Monsen, 1975; Björn-Rasmussen et al., 1976; Martinez-Torres and Layrisse, 1973).

This becomes an added problem when one is considering the potential advantages and disadvantages of an iron-enrichment program, for different groups of people may have individual and unique dietary habits. Inclusion of meats may enhance iron absorption for one group, while cereal products and milk may impair absorption for others (Cook and Finch, 1975). Furthermore, addition of labeled iron to a single food may result in better absorption than addition to a balanced meal containing the same foods.

Food Sources. Food sources of iron vary from one nation to another depending on their economy (Dagg and Goldberg, 1973; Cowan and Bharucha, 1973; Shah and Belonje, 1976; Takkunen and Seppänen, 1975), according to a World Health Organization Report (1970) (Table 8–2). It is obvious that most of the people in the world rely largely upon plant foods to supply the major portion of their nutrients, including dietary iron. Even in the industrialized nations of Europe, as well as in the United States, nearly half of the intake of iron is derived from plant foods. This does not necessarily mean that we absorb large amounts of iron from plant foods. As noted above, many substances in plant foods may have an inhibiting effect on availability of iron. The superiority of animal foods, in terms of iron absorption, is well demonstrated in Figure 8–2 (from Martinez-Torres and Layrisse, 1973).

Physiologic Needs for Iron. In the foregoing discussion, attention was called to the high degree of prevalence of iron deficiency throughout the world and to recent evidence that such deficiency does impair physical performance and that it also lowers economic standards. In addition to the vital function of iron as part of the hemoglobin molecule, this nutrient also participates in the functions of numerous tissue enzymes such as catalase, cytochrome C, cytochrome oxidase, aconitase, succinic dehydrogenase, and perhaps glutamate formimino

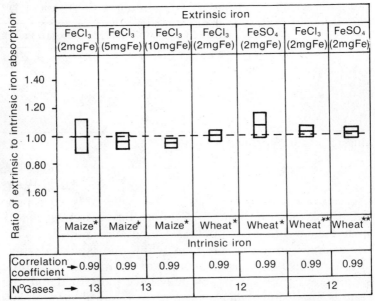

Figure 8–2 Effect of a complete meal on the absorption ratio between iron fortification (extrinsic tag) and vegetable foods (intrinsic tag). The symbol * indicates those studies in which enriched iron food was administered with a meal containing a large portion of meat, and ** indicates those in which the meal was administered without meat. It can be noticed that a complete meal does not disturb the ratio of extrinsic to intrinsic tag absorption, and the mean is close to unity in each study. There was no apparent difference in the amount absorbed from ferrous or ferric salt administered with a meal whether or not the meal contained meat.

transferase. Some authorities suggest that the fatigue of iron deficiency may result from enzymatic derangements, but this is speculative.

Iron Deficiency Anemia. Although this form of anemia is the most common of all, its causes and manifestations vary from one situation to another. In the foregoing discussion, the fact was established that iron deficiency of considerable severity generally precedes the onset of anemia. The actual *cause* of iron deficiency may be dietary or an inability to absorb or an excessive loss of iron as a result of bleeding. Whatever the cause, it would be most helpful to have some simple, inexpensive, non-invasive method for estimating total body stores of iron. Until recently it appeared that measurement of serum ferritin might serve this purpose, since this complex of iron represents a major storage mechanism (Avol et al., 1973; Christopher et al., 1975). Unfortunately, more recent evidence indicates that, although the level of ferritin in serum does correlate significantly with iron stores, it is not sufficiently specific and reliable to serve as a clinical guide in individual cases (Crosby, 1976; Ward et al., 1977). Thus it appears that estimates of iron stores must still be made on the basis of such time-tested procedures as serum iron and bone marrow stained with Prussian blue (Wallerstein, 1976; Cooperberg et al., 1977). Experimentally, the use of radioactive assays continues to provide a valid reference against which new tests and procedures can be evaluated.

Iron-deficiency anemia is most apt to occur at specific ages. A fetus can derive adequate iron from the mother, even though her own stores are depleted. And if the child is breast-fed, anemia is less likely to occur. But infants fed a cow's milk formula must be given iron supplements beginning at 3 months, since cow's milk is a very poor source of iron. Even in breast-fed infants, anemia in the first year of life is relatively common. After a child has begun to eat a variety of solid foods, its intake of iron increases. During the rapid-growing years both boys and girls need substantial amounts and adult women continue to need relatively large amounts until menopause. Oral contraceptive steroids decrease the amount of menstrual blood lost, whereas intrauterine devices increase the amount lost — but these differences are not great.

A strange habit called "pica" sometimes is associated with iron-deficiency anemia. Many authorities believe that pica (eating non-food substances) is a factor in causing iron deficiency, but Moore believed that iron deficiency created the desire to eat ice or clay or laundry starch. In any event pica is fairly common, particularly in black women living in the southeastern states of the United States.

Iron-deficiency anemia has an insidious onset. The patient may note some fatigue or palpitations with only moderate exertion. Headaches and "giddiness" may occur with severe anemia. Physical examination may reveal pallor of the skin and mucous membranes, angular lesions at the corners of the mouth, smoothness of the tongue with atrophy of filiform papillae, and in severe cases, a bounding pulse, a wide pulse pressure, and hemic murmurs over major arteries and along the left sternal border of the heart. Occasionally the spleen is enlarged. The fingernails may become indented or "spoon-shaped." Laboratory studies reveal an anemia of varying severity, accompanied by microcytosis and hypochromia. Common indices may show the following:

Mean Corpuscular Volume	(MCV)	$< 80 \ \mu^3$
Mean Corpuscular Hemoglobin	(MCH)	< 30 pg
Mean Corpuscular Hemoglobin Concentration	(MCHC)	$< 30\%$

Poikilocytosis is common. About half the patients have gastric achlohydria and a few will show esophageal dysfunction by X-ray (Plummer-Vinson syndrome).

Serum iron values will be low and the degree of saturation of transferrin may be less than 10 per cent. Prussian-blue stains of bone marrow will usually show absence of siderotic granules. (Normally about one-third of bone marrow normoblasts contain stainable granules).

Treatment of iron-deficiency anemia is simple and inexpensive (Perillie, 1977). Once the diagnosis has been made by laboratory tests, the patient should be given one of several forms of ferrous iron. Ferrous sulfate is effective and inexpensive, but some patients complain of unpleasant digestive tract symptoms. Ferrous gluconate or fumarate are less irritating, but also are less well absorbed. Recent studies of various chelated or complexed forms of iron suggest that oral iron therapy may become more effective in the future. These compounds include ferric citrate, ferric ascorbate, ferric fructose, and others, but Saltman's group prefers the fructose form because of its taste, effectiveness, and compatibility with various foods. Their studies indicate that, in guinea pigs, ferric fructose is absorbed twice as well as ferrous sulfate (Bates et al., 1972; Christopher et al., 1974; Saltman et al., 1976) (Figure 8–3).

A dose of 200 to 300 mg of ferrous sulfate or its equivalent three times daily will be ample. But the patient must be advised to eat a

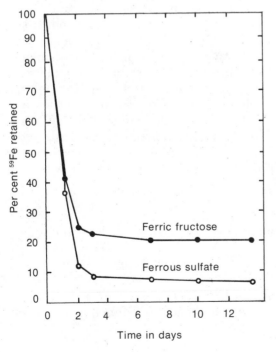

Figure 8–3 Kinetic pattern of ^{59}Fe retention by guinea pig given single initial dose of isotope per *os.*

nutritious diet (ask a dietitian to take a diet history and make specific suggestions to correct obvious defects), and a multiple vitamin supplement should be given daily for one month. The iron therapy may have to be continued for several months. Hematologic progress should be evaluated each month until normal values are achieved.

In some instances, parenteral iron may be necessary (Leavell and Thorup, 1971a). Saccharated iron can be given intravenously in a dose of 20 to 50 mg. This should be given slowly (at least 5 minutes) because vascular collapse may occur in rare cases. Later, the patient may tolerate doses of 100 to 200 mg intravenously once each week. Intramuscular administration of 100 to 500 mg given weekly can replace the intravenous therapy. The total amount of iron given parenterally throughout the course should not exceed 1500 to 5000 mg. There is a very slight risk of neoplasia at the site of intramuscular injection and a similar risk of anaphylactoid reaction from intravenous therapy. Obviously, the oral route is preferable if there are no contraindications.

Meanwhile, the physician should investigate the causes of any patient's anemia and attempt to find ways of preventing its recurrence. The fact that iron-deficiency anemia can result from occult loss of blood into the digestive tract or elsewhere must not be forgotten. Ulceration, neoplasia, and blood clotting disorders may be discovered in these patients.

Folic Acid Deficiency Anemia

The second commonest form of anemia in the United States results from folic acid deficiency. This water-soluble vitamin was named "folic" acid because it occurs in leafy foods, but it is even more abundant in liver and in yeast. Some folic acid is thought to be synthesized by bacterial growth in the bowel, but its availability is highly speculative. Folic acid is a heat-labile substance — hence, some is lost in cooking.

One of the problems in assessing folic acid nutrition arises from the methods of assay and from the fact that the term "folates" refers to a *group* of substances, pteroylglutamates, varying in the number of glutamate radicals attached. The bowel mucosa contains an enzyme (conjugase) that can remove glutamates, but the efficiency varies and may be impaired by common drugs, such as alcohol, anticonvulsants, and oral contraceptive steroids. For human beings, the monoglutamate form of folic acid appears to be most readily absorbed, but the bacteria used for assay of folic acid can grow with any of the folates. For this reason, it has become customary to assume that about one-fourth of the bacterial folic acid value of a food is available for human use. The average American diet contains about 100 to 200 μg daily (defined as folate available to the assay organism, *Lactobacillus casei*). This is marginal, since the recommended dietary allowance is 400 μg/d for most people and 800 during pregnancy. Despite this, frank folic acid deficiency occurs uncommonly unless a patient is taking a substance that interferes with absorption.

The usual causes of folate deficiency are: a poor diet, overcooked food — especially if cooking water is discarded — inadequate absorption, inadequate utilization, or increased requirements. Any process that is accompanied by rapid formation of new cells will increase the need for folates. These include pregnancy, infancy, injury to skin (burns, measles, chicken pox), injury to intestinal mucosa (dysentery, caustic chemical damage), and rapid destruction of red blood cells as in hemolytic anemia or in patients with certain types of artificial heart valves. Until authorities can agree to use a *single* assay method for folic acid in foods and in biological fluids, some degree of controversy will continue. At present, it appears that the folate content of the *average* American diet is marginally adequate *unless* food has been overcooked or kept hot for a prolonged period. (One wonders what the folate content is of foods served by various "fast food" establishments that are so popular in this country.)

Absorption of folic acid occurs chiefly in the proximal portion of the jejunum, primarily as the monoglutamate form (Leavell and Thorup, 1971b). Not only can ingestion of certain drugs, listed above, impair folate conjugase actively and interfere with absorption, but any form of intestinal malabsorption can impair folate absorption and lack of folate can, in itself, cause further malabsorption (Lien-Keng, 1957).

Once folic acid is absorbed, its utilization can be impaired by certain drugs and medications. These include ethanol, antifolates, antimalarials and protozoacides. Utilization also may be affected by deficiency of ascorbic acid, or vitamin B_{12} (Cowan and Bharucha, 1973; Shah and Belonje, 1976; Takkunen and Seppänen, 1975).

The amount of folic acid stored in the liver of a healthy, well-fed adult can prevent deficiency anemia for about 4 to 5 months in an individual with an intake of only 5 μg/d. The first manifestation of deficiency is a lowering of serum folate levels (normal = 6–20 ng/ml). Next, there is hypersegmentation of polymorphonuclear leukocytes. A metabolite, formiminoglutamic acid (FIGLU) appears in the urine in abnormal amounts, then in rapid succession there is a fall in the folate content of red blood cells (RBCs), a macro-ovalocytosis of RBCs, development of a megaloblastic bone marrow, and finally, frank anemia. The bone marrow discloses megaloblastic arrest, suggesting either folate or vitamin B_{12} deficiency. Clinical symptoms and signs of folate deficiency are few and nondescript. They do not differ substantially from those of iron deficiency anemia.

Therapy of folate deficiency necessitates a search for the cause. If it resulted from poor dietary habits, then personal instruction in diet plus dietary supplements may suffice. But some patients may be having an adverse reaction to medications. Others may have an undiscovered neoplasm or increased metabolic needs as in thyrotoxicosis. Thus it is not sufficient to give replacement therapy without a careful medical examination. Furthermore, the similarities between deficiencies of vitamin B_{12} and folic acid are close enough to mandate a search for undetected pernicious anemia. Folate therapy without adequate vitamin B_{12} reserves can result in a rapidly progressive form of subacute combined degeneration of the spinal cord with a potential for irreversible neurologic deficits.

When therapy of folate deficiency is undertaken, a dose of 100 μg of folic acid is given orally each day. This should result in a prompt hematologic response (the rise in reticulocytes reaching a peak about the seventh day). If folate deficiency is thus confirmed, a maintenance level of 500 μg daily should be given (Food and Agriculture Organization/World Health Organization, 1970).

Vitamin B_{12} Deficiency

Vitamin B_{12} is one of the most active substances required by man. A daily dose as low as 1 μg seems to meet all requirements (Committee on Dietary Allowances, 1974; Leavell and Thorup, 1971b), but 3 μg are recommended (four for pregnant or lactating women). This vitamin, unlike folic acid, is stored in the liver in sufficient amounts to last 1 to 2 years or longer, even if none is absorbed from the diet.

Historically, as every medical student has learned, Addisonian pernicious anemia was very well characterized long before the discovery of vitamin B_{12}. The disease begins insidiously with gradually progressing weakness, fatigue, and breathlessness. Slight exertion causes palpitations and dyspnea. Soreness of the tongue and "indigestion" are common but weight loss is modest. Numbness and tingling of fingers and toes progresses proximally and there is loss of position sense, so walking in the dark becomes difficult. Eventually, there is loss of ability to perform fine tasks with the hands (buttoning of clothing) or to walk without support. Loss of control of bowels and bladder often coincides with the onset of mental confusion, disorientation, delusions, and hallucinations.

Physical examination reveals an individual (usually elderly) who appears pale and somewhat yellow, often with white hair. The tongue usually is pale, and there is smoothness of the tip and lateral margins. The heart may be overactive and hemic murmurs are common. Splenomegaly is also common. There is abundant neurological evidence of sensory abnormalities, but vibratory and position senses are most affected. Light touch and 2-point discrimination are defective on the hands and feet.

Laboratory studies classically disclose a very severe degree of anemia with macrocytosis and hyperchromia. There also are poikilocytosis and polychromasia. Hypersegmentation of polymorphonuclear leukocytes also occurs and there is a moderate leukopenia with thrombocytopenia. Gastric analysis reveals achlorhydria which is histamine-fast. Examination of the bone marrow shows the classical megaloblastic arrest that is characteristic of deficiency of either vitamin B_{12} or folic acid.

The diagnosis can be suspected by finding low serum vitamin B_{12} levels and confirmed by performing a Schilling test to ascertain whether there is intrinsic factor (IF) in the gastric juice. This is performed by giving 0.5 μCi of ^{57}Co vitamin B_{12} by mouth. Two hours later, 1000 μg of non-radioactive vitamin B_{12} are injected intramuscularly. This serves to "flush out" the radioactive vitamin B_{12} that was absorbed in combination with IF. Urine is then collected for 24 hours and the amount of ^{57}Co contained therein is measured. If the test is abnormal, the patient is given 60 mg of IF orally and the entire test is repeated. This should result in a normal response unless the patient has a malabsorption defect involving the terminal ileum or unless there is a "blind loop" syndrome. In the latter instance, therapy with tetracycline, 250 mg q.i.d. × 10 days, should result in a normal response to a repeat Schilling test. With a normal response there is excretion of 77 per cent of the administered radioactivity in 24 hours. Treatment of pernicious anemia with injections of vitamin B_{12} has become standard practice, usually with a dose of 1000 μg the first week, then 500 μg the second week, followed by 50 μg doses weekly for two more weeks, then 100 μg each month thereafter.

But deficiency of vitamin B_{12} (serum levels below 160 μg/l) (normal range 160–1000) may result from a variety of causes. Surgical removal of most of the stomach may reduce the amount of intrinsic factor secreted, or surgical loss of the terminal portion of the ileum may result in failure to reabsorb intrinsic factor along with the vitamin B_{12} attached to it. The peculiar "blind loop syndrome" described above develops in some patients who have a segment of bowel which forms a cul-de-sac in which microorganisms can grow without being swept away by the passing food stream. Somehow this situation leads to depletion of vitamin B_{12}. Administration of antibiotics retards the growth of organisms and allows the patient to absorb vitamin B_{12}. A rare cause of vitamin B_{12} deficiency is the fish tapeworm, *Diphilobothrium latum* which competes with its host for this nutrient. Since eating raw fish is not very popular in the United States, this syndrome is seldom encountered.

Trace Mineral Deficiency

People living in the United States have little likelihood of developing deficiency of any of the trace minerals *unless* they have one of the malabsorption syndromes. The trace minerals of greatest interest from the standpoint of hematopoiesis are copper and zinc. In subhuman animals, copper deficiency occurs with some frequency, but in our society there are many opportunities for copper to "contaminate" our food or water. Most pasteurized milk has been in contact with copper pipes and has increased its copper content thereby. Much of our domestic water supplies likewise acquire a higher content of copper by virtue of passing through copper pipes. Many foods contain an abundance of copper and this may be further enhanced by use of cooking utensils made of copper. The author has seen only a few cases of copper deficiency and anemia; one was in a woman with sprue, the others were in patients treated with Total Parenteral Nutrition who developed deficiencies of both copper and zinc. But these patients were anemic before they received this form of therapy. The true incidence of copper deficiency as a cause of anemia must be very low (Fleming et al., 1976).

Copper is essential for normal absorption of iron from the gastrointestinal tract. Anemia develops in many species of animals deprived of copper. No doubt more attention will be paid to the hematologic effects of this metal in the future.

Zinc received a great deal of attention as a result of reports that lack of this element leads to anemia, dwarfism, and hypogonadism in young men in Near-Eastern countries. Their traditional diets were not only low in zinc but high in phytates, which are present in unleavened bread and can bind divalent cations, such as zinc.

Zinc is an essential component of many metalloenzymes and metalloproteins. Deficiency of zinc can impair growth of hair and fingernails, delay wound healing, cause sterility, and cause anemia. There is still some controversy about the mechanism or indeed the fact of zinc-deficiency anemia. It may be that zinc deficiency has an adverse effect upon iron metabolism or it is possible that impairment of enzymatic function causes hematopoietic inhibition.

Little-Known Causes of Anemia

Although the most common causes of anemia are deficiencies of iron, folic acid, or vitamin B_{12}, every physician knows how frequently patients with any form of chronic debilitating disorder become anemic. This type (or group) of anemias usually defies therapy, either with diet or medications. Sporadic reports suggest that there are other nutrients essential for hematopoiesis. Most of these may not be useful in treating patients but an awareness of their *potential* benefit is important.

Ascorbic acid deficiency usually results in classical scurvy within 3 months and soon thereafter the disease is likely to be either treated or fatal. There are, however, instances of "chronic scurvy" in which patients have subsisted on inadequate amounts of vitamin C and became anemic. Ascorbic acid does facilitate iron absorption and it also plays a role in conversion of folic acid to its active form, folinic acid or citrovorum factor (5-formyl-tetrahydrofolic acid). But deficiency of ascorbic acid in subjects fed an otherwise adequate diet does not usually result in anemia.

Nicotinic acid is essential not only for prevention of pellagra but also as a coenzyme in the formation of erythrocytes. In the past, patients with pellagra often had an anemia which might be macrocytic and responsive to folic acid or microcytic and responsive to iron. It is likely that they had multiple deficiencies.

Pyridoxine-responsive Anemia. Although experimental deficiency of vitamin B_6 results in leukopenia, it does not often produce anemia. But a peculiar condition known as "pyridoxine-responsive anemia" has been described, and the dose of pyridoxine necessary to correct this form of anemia is much larger than that required by most persons (Chillar et al., 1976).

Vitamin E–Deficiency and Hemolytic Anemias. Since the classical report of Horwitt demonstrating vitamin E deficiency in subjects fed a deficient diet for several years, there has been interest in the effect of vitamin E deficiency upon erythropoiesis and more particularly upon RBC survival. Horwitt demonstrated that the red blood cells of his volunteers were abnormally susceptible to chemical hemolysis (with H_2O_2 or dialuric acid). This has become a standard test for adequacy of vitamin E nutrition. Since that time a number of reports have appeared of hemolytic anemia in premature infants. This form of anemia is aggravated by oral iron therapy, presumably because iron destroys vitamin E in the digestive tract. Treatment of other forms of hemolytic anemia with large doses of vitamin E is useless.

Vitamin A–Deficiency Anemia. The author has observed a form of iron-deficiency anemia developing in a group of healthy, middle-aged men who participated in a study of vitamin A deficiency. This anemia was accompanied by hypoferremia and low iron binding capacity. It did not respond well to oral administration of medicinal iron until *after* vitamin A had been restored to the diet. A search of the library revealed numerous references to vitamin A and anemia throughout the past 50 years, but the mechanisms involved are yet to be elucidated (Mejia et al., 1977; Hodges et al., 1978).

The Anemia of Chronic Illness. Many physicians have attempted to correct the anemia which chronically ill patients so often develop. Recent studies have shown that there is no statistical correlation between the severity of this type of anemia and any of the nutrients usually associated with hematopoiesis. There is, however, a significant correlation between hemoglobin levels and albumin concentration, suggesting that the common denominator may well be the rate of protein synthesis. Indeed the results of studies of patients treated vigorously with Total Parenteral Nutrition confirms an apparent relationship between correction of hypoalbuminemia and of anemia.

SUMMARY

Virtually every phase of blood formation, function, and degradation is closely linked to essential nutrients. A working knowledge of the role of food and nutrition in the management of hematologic disorders should be helpful to physicians who deal with these problems.

REFERENCES

Anonymous Editorial: Undernutrition in Massachusetts. *New Eng. J. Med.* 287:886, 1972.

Avol, E., Carmichael, D., Hegenauer, J., and Saltman, P.: Rapid induction of ferritin in laboratory animals prior to its isolation. *Preparative Biochemistry* 3:279, 1973.

Bates, G. W., Boyer, J., Hegenauer, J. C., and Saltman, P.: Facilitation of iron absorption by ferric fructose. *Amer. J. Clin. Nutr.* 25:983, 1972.

Bates, G., Hegenauer, J., Renner, J., Saltman, P., and Spiro, T. G.: Complex formation, polymerization, and antoreduction in the ferric fructose system. *Bioinorganic Chemistry* 2:311, 1973.

Björn-Rasmussen, E., Hallberg, L., Magnussen, B., Rossander, L., Svanberg, B., and Arvidsson, B.: Measurement of iron absorption from composite meals. *Amer. J. Clin. Nutr.* 29:772, 1976.

Butterworth, C. E., Jr.: Iron "undercontamination" (Editorial). *J.A.M.A.* 220:581, 1972.

Carmichael, D., Christopher, J., Hebenauer, J., and Saltman, P.: Effect of milk and casein on the absorption of supplemental iron in the mouse and chick. *Amer. J. Clin. Nutr.* 28:487, 1975.

Charlton, R. W., Bothwell, T. H., and Seftel, H. C.: Dietary iron overload. *In Clinics in Hematology, Volume 2.* S. T. Callender (ed.). W. B. Saunders Company, Ltd., London, 1973, pp. 383–403.

Chillar, R. K., Johnson, C. S., and Beutler, E.: Erythrocyte pyridoxine kinase levels in patients with sideroblastic anemia. *New Eng. J. Med.* 295:881, 1976.

Christopher, J. P., Hegenauer, J. C., and Saltman, P. D.: Iron metabolism as a function of chelation. *In Trace Element Metabolism in Animals.* W. G. Hoekstra, J. W. Suttie, H. E. Ganther, and W. Mertz (eds.). Butterworths, London, 1974, pp. 133–145.

Christopher, J., Hatlen, L., Hegenauer, J., Ripley, L., Saltman, P., and Ward, C.: Radioimmunoassay of ferritin in rat serum: correlation of serum ferritin with liver ferritin iron stores. In *Proteins of Iron Storage and Transport in Biochemistry and Medicine*. R. R. Crighton (ed.). North Holland Publishing Company, Amsterdam, 1975, pp. 411–416.

Committee on Dietary Allowances: Recommended Dietary Allowances. Eighth Revised Edition. Food and Nutrition Board, National Research Council — National Academy of Sciences, Washington, D.C., 1974. Iron, pp. 92–94.

Cook, J. D., and Finch, C. A.: Iron nutrition (Medical Progress). *West. J. Med. 122*:474, 1975.

Cook, J. D., and Monsen, E. R.: Food iron absorption: 1. Use of a semisynthetic diet to study absorption of nonheme iron. *Amer. J. Clin. Nutr. 28*:1289, 1975.

Cook, J. D., and Monsen, E. R.: Vitamin C, the common cold, and iron absorption. *Amer. J. Clin. Nutr. 30*:235, 1977.

Cooperberg, A. A., Rosenberg, A., and Schwartz, J. P.: Diagnostic value of bone marrow iron deposits in idiopathic hemochromatosis. *Arch. Int. Med. 137*:748, 1977.

Council on Foods and Nutrition. White, P. L. (secretary). Iron in enriched wheat flour, farina, bread, buns, and rolls. *J.A.M.A. 220*:855, 1972.

Cowan, B., and Bharucha, C.: Iron deficiency in the tropics. In *Clinics in Hematology, Volume 2*. S. T. Callender (ed.). W. B. Saunders Company, Ltd., London, 1973, pp. 353–363.

Crosby, W. H.: Improving iron nutrition (Editorial). *West. J. Med. 122*:499, 1975.

Crosby, W. H.: Serum ferritin fails to indicate hemochromatosis — nothing gold can stay (editorial). *New Eng. J. Med. 294*:333, 1976.

Dagg, J. H., and Goldberg, A.: Detection and treatment of iron deficiency. In *Clinics in Hematology, Volume 2*. S. T. Callender (ed.). W. B. Saunders Company, Ltd., London, 1973, pp. 365–380.

Finch, C. A., and Monsen, E. R.: Iron nutrition and the fortification of food with iron. *J.A.M.A. 219*:1462, 1972.

Fleming, C. R., Hodges, R. E., and Hurley, L. S.: A prospective study of serum copper and zinc levels in patients receiving total parenteral nutrition. *Amer. J. Clin. Nutr. 29*:70, 1976.

Food and Agriculture Organization/World Health Organization: Requirements of ascorbic acid, vitamin D, vitamin B_{12}, folate, and iron. World Health Organization Technical Report Series No. 452, Geneva, 1970.

Food and Nutrition Board, National Academy of Sciences — National Research Council, Washington, D.C. General policies in regard to improvement of nutritive quality of foods. Enrichment Policies, 1973.

Gardner, G. W., Edgerton, V. R., Senewiratne, B., Barnard, R. J., and Ohira, Y.: Physical work capacity and metabolic stress in subjects with iron-deficiency anemia. *Amer. J. Clin. Nutr. 30*:910, 1977.

Goldsmith, G. A.: Iron enrichment of bread and flour. *Amer. J. Clin. Nutr. 26*:131, 1973.

Greenberger, N. J.: Effects of antibiotics and other agents on the intestinal transport of iron. *Amer. J. Clin. Nutr. 26*:104, 1973.

Helbock, H. J., and Saltman, P.: The transport of iron by rat intestine. *Biochim. Biophys. Acta 135*:979, 1967.

Hodges, R. E., Sauberlich, H. E., Canham, J. E., Wallace, D. L., Rucker, R. B., Mejia, L. A., and Mohanram, M.: Hematopoietic studies in vitamin A deficiency. *Am. J. Clin. Nutr. 31*:876, 1978.

Hofvander, Y.: Hematological investigations in Ethiopia with special reference to a high iron intake. *Acta Med. Scand. Supp. 494*:1, 1968.

Interdepartmental Committee on Nutrition for National Defense. *Ethiopia Nutrition Survey*. Washington, Government Printing Office, 1959.

Jacobs, A.: The mechanism of iron absorption. In *Clinics in Hematology, Volume 2*. S. T. Callender (ed.). W. B. Saunders Company, Ltd., London, 1973, pp. 323–337.

Jenkins, D. A. J., Hill, M. S., and Cummings, J. H.: Effect of wheat fiber on blood lipids, fecal steroid excretion, and serum iron. *Amer. J. Clin. Nutr. 28*:1408, 1975.

Leavell, B. S., and Thorup, O. A., Jr.: Disorders of iron metabolism. In *Fundamentals of*

Clinical Hematology. W. B. Saunders Company, Philadelphia, 1971a, pp. 116–155.

Leavell, B. S., and Thorup, O. A., Jr.: Disorders of vitamin B_{12} and folic acid metabolism. In *Fundamentals of Clinical Hematology*. W. B. Saunders Company, Philadelphia, 1971b, pp. 86–115.

Lien-Keng, K.: Erythroblastopenia with giant pro-erythroblasts in kwashiorkor. *Blood* 12:171, 1957.

Margo, G., Baroni, Y., Green, R., and Metz, J.: Anemia in urban underprivileged children. Iron, folate, and vitamin B_{12} nutrition. *Amer. J. Clin. Nutr.* 30:947, 1977.

Martinez-Torres, C., and Layrisse, M.: Nutritional factors in iron deficiency: Food iron absorption. In *Clinics in Hematology, Volume 2*. S. T. Callender (ed.). W. B. Saunders Company, Ltd., London, 1973, pp. 339–351.

Mejia, L. A., Hodges, R. E., Arroyave, G., Viteri, F., and Torún, B.: Vitamin-A deficiency and anemia in Central American children. *Amer. J. Clin. Nutr.* 30:1175, 1977.

Monsen, E. R., and Cook, J. D.: Food iron absorption in human subjects. IV. The effects of calcium and phosphate salts on the absorption of nonheme iron. *Amer. J. Clin. Nutr.* 29:1142, 1976.

Moore, C. V.: The importance of nutritional factors in the pathogenesis of iron deficiency anemia. *Amer. J. Clin. Nutr.* 3:3, 1955.

Moore, C. V.: Iron nutrition and requirements. *Series Haematologica* 6:1, 1965.

Perillie, P. E.: Cost of iron therapy (Letter to Editor). *Ann. Int. Med.* 86:364, 1977.

Saltman, P., Hegenauer, J., and Christopher, J.: Tired blood and rusty livers. *Ann. Clin. Lab. Med.* 6:167, 1976.

Schaefer, A. E.: Iron deficiency anemia (Editorial). *Biomedical News*, p. 2, Sept. 1972.

Shah, B., and Belonje, B.: Liver storage iron in Canadians. *Amer. J. Clin. Nutr.* 29:66, 1976.

Spiro, Th. G., and Saltman, P.: Polynuclear complexes and their biological implications. In *Structure and Bonding, Volume 6*. P. Hemmerich, C. K. Jørgensen, J. B. Neilands, S. R. S. Nyholm, D. Reinen, and R. J. P. Williams (eds.). Springer-Verlag, New York, 1969, pp. 115–156.

Takkunen, H., and Seppänen, R.: Iron deficiency and dietary factors in Finland. *Amer. J. Clin. Nutr.* 28:1141, 1975.

Ten State Nutrition Survey 1968–1970. Department of Health, Education, and Welfare. Publication No. (HSM) 72–8132, 4:3, 1972.

Wallerstein, R. O.: Role of the laboratory in the diagnosis of anemia. *J.A.M.A.* 236:490, 1976.

Ward, C., Saltman, P., Ripley, L., Ostrup, R., Hegenauer, J., Hatland, L., and Christopher, J.: Correlation of serum ferritin and liver ferritin iron in the anemic, normal, and iron-loaded rat. *Amer. J. Clin. Nutr.* 30:1054, 1977.

White, H. S.: Current use and change in use of cast iron cookware. *J. Home Economics* 60:724, 1968.

Wintrobe, M. M., Lee, G. R., Boggs, D. R., Bithell, T. C., Athens, J. W., and Foerster, J.: Anemias characterized by impaired iron metabolism. In *Clinical Hematology, Seventh Edition*. Lea and Febiger, Philadelphia, 1974, pp. 621–692.

9

NUTRITION
AND INFECTION

Robert E. Hodges, M.D.

Most of us who live in the prosperous environment of our industrialized nations fail to appreciate the clinical and epidemiologic importance of interactions between malnutrition and infectious diseases. This, according to Gordon (1976), results from the high standard of living, the good state of nutrition, and the relatively infrequent occurrence of severe infections in our own communities.

But Suskind and colleagues (1977a) cited evidence from a recent study of children living in Latin American cities, to indicate that malnutrition was and presumably still is directly or indirectly responsible for more than half of the deaths of children under five years of age. And Gontzea (1974) remarked that famine was accompanied by two consequences that "appear as twins:" an increase in the incidence of infectious illnesses and an increase in the severity of these infections. Scrimshaw and others (1968) also noted an association between famine and pestilence and they stated that ". . . commonly occurring interrelationships between infection and malnutrition are direct and causal." These interactions are of two kinds; malnutrition alters the resistance of individuals to infection, and the infection exaggerates the malnutrition. Little wonder that the result is a high incidence of deaths, especially among children who have not yet acquired substantial immunity to the common pathogenic organisms of their environment.

In the following pages, the factors which normally protect us from infections will be examined with regard to the possible mechanisms whereby malnutrition impairs natural immunity. These include the skin and mucous membranes, the phagocytic cells, circulating antibodies and systemic responses to infection such as fever, ketosis, and levels of circulating nutrients.

220

NORMAL MECHANISMS OF RESISTANCE TO INFECTION

Despite an environment teeming with microorganisms, the human body manages to maintain nearly complete sterility of all save one of its internal compartments. The obvious exception is the digestive tract, and even here the types of microorganisms that predominate are closely regulated by a combination of factors: pH, digestive enzymes, and nutrients.

By far the greatest degree of protection is afforded by mechanical barriers — the skin and the mucous membranes — but these structures provide additional protection by virtue of their secretions. Fatty acids and organic acids in cutaneous secretions have bacteriostatic and bactericidal effects. And the mucus secreted by goblet cells in various epithelial surfaces provides a sticky coating that mechanically traps many microorganisms. In the respiratory tract, the columnar epithelial cells have cilia that "beat" rhythmically and propel the mucus blanket that covers the epithelial surfaces in the direction of the pharynx. As a result, most bacteria and other microorganisms that are inhaled into the tracheobronchial tree become trapped and are slowly expelled into the pharynx where the mucoid secretions are either swallowed or expectorated.

Many microorganisms that are swallowed cannot survive the low pH and the digestive enzymes of the stomach. A notable example is the higher-than-average incidence of tuberculosis in patients who have had a gastrectomy or who are achlorhydric for any other reason.

Once bacteria or other microorganisms gain access to the interior, they may be destroyed promptly or they may proliferate and cause clinical disease. Phagocytosis of microorganisms by polymorphonuclear leukocytes, by certain lymphocytes, and by tissue phagocytes represents a potent "second line of defense" against infection. And if the foreign protein introduced by invading microorganisms reaches a certain critical mass, the lymphoid cells respond and produce humoral substances or antibodies. These immune globulins (Ig) serve a variety of functions and have been named IgG, IgA, IgM, IgD, and IgE. By far the most abundant and longest lasting member of this group is IgG, which has antibacterial, antiviral, and antitoxic properties (Wehrle and Haddad, 1976). Its major roles appear to be neutralizing bacterial toxins and binding microorganisms, thereby facilitating phagocytosis.

The second most abundant immunoglobulin in the serum is IgA but it is more concentrated on the surface of mucous membranes where it exerts its protective effects against viruses. Production of IgA is stimulated by direct contact between a virus or its antigen and the surface of the mucous membrane.

IgM is the principal antibody formed by newborn children and it may also be the primary antibody formed by persons of any age when first exposed to an antigenic stimulus. The transient IgM response is soon replaced by IgG, which persists much longer. But IgM may be of major importance in agglutination and cytolysis of bacteria and it also includes the isohemagglutinins, Anti A and Anti B.

IgD has been found on the surface of cord blood lymphocytes but its functions are not well delineated.

IgE is termed the reaginic antibody and is present in only minute amounts in serum. It can also be found in the respiratory mucosa and on the surface of tissue mast cells. Combination of antigens with IgE on mast cells causes release of chemical mediators (histamine, serotonin, bradykinin, and slow-reacting substance of anaphylaxis) which produce the allergic response (Steihm, 1977). It appears that T-cells are important regulators of IgE production. In malnourished children with intestinal parasitism, serum levels of IgE may become markedly elevated. By contrast at least some of the immunoglobulins may be depressed by malnutrition, specifically by deficiencies of one or several vitamins (Axelrod et al. 1947).

EFFECTS OF NUTRITIONAL STATUS ON RESISTANCE TO INFECTION

Evidence has been presented that malnutrition, particularly in growing children, leads to more frequent and more severe infections. But specific types of malnutrition seem to have more or less specific effects on resistance to infection. Available information does not yet clearly identify precise mechanisms but the trends are quite apparent.

Protein-calorie malnutrition, including marasmus or general starvation, and kwashiorkor or protein deficiency, is most commonly seen in children less than three years of age. Associated deficiencies of vitamins are common (Suskind et al., 1977). Resistance to infections, especially of the respiratory tract and of the digestive tract, is low and death rates from infections of these systems are high. Although some of this may be attributed to poor living conditions, inadequate sanitation, crowding, and ignorance, malnutrition also contributes to the outcome. Indeed, as noted previously, Scrimshaw and colleagues (1968) not only presented abundant evidence that poor nutrition impairs resistance to infection but also showed that infections result in even worse malnutrition. It is a peculiar fact that, in many developing societies, sick people, and especially sick children, are so often fed a liquid diet that is lacking in protein and most other essential nutrients.

Scrimshaw and his group (1968) tabulated many reports of the effects of specific types of deficiency on the host's response to a wide variety of specific pathogens. Their results are briefly summarized in the following pages.

Multiple nutritional deficiencies in man as well as in several other species were found to have a "synergistic" or worsening effect on tuberculous and enteric infections. Only in a few instances did malnutrition have an antagonistic or protective effect and this occurred chiefly in experimental animals. The effects of deficiencies of protein and amino acids also were synergistic in most instances where the infectious agent was *Mycobacterium tuberculosis.* In several animal studies, a very high intake of protein had an adverse effect on experimental tuberculosis. In general, lack of adequate amounts of protein in the diet impaired resistance to infection with bacteria, viruses, protozoa, and helminths. In a few instances, protozoan infections in animals were antagonized by low-protein diets but this was not the rule. Tryptophan deficiency in mice and rats gave some protection against viral infections.

Deficiency of vitamin A was found to be synergistic with almost every known infectious disease and in almost every species studied.

By contrast, deficiency of vitamin D, even to the point of rickets, had no effect on resistance to infection in at least half of the studies reviewed by Scrimshaw and colleagues. Deficiency of vitamin E was synergistic for experimental infections with a bacterial and with a viral agent but antagonistic to infestation with *Trichinella spiralis.*

Ascorbic acid has been widely hailed by some as a potent antiinfectious agent and rejected by others who feel it is useless. Perhaps the source of disagreement is failure to recognize the difference between physiologic doses that will prevent scurvy in susceptible species and pharmacologic doses that may induce a variety of changes. The minimal daily requirement for ascorbic acid in healthy adults is about 10 mg and the recommended daily allowance varies from one country to another. The United Nation's World Health Organization has established 30 mg as a suitable level of intake, and in the United States the recommendation (as of 1974) was 45 mg per day. Although some persons suggest that doses ten to one hundred times larger may be beneficial, the available evidence for such conclusions leaves much to be desired. Scrimshaw and his group report that deficiency of ascorbic acid is synergistic with all infectious diseases studied with the exception of a single report of antagonism in monkeys with malaria. Unfortunately, few studies have been made of viral infections in scorbutic animals.

Deficiencies of one or more members of the vitamin B complex have been noted to increase the fatality rate of many infections. Lack of thiamin is generally synergistic with infectious diseases of bacterial origin and often antagonistic with diseases of viral origin. And lack of riboflavin is synergistic with most infectious diseases of any type. Niacin deficiency seems to have less influence on infection than any nutrient discussed above.

Pyridoxine deficiency, like pantothenic acid deficiency, has a variety of effects ranging from synergism with some infections to antagonism with others. In a number of studies of pyridoxine deficiency there was no effect on experimental infections. And the effects of pantothenic acid deficiency were about evenly divided between synergism (chiefly bacterial infections) and antagonism (especially with protozoal infections). These results are somewhat surprising in view of the well-established effects of deficiencies of these two vitamins on antibody formation. Axelrod and colleagues (1947), and Axelrod (1971), in a series of studies in experimental animals, demonstrated that many of the vitamins were essential for normal production of antibodies, and deficiency of two, pantothenic acid and pyridoxine, caused complete immunologic paralysis as judged by methods then available. Hodges and others (1962) repeated Axelrod's animal studies in humans and confirmed his observations that simultaneous deficiency of pantothenic acid and pyridoxine did result in virtually complete failure of immunologic responses to the antigens of typhoid and tetanus. But these same subjects responded well to killed polio virus antigen and they had no loss of isohemagglutinins A or B. The objective of these studies was to evaluate the possibility of inhibiting the rejection phenomenon, thus making organ transplantation feasible. At that time, little was known about cellular immunity and no studies were made of tissue reactivity.

Deficiencies of folic acid appear to protect experimental animals against certain viral diseases, but children lacking this vitamin are found to have more severe diarrhea, which may itself contribute to the deficiency of folic acid.

Data concerning the effects of deficiencies of biotin, inositol, and choline are limited and in many instances show no effect. There does appear to be some synergism between lack of biotin and infections with viruses and protozoa. Deficiency of para-amino benzoic acid may provide some protection against protozoal infections.

Deficiencies of minerals may also have an effect on resistance to infection. And the possibility that an excess of some minerals, notably iron, may impair resistance will be discussed later. Scrimshaw observed that deficiencies of calcium and phosphorus had variable effects on viral infections: some antagonism, some synergism. But lack of these minerals had a synergistic effect on helminthic infestations. Lack of sodium and potassium and chloride had variable effects but lack of magnesium had an antagonistic effect on bacterial infections and helminthic infestations.

Iron deficiency, which is so prevalent in many parts of the world, and especially in economically depressed areas, has long been said to lower resistance to infection. Srikantia and others (1976) studied anemic young children in India and found that both their cell-mediated immune response and the bactericidal activity of their polymorphonuclear leukocytes were impaired when levels of hemoglobin fell to 10 gm/dl or less. Studies of iron metabolism in these anemic children disclosed that transferrin saturation was less than 15 per cent in 36 of 46 patients. Furthermore the per cent of T lymphocytes was significantly lower than normal in the anemic children.

Along similar lines, Bhaskaram and others (1977) not only confirmed these observations but showed that treatment of anemic children with iron increased their hemoglobin values from an average of 10.3 to 12.7 gm/dl and doubled the per cent of transferrin saturation. This significantly increased the bactericidal activity of their leukocytes, the percentage of T lymphocytes, and the incorporation of tritiated thymidine into peripheral blood lymphocytes. These studies appear to confirm the clinical impression that iron-deficiency anemia impairs immune mechanisms, at least in children.

But other lines of investigation seem to cast doubt on the concept that iron deficiency impairs immunity in children. Suskind and colleagues (1977) studied the immune responses of children in Thailand who were severely anemic as a result of iron deficiency. They found that stimulation of peripheral lymphocytes with phytohemagglutinins resulted in a normal rate of conversion to blast forms. Similarly, the bactericidal activity of leukocytes was normal in seven of eight children. Thus, the controversy persists at the clinical level.

Even in the laboratory, there is strong disagreement among experts. Weinberg (1966; 1971) has shown that many microorganisms require iron and other metallic ions for normal growth and metabolism. A host factor, "paciferin," protects mice against *Salmonella typhimurium*. This substance has a strong affinity for ferrous iron and apparently adjusts the available concentration of this element in such a way as to favor the growth of non-virulent organisms while virulent organisms are retarded. Normal serum has considerable bactericidal power, partly as a result of unsaturated transferrin, but this can be depressed by ferrous iron. Other ions, including calcium, magnesium, and copper, play important roles in these host-parasite interactions: Weinberg has summarized the roles of iron in these interactions as including: "(1) stimulation of growth of bacterial or fungal pathogens, (2) inhibition of bactericidal proteins of leukocyte lysosomes, (3) enhancement or suppression of bacterial secondary metabolism, and (4) detoxification of factors of virulence." He believes that the iron-binding proteins are effective antibiotics, and that administration of iron preparations can inhibit this protective effect. This view is shared by Elin and Wolff (1973), who found that *in vitro* growth of *Candida albicans* was markedly inhibited by normal serum, but that this inhibition was progressively diminished by addition of iron or by lowering pH.

A different interpretation is given by Hegenauer and Saltman (1975), who have studied many aspects of iron metabolism. They agree that transferrin is bacteriostatic and that saturation of transferrin would negate this effect. But they point out that orally administered iron will *not* fully saturate transferrin in the serum. Indeed the normal range of saturation of transferrin is only 20 to 45 per cent and orally administered iron does not result in greater-than-normal levels of saturation. Accordingly, it seems reasonable to conclude that there is considerable clinical evidence suggesting (and some evidence to the contrary), that iron-deficiency anemia in children reduces their resistance to infection. And there is almost no clinical evidence that oral administration of iron has an adverse effect on resistance to infection, whereas there is some evidence of a favorable effect. On the basis of these findings, the author favors prevention or treatment of iron deficiency by giving adequate amounts of this substance either in food or as supplements to the diet.

The effect of inanition from limitation of food has mostly synergistic actions on bacterial infections but antagonistic effects on viral and protozoal infections.

Scrimshaw and colleagues, after studying hundreds of reports, drew some general conclusions. "Synergism is the characteristic reaction with infectious agents such as bacteria, rickettsiae, intestinal protozoa, and intestinal helminths." They recorded over 150 instances of synergism and only 13 of antagonism. But they also stated ". . . On the other hand, antagonism is relatively common with viruses, which are intracellular and highly dependent upon the metabolism of the cell."

EFFECTS OF INFECTION ON NUTRITIONAL REQUIREMENTS

According to Scrimshaw and colleagues (1968), all infectious diseases have direct, adverse metabolic effects and they may also influence the amount and kind of food consumed. Although most of the evidence is based on studies in animals, a number of metabolic studies in humans provide supportive data. Furthermore, information on morbidity and mortality of specific infectious diseases in populations clearly supports the concept that infection increases nutritional needs, but often decreases food consumption. Specific examples include enteric infections that lead to diarrhea and malabsorption of protein and other nutrients. In addition, most febrile illnesses cause an increase in urinary excretion of nitrogen. This was formerly attributed to an increased rate of protein catabolism but more recent evidence suggests that the defect is one of impaired synthesis in the face of continuing breakdown of protein.

Tuberculosis also results in an increase in urinary excretion of nitrogen accompanied by anorexia and a decreased intake of food. In most chronic infectious diseases there is a marked decrease in levels of albumin in serum. This is a reflection of the short half-life of this protein and the marked impairment of protein synthesis that accompanies any catabolic state, whether it results from infection, injury, or operation.

Some viral infections, particularly measles, impose a very severe nutritional stress on an individual. Measles is a common precursor of kwashiorkor in undernourished children in many of the developing nations. Children who have lost weight from an infection need more protein to compensate for growth lost during the illness (Whitehead and Biol, 1977).

Helminthic infestations may interfere with absorption of protein and other essential nutrients. Hookworm infestations may not cause as much bleeding as was once believed, but they result in surprisingly great losses of albumin into the lumen of the bowel.

Acute infectious illnesses, especially in children, may result in substantial lowering of the concentration of vitamin A in plasma. Infection can precipitate acute nutritional deficiencies of vitamin A in persons with latent deficiency. This is still an important cause of blindness in children living in Indonesia and other countries where deficiency of vitamin A is common: And vitamin-A deficiency impairs protein synthesis and may also contribute to the anemia (Hodges et al., 1977).

Infection can also affect thiamin metabolism. Individuals who chronically consume less than adequate amounts of thiamin may develop acute beriberi following the onset of a febrile infectious illness. Presumably, the added nutritional needs imposed by fever result in metabolic decomposition of thiamin-dependent enzyme systems.

Folic acid deficiency may be precipitated by acute respiratory infections in children who have less than adequate intakes of this vitamin. Animal studies have confirmed this relationship between intercurrent infection and precipitation of megaloblastic anemia in monkeys fed a diet low in folic acid.

In children who are deficient in vitamin D, the calcium level in serum may be normal or slightly low, but classically the level of phosphorus is low. These children may have a calcium balance that is precarious and easily upset. They are not able to mobilize calcium from bone as rapidly as normal and they have little Ca^{++} reserve. Consequently, the metabolic trauma of an acute infection can cause a rapid fall in serum levels of calcium. This is particularly apt to occur in premature infants.

CELL-MEDIATED IMMUNITY

It is now well established that many of the functions of the immunologic system are performed by specialized cells. The most abundant of these are called "T-cells" and are lymphocytes that were formed in bone marrow and transformed in the thymus. They constitute about 60 per cent of circulating lymphocytes. Cell-mediated immunity (CMI) is defined as "that particular response of the immune system which requires previously sensitized thymus-derived lymphocytes and is independent of circulating antibody" (Wing and Remington, 1977). CMI is of major importance in resistance to a variety of intracellular organisms as well as foreign cells including allografts and malignant tumors. CMI is responsible in part for the phagocytic activities of macrophages, and for synthesis of interferon and other nonspecific defense factors. CMI activity can be estimated by a variety of tests: a delayed hypersensitivity test, a lymphocyte transformation test, and a mixed lymphocyte reaction.

Patients who are severely malnourished, including children with kwashiorkor (Edelman, 1977), and especially patients with disseminated malignant disease, may have lost most or all of their CMI. Immunosuppressive measures, of course, inhibit CMI as their primary action. Souchon and others (1975) have shown that although many patients with disseminated malignant disease lack CMI, restoration of their nutritional state by parenteral feeding often restores their CMI. This is associated with a better prognosis for response to other forms of anticancer treatment.

Kwashiorkor is known to impair polymorphonuclear neutrophil function in children (Schopfer and Douglas, 1976). This form of cellular immunity is more directly related to microbicidal activity and may be completely absent in this form of malnutrition. These authors estimated that there are more than 350 million children in the world who are suffering from some degree of protein-calorie malnutrition. Marasmus represents one end of the spectrum (lack of protein *and* calories), and kwashiorkor the other end (primary protein deficiency with some calories). Other deficiency syndromes may impair the functions of polymorphonuclear neutrophils but presumably lack of protein leads the list.

SURPLUS OF NUTRIENTS

It seems to be human nature to be gullible, and scientists are no exception. The fact that deficiency of a specific nutrient results in increased susceptibility to infection seems to suggest that very large amounts of the same substance should give greater-than-normal protection against infection. This type of reasoning has led to a series of trials of one vitamin after another in the hope of preventing or curing infections.

In the 1930's there was a wave of enthusiasm for giving cod liver oil to prevent or treat respiratory infections. Beard (1934) gave vitamins A and D to subjects and reported not only a 50 per cent reduction in the number of colds but also two-thirds of the colds contracted were "mild."

Cameron (1935) gave cod liver oil or other forms of vitamin A to subjects and failed to find convincing evidence of a reduction in the number of colds but the duration of colds was reduced by "five to ten days" and 60 per cent of those with colds were "improved" by the treatment.

Holmes and others (1936) performed a five-year study in an industrial plant. More than 3000 subjects were followed throughout the five years. Half received a tablespoonful of cod liver oil daily, five times each week. The results were difficult to evaluate, but the authors stated that throughout the five years, the treated subjects had about 30 per cent less absenteeism caused by colds or influenza. But now, forty years later, we recognize that neither vitamin A nor vitamin D will prevent colds and either may be toxic if given in excessive doses.

The concept of advocating very large doses of vitamin C for the general public in the hope of preventing or ameliorating colds will be discussed in more detail in the chapter on "Food.Fads and Megavitamin Therapy." It is sufficient to quote the opinion of Dykes and Meier (1975), who reviewed all pertinent publications on this subject and concluded, in part: (1) There is little convincing evidence to support the claims. (2) The most convincing evidence was reported by Anderson and colleagues but their second study failed to confirm the first. (3) Even if ascorbic acid were shown statistically to be effective in reducing the incidence or severity of colds, it still would be necessary to establish its therapeutic role. (4) Until such time as pharmacologic doses of ascorbic acid have been shown to have an obvious and important clinical value, we cannot advocate its unrestricted use for such purposes.

Since that was published, there have been additional adverse reports in the form of therapeutic failure and in the form of disturbing toxicity. The author does not advocate the use of ascorbic acid as a preventive of the common cold.

SUMMARY

Nutrition has, in many ways, an important impact on resistance to and recovery from infection. Most of the supporting evidence describes the adverse effects of deficiency of one or more essential nutrients. Some deficiencies are "synergistic" with infectious agents and either weaken the host's resistance or facilitate growth of the invading organism. In a few instances, a nutritional deficiency is actually antagonistic in that it protects the host or impairs the growth of the infecting organism.

Many years ago it was found that deficiencies of certain nutrients impaired formation of circulating antibodies. Now it is recognized that cell-mediated immune mechanisms also can be inhibited by certain types of malnutrition. This is an exciting finding in view of the role of cell-mediated immune mechanisms in inhibiting growth of malignant cells.

Nutrition is still in its infancy but already it appears to be highly important in the clinical setting as well as in preventive medicine.

REFERENCES

Axelrod, A. E.: Immune processes in vitamin deficiency states. *Amer. J. Clin. Nutr.* 24:265, 1971.

Axelrod, A. E., Carter, B. B., McCoy, R. H., and Geisinger, R.: Circulating antibodies in vitamin-deficiency states. I. Pyridoxine, riboflavin and pantothenic acid deficiencies. *Proc. Soc. Exper. Biol. Med.* 66:137, 1947.

Beard, H. H.: The prophylactic effect of vitamins A and D upon the prevention of the common cold and influenza. *J. Amer. Dietet. Assoc.* 10:193, 1934.

Bhaskaran, P., Prasad, J. S., and Krishnamachari, K. A. V. R.: Anaemia and immune response (Letter to the Editor). *Lancet* 1:1000, 1977.

Cameron, H. C.: The effect of vitamin A upon incidence and severity of colds among students. *J. Amer. Dietet. Assoc.* 11:189, 1935.

Dykes, M. H. M., and Meier, P.: Ascorbic acid and the common cold. Evaluation of its efficacy and toxicity. *J.A.M.A.* 231:1073, 1975.

Edelman, R.: Cell-mediated immune response in protein-calorie malnutrition — A Review. In *Malnutrition and the Immune Response*, Robert M. Suskind (ed.). New York, Raven Press, 1977, pp. 47–75.

Elin, R. J., and Wolff, S. M.: Effect of pH and iron concentration on growth of *Candida albicans* in human serum. *J. Infect. Dis.* 127:705, 1973.

Faulk, W. P., and Vitale, J. J.: Immunology. In *Nutritional Support of Medical Practice*, Howard A. Schneider, Carl E. Anderson, and David B. Coursin (eds.). New York, Harper & Row, 1977, pp. 341–346.

Gontzea, I.: II. The effects of underfeeding (undernutrition), pp. 20–55; III. Importance of protein intake, pp. 59–99; VI. Importance of vitamins, pp. 110–166. In *Nutrition and Anti-infectious Defence*, 2nd edition, Iancu Gontzea, and Florin R. Jantea (eds.). Basesl, S. Karger, 1974.

Gordon, J. E.: Synergism of malnutrition and infectious disease. In *Nutrition in Preventive Medicine*, G. H. Beaton, and J. M. Bengoa (eds.). Geneva, World Health Organization Monograph 62, 1976, pp. 193–209.

Hegenauer, J., and Saltman, P.: Iron and susceptibility to infectious disease. *Science* 188:1038, 1975.

Hodges, R. E., Bean, W. B., Ohlson, M. A., and Bleiler, R. E.: Factors affecting human antibody response: V. Combined deficiencies of pantothenic acid and pyridoxine. *Amer. J. Clin. Nutr.* 11:187, 1962.

Hodges, R. E., Sauberlich, H. E., Canham, J. E., Wallace, D. L., Rucker, R. B., Mejia, L. A., and Mohanram, M.: Hematopoietic studies in vitamin A deficiency. *Amer. J. Clin. Nutr.* (in press), 1977.

Holmes, A. D., Pigott, M. G., Sawyer, W. A., and Comstock, L.: Cod liver oil — A five-year study of its value for reducing industrial absenteeism caused by colds and respiratory diseases. *Industrial Med. Surg.* 5:359, 1936.

Schneider, J. A., Weller, M., Gersh, E. S., Trauner, D., and Nyhan, W. L.: Rickets. *West. J. Med.* 125:203, 1976.

Schopfer, K., and Douglas, S. E.: Neutrophil function in children with kwashiorkor. *J. Lab. Clin. Med.* 88:450, 1976.

Scrimshaw, N. S., Taylor, C. E., and Gordon, J. E.: I. Basic principles and considerations, pp. 11–23; II. Effect of infection on nutritional status, pp. 24–59; III. Effect of malnutrition on resistance to infection, pp. 60–142. In *Interactions of Nutrition and Infection.* Geneva, World Health Organization, 1968.

Souchon, E. A., Copeland, E. M., Watson, P., and Dudrick, S. J.: Intravenous hyperalimentation as an adjunct to cancer chemotherapy with 5-fluorouracil. *J. Surg. Res.* 18:451, 1975.

Srikantia, S. F., Prasad, J. S., Bhaskaram, C., and Krishnamachari, K. A. V. R.: Anemia and immune response. *Lancet* 1:1307, 1976.

Stiehm, E. R.: Biology of immunoglobulins: humoral and secretory — A Review. In *Malnutrition and the Immune Response,* Robert M. Suskind (ed.). New York, Raven Press, 1977, pp. 141–168.

Suskind, R. M., Thanangkul, O., Damrongsak, D., Leitzmann, C., Suskind, L., and Olson, R. E.: The malnourished child: clinical, biochemical, and hematological changes. In *Malnutrition and the Immune Response,* Robert M. Suskind (ed.): New York, Raven Press, 1977a, pp. 1–8.

Suskind, R. M., Kulapongs, P., Vithayasi, V., and Olson, R. E.: Iron deficiency anemia and the immune response. In *Malnutrition and the Immune Response,* Robert M. Suskind (ed.). New York, Raven Press, 1977b, pp. 387–393.

Wehrle, P. F., and Haddad, Z. H.: Infection and immunity. In *Communicable and Infectious Diseases,* Franklin H. Top, Sr., and Paul F. Wehrle (eds.). St. Louis, C. V. Mosby, 1976, pp. 1–7.

Weinberg, E. D.: Roles of metallic ions in host-parasite interactions. *Bacteriol. Rev.* 30:136, 1966.

Weinberg, E. D.: Roles of iron in host-parasite interactions. *J. Infect. Dis.* 124:401, 1971.

Whitehead, R. G., and Biol, F. I.: Protein and energy requirements of young children living in the developing countries to allow for catch-up growth after infections. *Amer. J. Clin. Nutr.* 30:1545, 1977.

Wing, E. J., and Remington, J. S.: Cell-mediated immunity and its role in resistance to infection. *West. J. Med.* 126:14, 1977.

10

NUTRITION AND THE KIDNEY

*Raymond D. Adelman, M.D.,
and Robert E. Hodges, M.D.*

In the short span of half a century, the outlook for the patient with serious renal disease has improved dramatically, largely as a result of a fortunate coincidence of events: a growing understanding of renal physiology, new knowledge of immune mechanisms, the discovery of effective antibiotics, new technology of both peritoneal and hemodialysis, and ultimately, renal transplantation. With these new-found opportunities to restore many patients to comfortable, useful lives, it has become mandatory that physicians utilize all available knowledge and skills to improve the nutritional state of patients with renal disease. What once was little more than a means of delaying inevitable death has now become a method of improving the quality of life, reducing the frequency of dialysis, and in many instances, preparing a patient for renal transplantation. This chapter will briefly review renal physiology, view the role of the kidney in nutritional diseases, and then discuss nutritional management of the following renal disorders: acute glomerulonephritis, nephrotic syndrome, chronic renal failure, acute renal failure, and urolithiasis.

PHYSIOLOGY OF THE KIDNEY

As Homer W. Smith (1951) indicated many years ago, the kidney maintains an internal environment compatible with life outside the sea. Actually, the kidney serves four major functions. First, it is responsible for maintaining proper volume and composition of body fluids, especially the extracellular fluid which bathes cells and cushions them from abrupt physiochemical changes. Extracellular fluid in the circulatory system and in the digestive tract plays a key role in the transportation of nutrients to and removal of products from cells. Extracellular fluid volume is regulated primarily through variations in renal conservation and excretion of sodium, chloride, and water. Second, the kidney excretes hydrogen ions, which normally accumulate in the body at a rate of about 50 to 100 mEq per day in the adult and 2 to 3 mEq/kg/day in the child. Renal acid-base regulation is primarily accomplished by resorption of filtered bicarbonate, formation of ammonium, and titration of acids, especially phosphates. Third, the kidney acts as an endocrine organ. It synthesizes erythropoietin, which stimulates erythropoiesis in bone marrow; renin, which influences blood pressure; and 1,25-dihydroxycholecalciferol, which is the most active form of vitamin D. Other hormones such as prostaglandins and somatomedin are also synthesized by the kidney. Fourth, the kidney, by filtration of plasma and formation of urine, eliminates wastes and surplus compounds such as urea, creatinine, uric acid, phosphates, and sulfates.

The kidney may, in fact, be considered an organ of nutrition. It allows the normal individual to consume a wide variety of foods and compensates with remarkable efficiency for transient dietary binges or privations. Hence, diuresis follows overhydration and antidiuresis follows underhydration. Ingestion of highly salted foods results in increased urinary sodium excretion, whereas absence of dietary salt is accompanied by virtual cessation of renal sodium excretion. Similar adjustments in urinary excretion may occur with varying dietary loads of acid, alkali, potassium, and many other substances. The remarkable manner in which our body adapts to the tortures of freak diets and Brobdingnagian dosages of vitamins hinges to a large degree on renal adaptation. But even the kidney is limited in its adaptive powers; and these limits become much more apparent in the presence of renal disease.

THE KIDNEY IN NUTRITIONAL DISEASES

Malnutrition. Severe disturbances in nutrition may have a pronounced effect upon renal function and morphology. Children with protein-calorie malnutrition have glomerular filtration rates, as measured by inulin clearance, that are only about one-half to one-third of normal. Similar findings have been reported in adults, although reports have been conflicting (Klahr and Alleyne, 1973). Why this occurs is unclear: it may be related to hypoalbuminemia, decreased effective plasma volume, decreased cardiac output, decreased renal blood flow, or some combination of these. Interestingly, although urea clearance is normally 60 per cent of inulin clearance in the well-nourished individual, urea clearance in malnutrition often falls to less than 25 per cent of inulin clearance values, regardless of glomerular filtration rate or state of hydration. This may reflect increased or even active tubular resorption of urea, perhaps a compensatory mechanism for conservation of nitrogen in the face of nitrogen deficiency from inadequate protein intake (Klahr and Alleyne, 1973). Gallina and Dominguez (1971) observed that when obese humans were fed a low calorie diet, they could utilize urea in lieu of a portion of their dietary protein if their diet contained adequate amounts of carbohydrates. They could not utilize urea when there was a carbohydrate deficit. Thus decreased dietary protein and the possible utilization of urea as a nitrogen source for anabolism may explain the low blood urea levels commonly seen in undernutrition. Low creatinine levels are also common, a result of decreased muscle mass from which creatinine is derived. Hence, in the malnourished patient, urea nitrogen and creatinine levels may appear deceptively normal despite substantially diminished renal function.

Malnourished patients commonly have an abnormality of urine concentration and may present clinically with polyuria, polydipsia, and nocturia (Klahr and Alleyne, 1973). This does not appear to be an antidiuretic hormone deficiency or insensitivity since these subjects will secrete antidiuretic hormone in response to an appropriate stimulus such as infusion of hypertonic saline and they also will respond to pitressin administration. One likely explanation is that the renal medulla in malnourished individuals is not sufficiently hypertonic to allow for adequate concentration of urine. Diminished medullary tonicity may result from decreased medullary urea concentration from low protein intake. Animals fed low protein diets develop the same phenomenon. Malnourished humans show a return of renal concentrating ability after blood urea levels rise in response to either protein repletion or short-term parenteral infusion of urea.

The defect in urinary acidification which occurs in malnutrition does not, under ordinary circumstances, lead to difficulty since it is balanced by a decrease in acid formation resulting from reduced net protein degradation. Malnourished individuals, however, when stressed with acid loads become acidotic, primarily because of a blunted rise in titratable acid which results from low serum phosphate levels and thus reduced filtered phosphate (Klahr and Alleyne, 1973).

Druing prolonged starvation the kidney, unlike other organs, is metabolically very active. Oxygen consumption increases and various substrates such as lactate, pyruvate and fatty acids are utilized, resulting in increased renal production of glucose and acetoacetate. During starvation the kidney is actually responsible for almost half the total glucose synthesized daily.

TABLE 10-1 COMMON CAUSES OF POTASSIUM DEFICIENCY

GASTROINTESTINAL LOSSES
  Diarrhea, vomiting, use of purgatives, malabsorption (including Crohn's Disease and ulcerative colitis)

URINARY LOSSES
  Hyperaldosterone — primary or secondary, Cushing's Syndrome, diabetes mellitus, renal tubular dysfunction, chronic renal failure, abuse of steroids, overdose of diuretics

Potassium Deficiency. Potassium deficiency can lead to functional and structural disturbances of the kidney that may, if the deficiency is severe and prolonged, become permanent. Potassium depletion itself (Table 10–1) may result from gastrointestinal losses due to diarrhea, vomiting, fistula drainage, extensive use of purgatives, and malabsorption or from urinary losses due to primary or secondary hyperaldosteronism, Cushing's syndrome, diabetes mellitus, renal tubular dysfunction, and chronic renal failure with salt wasting. Abuse of steroids and overuse of diuretics are perhaps the most frequent causes of potassium deficiency today. Symptoms of potassium deficiency include polydipsia, nocturnal frequency, polyuria, fatigue, and weakness of the limbs (Black, 1967). Electrocardiographic changes include an apparent prolongation of the Q-T interval, flattening and inversion of T-waves, and prominent U-waves. Mental disturbances are common, though they may be overlooked. Histologic changes in the kidneys include striking vacuolization of the proximal and distal convoluted tubules, and after a time, development of interstitial fibrosis. Functional abnormalities include vasopressin-resistant hyposthenuria and isosthenuria (inability to concentrate), an inability to acidify the urine maximally, and rarely, an inability to void as a result of muscular paralysis of the bladder (Black, 1967). Patients likely to develop potassium deficiency, especially those receiving steroids or diuretics, must be given an adequate oral intake of potassium (Milne et al., 1957; Macpherson and Pearse, 1957). Often, potassium supplements, in the form of potassium gluconate, potassium citrate, potassium carbonate, or potassium acetate, are necessary, since patients may lapse in following dietary instructions which encourage daily intake of fruits and vegetables that are high in potassium (see Table 10–2). Enteric-coated potassium chloride tablets must be avoided because they can cause ulceration or even perforation of the bowel.

Other Nutritional Disturbances and the Kidney. In animal models, deficiencies of vitamins C, K, A, and E, linoleic acid, choline, magnesium, and chloride all have been associated with renal structural changes, most notably in the tubules. Human counterparts to these experimental states have not been reported. On the other hand,

TABLE 10–2

FRUITS AND VEGETABLES WITH HIGH POTASSIUM CONTENT
Banana, watermelon, cantaloupe, oranges, apricots, tomatoes, dried fruits (raisins, prunes, dates, figs), potatoes, broccoli, spinach

POTASSIUM CONTENT OF BEVERAGES

per 8 oz. serving	*k mEq*
prune juice	16.0
tomato juice	14.2
skim milk (fortified)	12.3
cocoa	10.5
orange juice	11.7
grapefruit juice	9.2
whole milk	8.6
pineapple juice	8.6
grape juice	7.4
apple cider	6.1
instant coffee	6.1
drip coffee	4.9
Coca Cola	3.2
Pepsi Cola	0.2
Koolade	0

several cases of vitamin D excess have been reported in man. These have led to hypercalcemia, hypercalciuria, nephrocalcinosis, nephrolithiasis, and in some cases, renal insufficiency (Yendt, 1972). An early sign of hypervitaminosis D is impaired concentrating ability, resulting in polyuria and polydipsia. One child, immobilized with Crohn's disease, developed hypercalciuria and renal stones while receiving total parenteral nutrition solutions containing a high concentration of calcium (Adelman et al., 1977).

NUTRITION IN KIDNEY DISEASE

Acute Glomerulonephritis. Traditional treatment of acute glomerulonephritis emphasized the need for protein restriction to "rest" the kidney from what was thought to be its chief metabolic task, namely the transport of urea. It is now apparent that a substantial part of the energy required by the kidney is consumed by the convoluted tubules in the act of transporting electrolytes, and not in the movement of urea. Hence, protein restriction *per se* is not required in acute glomerulonephritis unless patients exhibit oliguria and anuria with rising blood urea nitrogen and creatinine levels, in which case the regimen for acute renal failure (see page 245, below) should be instituted. Clinical studies have not shown protein restriction in cases of mild to moderately severe acute glomerulonephritis to be of any benefit, either in the short-term or in the long-term analysis.

Patients who develop edema and hypertension do require sodium restriction, since they suffer from an expanded extracellular fluid space which may progress, if unchecked, to congestive heart failure, pulmonary edema, seizures, cerebral vascular accidents, and death. Dietary sodium may be reduced in adults to 40 milliequivalents* a day and in children to a "no added salt" diet. With severe edema and hypertension, daily sodium intake may be reduced to 20 milliequivalents for adults and 5 milliequivalents for children. In actual practice, such severe reduction may prove unacceptable to patients because of its effect on the palatability of the diet.

It is prudent to restrict the intake of foods high in potassium (Table 10-2) until it is apparent that the urine output is adequate, because hyperkalemia can develop rapidly in these patients.

Nephrotic Syndrome. The nephrotic syndrome is characterized by heavy proteinuria (usually greater than 3.5 gm per $1.73M^2$ per day), hypercholesterolemia, hypoalbuminemia, and, usually, edema. Urinary protein losses may be massive, greater than 25 gm per day in some nephrotic patients. Albumin is the major protein lost in the urine, but other important plasma proteins such as ceruloplasmin, transferrin, immune globulins, and thyroid binding protein may also be lost. Increases in serum lipids, including cholesterol, triglycerides, and phospholipids, are usually seen. If sufficiently large protein losses persist, edema accompanied by avid sodium and water retention will result. The overall effect of continued protein losses on an individual is predictable. Considerable wastage occurs, not only of plasma proteins, but also of body tissues, especially muscle and cartilage. The net result is malnutrition. Edema may round out body contours and obscure the miserable condition of these patients. The physician may be startled by the appearance of extreme cachexia that becomes apparent only after removal of edema fluid.

The primary goals of dietary management of the nephrotic syndrome are: salt restriction, adequate protein intake, and abundant caloric intake. A state of avaricious sodium retention obligates the restriction of dietary sodium to retard further accumulation of edema fluid. Low-sodium milk products (such as Lonalac) and low electrolyte caloric supplements (such as Contralyte, Cal-Power, Hycal, Polycose) may be especially useful in providing calories without the usual component of sodium. Diuretics may be needed for relief of symptomatic edema, although they must be used with caution, for they do not affect the underlying process and may cause hypokalemia, volume depletion, and even shock (Yamauchi and Hopper, 1964).

Protein intakes of 100-150 gm per day for the average adult

---

*sodium in milliequivalents $\times$ 57 = NaCl in mg: 20 mEq = 1140 mg NaCl; 5 mEq = 285 mg NaCl patient and 2 to 3 gm/kg for the child should be encouraged in order to compensate for the excessive urinary losses and to allow for repletion of body protein deficits. Despite continuing proteinuria, patients who consume high protein diets may show positive nitrogen balances reflecting net retention of protein. Rises in serum protein may be accompanied by increased proteinuria. This is usually no cause for alarm because it merely reflects the increased amount of protein filtered by the kidney and is not necessarily an indication of renal deterioration. It is preferable to replace urinary protein losses with an equivalent amount of protein of high biological value (see below) such as milk, meat, fish, fowl, and egg protein.

An essential and often neglected point is that a high caloric intake must be maintained during a high protein diet to minimize the amount of protein catabolized by the body for energy needs. Patients receiving steroid therapy usually have good caloric intakes because of drug-induced hyperphagia.

The presence of hyperlipidemia in most nephrotic patients and the evidence that these patients have a substantially greater incidence of coronary heart disease has led some nephrologists to recommend measures to decrease lipidemia, such as the use of hypocholesterolemic agents and unsaturated fats in the diet. However logical this may seem, the actual benefit of this approach has yet to be demonstrated.

Chronic Renal Failure. Renal failure, an ill-defined term implying a marked inability to perform renal function adequately, is accompanied by retention of nitrogenous wastes, acidosis, and abnormalities in electrolyte balance. Clinical manifestations of chronic renal failure include fatigability, hypertension, bone disease, and, in children, poor growth. In its more severe state, uremic poisoning ensues with lassitude, nausea, vomiting, pruritus, muscle twitching, paresthesias, convulsions, easy bruising, and congestive failure.

Anemia is present due to impaired production of erythropoietin, shortened red blood cell survival time, and often deficiencies of iron, folates, and perhaps other essential nutrients, including protein (Siddiqui and Kerr, 1971) and histidine (Kopple and Swendseid, 1975). In addition, blood loss may occur through the GI tract and externally with hemodialysis. Glucose metabolism becomes impaired as manifested by elevated fasting blood glucose levels and abnormal glucose tolerance curves, but frank diabetes mellitus seldom develops (Cohen, 1962). Insulin requirements in the diabetic may lessen owing to decreased renal insulin degradation. Hypercholesterolemia and hypertriglyceridemia are common in chronic renal failure, yet the mechanism remains obscure (Gutman et al., 1973).

When renal function is totally gone or severely compromised, food that could formerly be eaten because of renal "balancing" of body needs may no longer be tolerated. If body composition is to be maintained in a normal or near normal state, dietary intake must be adjusted. These adjustments concern protein, calories, fluids, minerals, and vitamins, and may also involve the use of oral medications.

The first and most important goal of diet therapy is to relieve unpleasant symptoms. Although some patients have few complaints, they may, after adopting a therapeutic diet, remark that they "feel much better" or have "regained my appetite." Perhaps the most important symptom to be relieved is the patient's conviction that he or she is doomed to a progressively more miserable existence until death arrives. When the patient learns that diet can lessen his or her distress in several ways and lead to better preparation for dialysis or renal transplantation, this patient's attitude may improve considerably.

The physician should aim toward minimizing the breakdown of body protein, normalizing electrolyte and water balance, and managing the bone disease and hypertension. It is extremely important that the physician work closely with a skilled dietitian to optimize dietary therapy by reducing monotony, increasing variety, and selecting high quality foods compatible with the patient's own preference and budget. Additional dietary information is available at local chapters of the Kidney Foundation and in an excellent source book, the *Mayo Clinic Renal Diet Cook Book* (Margie, J. D. et al., Western Publishing Co., New York, 1975).

Protein. Any discussion of protein requirement in renal failure requires a brief explanation of three important concepts: essential amino acids, nitrogen balance, and biological value.

There are eight essential amino acids required in the diet of normal adults: tryptophan, isoleucine, leucine, phenylalanine, threonine, methionine, valine, and lysine. Histidine appears to be essential in the diet of infants and uremic patients (Kopple and Swenseid, 1975). Some evidence suggests arginine also may be essential in uremia (Featherston et al., 1973). Amino acids are essential simply because their carbon skeletons cannot be adequately synthesized within the body. They must be ingested. Nonessential amino acids, on the other hand, can be formed *in vivo* using endogenous carbon skeletons and a nitrogen source. In uremia, urea may serve as a nitrogen source. In situations where rapid growth or acquired illness increases the need for the rate of protein synthesis, certain other amino acids become relatively essential, simply because the body cannot synthesize their carbon skeletons at a sufficient rate.

Nitrogen balance is the difference between nitrogen intake and nitrogen loss. In healthy persons consuming an average diet, three-fourths of nitrogen loss is urinary, the rest being fecal and epithelial. Positive nitrogen balance occurs with growth or with repletion of a protein deficit. A negative nitrogen balance implies loss of lean body mass that is being broken down in the absence of adequate protein synthesis. This, in turn, may result from lack of an adequate protein intake, lack of sufficient caloric energy to protect dietary proteins, or from a catabolic state resulting from severe illness or injury.

Biological value is defined as nitrogen retained/nitrogen absorbed. Foods of high biological value have: (1) most nitrogen present as essential amino acids; (2) all of the essential amino acids present; and (3) concentrations of the essential amino acids approximately proportional to minimal daily dietary requirement. Using the highest biological value proteins, such as eggs, milk, fowl, meat, and fish, it is possible to reach the minimal protein intakes consistent with nitrogen balance and still limit the total nitrogen load.

Giordano (1963) and Giovannetti and Maggiore (1964) used high-biological-value protein to study the incorporation of urea into protein in uremic subjects. They prepared low-protein pastas and bread substitutes together with essential amino acids either in pure form or as supplied by egg protein and demonstrated that nonessential amino acids could be synthesized by siphoning nitrogen from accumulated urea. This diet resulted in improvement in uremic symptoms, together with considerable reduction of some blood abnormalities. The Giordano-Giovannetti diet has, with some modifications, been widely used. These diets generally follow the pattern of essential amino acids as delineated by Rose (1928). Berlyne and others (1965) modified the Giordano-Giovannetti diet to suit British tastes. Their diet contained 18 to 20 gm of high-biological-value protein plus 0.5 gm of methionine. An important aspect of these diets was a high caloric intake of non-protein foods.

The level of renal impairment at which dietary protein restriction should begin is controversial. Some feel that restriction should be started early to prevent "trade offs" when metabolic adjustments are called into play to correct one abnormality (for example, hyperphosphatemia) but cause another (excess parathormone production). Other clinicians feel it is wise to wait until blood urea nitrogen reaches a level of 100 mg/dl or until uremic symptoms begin. Elevated blood urea nitrogen is a marker for retention of nitrogenous wastes contributing to the uremic syndrome. It is questionable to what extent urea itself contributes to uremic symptoms. Johnson and others (1972) studied urea-loaded patients with far advanced renal failure and observed that concentrations of blood urea of less than 300 mg/dl were well tolerated. (Since the molecular weight of urea is 60 and the urea molecule contains two nitrogen atoms with a total weight of 28, the "blood urea" value is approximately double the "BUN" value.) These authors concluded that urea is the least toxic of the various nitrogenous substances which accumulate in body fluids of the uremic patient. Rapid changes in urea concentration were, however, accompanied by headache, nausea, and tremor. The guidelines described by Anderson and colleagues (1973) appear to be reasonable approximations of dietary protein restriction in uremia:

Creatinine Clearance (ml/min/1.73M^2)	Grams/kg body weight/day
30–20	0.7–0.5
19–5	0.38
< 5	0.26

Studies by Kopple and colleagues (1968), however, indicate that daily protein restriction of less than 0.6 gram/kg body weight may not be necessary if 70 per cent of protein is of high biologic value. These figures are only estimates and each patient must be assessed individually with regard to blood urea nitrogen level, presence and severity of symptoms, willingness and ability of the patient to comply, the present state of nutrition, and special factors including growth needs in children, age, income, physical activity, and personality. One must avoid overzealous protein restriction, which may not be indicated and may result in malnutrition. Protein should be divided into meals and served with carbohydrate and fat.

Patients who are being treated with hemodialysis can and should receive higher levels of dietary protein (greater than 1.0 gm/kg/day) because of removal of protein-derived "wastes" by dialysis and because of large amino acid losses in the dialysate fluid (16–20 gm/6 hr). Peritoneal dialysis is also accompanied by nitrogen loss (1.65 gm albumin/1000 cc exchange) and dialyzed patients must have increased oral or intravenous protein intakes (1.5–2.0 gm/kg/day). Dietary protein may be increased gram per gram to match the urinary protein losses.

Essential amino acid supplementation of patients with chronic renal failure has been studied in several centers. Norée and Bergström (1975) gave 16 to 20 gm of unselected protein with oral supplementation of 14 to 21 gm of essential L-amino acids. Blood urea nitrogen fell, despite a doubling of nitrogen intake, and the general condition of patients improved. Josephson and others (1970) achieved positive nitrogen balance in uremic patients who received intravenous or oral essential amino acids along with low protein diets. Heidland and Kalt (1975) infused 17 grams of essential amino acids during the end of hemodialysis and noted rises in serum total protein, albumin, transferrin, and hemoglobin. Studies by Kopple and Swendseid (1977) and Pennisi and colleagues (1976) suggest that supplements of nonessential and essential amino acids are superior to essential amino acid supplements alone in promoting nitrogen balance. Metabolic abnormalities in uremia may increase dietary requirements of some or all essential and nonessential amino acids. There is evidence that tryptophan binding is reduced in uremic patients (Gulyassy et al., 1970; Gulyassy and De Torrente, 1975). Furthermore, the ability of the uremic patient to convert phenylalanine to tyrosine is impaired in renal failure, presumably because of reduced activity of the enzyme phenylalanine hydroxylase (Young and Parsons, 1971). Further studies in this area may more clearly define the role of amino acid supplementation in the management of the uremic patient.

Walser and others (1973) postulated that endogenous urea could be used for synthesis of essential as well as nonessential amino acids, provided the proper carbon skeletons were available. He administered such carbon skeletons in the form of α-keto analogues of the essential amino acids (valine, leucine, isoleucine, methionine, and phenylalanine, and in one instance, tryptophan and histidine) to ten severely uremic patients whose net nitrogen intake averaged 1.8 gm/day. In five subjects, there was improvement in uremic symptoms and a decline in the rate of appearance of urea nitrogen in the urine and body fluids. One totally anuric patient was maintained for almost a month on keto-acids, during which time blood urea nitrogen rose less than 1 mg/day while creatinine climbed from 14.4 to 29.6 mg/dl. There was no evidence of toxicity and no detectable accumulation of keto-acids in plasma or urine.

There is some controversy about the biochemical basis behind the effectiveness of the Giordano-Giovannetti diets. Since urea has recently been shown by Varcoe and colleagues (1975), in uremic and normal subjects, to contribute little of nitrogen for albumin synthesis, it is possible that low nitrogen diets reuse nitrogen primarily from reutilized amino groups before they are incorporated into urea (Kopple and Swendseid, 1977). Similarly, our understanding of the effectiveness of keto-acid supplementation is unclear since their nitrogen sparing action is greater than can be accounted for if all keto-acids are transaminated into essential amino acids (Richards, 1975). Furthermore, the effect of keto-acid supplementation on nitrogen balance persists several days after therapy is concluded.

Calorie Intake

Restoration of caloric balance is as important as limitation of protein intake. Most uremic patients have already restricted their food intake to such a degree as to superimpose starvation upon renal failure. Generous amounts of energy are needed to promote protein synthesis. The suggested level is 35 to 45 kcal/kg of normal body weight, but the optimal value for patients with renal failure appears to be perhaps 25 to 50 per cent higher, the precise amount depending upon weight, age, sex, physical activity, and degree of pre-existing undernutrition (Hyne et al., 1972). Calories can be provided through varied sources that are compatible with the personal and ethnic tastes of the patient, and with his or her budget. Giovannetti used as calorie sources butter, lard, vegetable oils, sugar, honey, maize starch, low protein wheat starch, tapioca, and alcohol. These ingredients were incorporated into soups, puddings, wafers, and spaghetti. Kark (1972) used ale, wine, avocado, sago, arrow root, and sherbets, meringues and nougats prepared with eggs. For patients who can tolerate sweets, there are many carbohydrate supplements, including gumdrops, popsicles, sugar, honey, and hard candy. For others, it is worth trying some of the commercial preparations, mentioned above, that provide calories without undue sweetness.

Water

Liberal fluid intake should be encouraged in the patient with chronic renal failure who does not have oliguria or anuria. Obviously excessive intake may lead to dilutional hyponatremia. However, deficient intake may result in dehydration and further impair renal function. Adults should be encouraged to drink around 2.5 liters of fluids/day and children around 100 ml/100 calories metabolized. Patients should be cautioned to increase fluid intake with fever or gastrointestinal upsets, and when in hot climates. In the hemodialysis patient, especially with volume dependent hypertension, fluids should be adjusted so as to prevent weight gains of greater than 1 kg between dialyses.

Sodium

Sodium requirements must be individualized for each patient. Arbitrary sodium restriction, especially in renal patients with pyelonephritis, analgesic abuse, medullary cystic disease, or hydronephrosis accompanied by considerable salt wasting, may lead to severe dehydration and pronounced deterioration of renal function. Excessive sodium intake can result in edema, hypertension, and congestive heart failure. Patients may be initially started on 50 to 75 mEq Na/day while 24-hour urinary sodium is measured. If sodium output equals intake dietary sodium may be gradually increased until sodium balance becomes positive or until evidence of mild edema occurs. Minimal obligatory sodium intake may be determined by cautiously lowering daily sodium intake until urinary sodium output exceeds oral intake or until signs of volume depletion occur. The patient is thus given a rough range of sodium intake adequate for his or her usual daily needs. Again gastrointestinal upsets and hot climatic temperatures are indications for liberalization of sodium intake. When salt requirements change as renal function deteriorates, further adjustments must be made.

Potassium

In general, potassium retention is not seen until the glomerular filtration rate falls below 5 ml/min. However, patients should be encouraged to avoid excessive intake of foods high in potassium (Table 10–2). Potassium-sparing diuretics such as spironolactone, transfusions with old blood, and large doses of such potassium salts as penicillin should be avoided.

Calcium and Phosphorus Balance. In the early phases of renal failure, calcium values may be mildly depressed and phosphorus slightly elevated, but with progressive failure there is more phosphate retention, leading to a reciprocal fall in serum calcium. In addition, there is poor gastrointestinal absorption of calcium from lack of $1,25(OH)_2CC$, often poor calcium intake, and calcium losses from bone buffering of hydrogen ion. Parathyroid hormone (PTH) is stimulated and osteodystrophy may ensue. Correction of calcium phosphorus imbalance is often difficult. Recent breakthroughs in the area of vitamin D metabolism suggest that hydroxylated derivatives of vitamin D may soon be readily available to the practitioner. Renal bone dystrophy can presently be effectively treated with massive doses of vitamin D, oral phosphate binding agents, and oral calcium supplements. Phosphate binding agents, such as aluminum hydroxide gels (e.g., Amphojel, 1 to 3 tsp/day [320–960 mg $Al(OH)_3$] for the infant or child and 50 to 100 ml/day [3200] for adults) may correct hyperphosphatemia.

In addition vitamin D is often needed for correction of osteodystrophy, but treatment with it should not be started until serum phosphorus levels are lowered. Start with 50,000 units of vitamin D daily by mouth and increase at monthly intervals until calcium and alkaline phosphatase levels normalize. Although some authorities have given very large doses, it probably is unnecessary to give more than 150,000 units daily. When bone pain is relieved, and chemical and radiologic findings have returned toward normal, the dose should be reduced to 50,000 units or less daily. Therapy may have to be continued for a year or longer before the desired result is achieved. One must keep in mind the risk of hypercalcemia with vitamin D therapy. Vitamin D activity persists for a long time, partly as a result of storage in body fat. Dihydrotachysterol has a shorter half-life and is preferable to vitamin D (1 mg dihydrotachysterol = 120,000 units vitamin D).

An important reason for disturbances of calcium and phosphorous metabolism in patients with chronic renal failure is the dependence of the body upon the kidney's ability to hydroxylate 25 OH-cholecalciferol into the most active form, 1,25-dihydroxy-cholecalciferol (Brickman et al., 1972). Administration of this highly potent vitamin (or hormone, as it is now called) to patients with advanced renal failure resulted in a rise in serum calcium, better absorption of radioactively labeled calcium, and a decrease in fecal calcium content. Since this compound is very difficult to produce other investigators sought to develop a synthetic substitute for it (Chalmers et al., 1973). 1,α-hydroxy-cholecalciferol was given to three patients with chronic renal failure. As little as 10 μg/day significantly increased calcium absorption, raised serum calcium levels, and reduced the alkaline phosphatase level. These compounds are being actively investigated in patients with renal failure (DeLucca, 1976). Oral calcium therapy may be used in conjunction with phosphate-binding gels and vitamin D therapy. Recommended dosages in adults are 5 to 10 grams of calcium carbonate.

Other Vitamin and Mineral Deficiencies. The anemia of renal failure is unique for two reasons: it is remarkably well tolerated and it is even more remarkably resistant to therapy. Probably all patients with chronic renal failure have some measure of nutritional deficiency and this is likely to become worse in those who undergo peritoneal dialysis or hemodialysis. Administration of a standard multivitamin preparation containing the recommended dietary allowance for each of the vitamins daily is sufficient to provide adequate amounts of most of these essential nutrients. But additional amounts of folic acid should be given because the quantity (400 μg) of mixed folates in most multiple vitamin preparations is meager. A daily dose of 500 μg of folic acid or four times this amount (2000 μg) of mixed folates is advised. In addition, serum concentrations of iron and transferrin should be measured to determine whether iron supplements are desirable. Small doses of ferrous gluconate or fumarate should be given orally three times daily until serum iron levels return to normal. There may be no measurable change in the hemoglobin or hematocrit values but iron deficiency affects several enzyme systems as well as hemoglobin synthesis.

For every patient, one must establish goals of therapy and set a plan of action. This will vary with each patient depending upon the type, severity, and duration of the renal disease. The patient with acute renal failure may die or begin to recover before any form of oral nutritional therapy can be instituted; but the patient with chronic renal disease may be followed over a period of several decades.

ACUTE RENAL FAILURE

The nutritional management of the patient in acute renal failure utilizes many of the principles already discussed. Protein intake is reduced to minimize urea formation and high caloric intake is encouraged for its protein sparing effect and for generally improved nutrition. High biological value protein .25 gm/kg of body weight/day in the adult, .5 gm/kg in the child, and 1 gm/kg in the infant should be provided with 35 to 45 calories/kg in the adult and 50 to 75 calories/kg in the child. Protein can be provided from food sources or essential amino acid preparations (such as Amin-Aid, which also contains nonprotein carbohydrate and fat calories). Additional calories can be provided through the use of fat substances and carbohydrate sources already mentioned (see Chronic Renal Failure). If oral intake is not possible due to vomiting, or to ileus or abdominal surgery, intravenous feeding can be provided with 10 per cent dextrose, Intralipid, and essential amino acid preparations such as Nephramine. If renal failure is non-oliguric (little or no decrease in urine volume but retention of waste products), fluids need not be restricted and adequate calories may be provided by intravenous solutions fed through a peripheral vein. In the patient with oligo-anuria, fluids should be restricted to insensible water loss plus urine output. Less fluid should be provided in the presence of edema or congestive heart failure. In the oligo-anuric patient parenteral nutrition through a central venous catheter or a Scribner shunt may be necessary to provide adequate calories. Abel and colleagues (1973) have shown improved survival and shortened duration of renal failure in patients with acute renal failure treated with intravenous essential L-amino acids and 57 per cent glucose. Toback (1977) has shown that infusions of amino acids in rats with mercuric chloride–induced acute renal failure increased the synthesis of choline-containing phospholipids for new membranes in regenerating tubular cells and decreased the level of renal insufficiency. Additional studies are needed to further define the role of parenteral nutrition in the management of acute renal failure.

The oligo-anuric patient should receive no sodium or potassium if possible. The physician should be aware of occult sodium sources, such as antibiotics, saline flushes of indwelling catheters, and sodium polystyrene sulfonate (such as Kayexalate). Large amounts of sodium bicarbonate therapy to completely normalize acidosis are unwise because of the sodium load entailed. Not infrequently, a salt-overloaded oligo-anuric patient will respond to a potent diuretic like furosemide. In a symptomatic patient diuretic therapy may be tried, but if a response is lacking, repeated or high dosages of furosemide, or both, should be avoided to prevent ototoxicity.

Hyperkalemia may occur despite rigid restriction of potassium intake, especially with acidosis, blood transfusions, or a highly catabolic state. Traditional measures for the treatment of hyperkalemia manifested by elevated serum potassium levels or electrocardiographic abnormalities include administration of hypertonic glucose with insulin, sodium bicarbonate, and calcium gluconate along with the oral or rectal administration, or both, of sodium polystyrene sulfonate.

Traditionally, dialysis has been instituted for severe hyperkalemia, acidosis, hypervolemia, azotemia, or signs of clinical deterioration. Early dialysis is now more frequently done because of the availability of facilities and trained personnel and the impression that early dialysis reduces morbidity and mortality in the patient with acute renal failure. The dialyzed patient may have protein intake liberalized (see discussion of "Protein," above). Additional carbohydrate calories become available from glucose present in peritoneal dialysate solutions. Food intake during peritoneal dialysis should be cautiously reduced or eliminated, since oral intake is frequently poorly tolerated.

NUTRITION IN CHILDREN WITH CHRONIC RENAL FAILURE

The concepts of protein restriction and of the Giordano-Giovannetti diet apply equally well to children and to adults. The physician should be aware that dietary therapy of uremic children requires tact, flexibility, ingenuity, and enormous patience. Generally, protein need not be restricted until glomerular filtration rates fall to the range of 5 to 20 ml/min/1.73 M^2. The decision as to when to restrict protein and to what extent is an arbitrary one. The physician must consider such factors as the presence or absence of uremic symptoms, the level of blood urea nitrogen, patient compliance, family economics and motivation, and the psychological profile of the patient. For example, uremic infants readily tolerate low-protein, low-phosphate milk formulas, but uremic adolescents with peer group diets of hamburgers and milkshakes often have great difficulty with severely curtailed "strange" diets. It isn't clear what protein allowance is best for optimal nutrition and growth in uremic children. It is probably reasonable not to restrict the diet of infants to less than 1.5 to 2.0 gm/kg of high quality protein nor to restrict older children and adolescents to less than 1 gm/kg. More severe protein restriction may be poorly tolerated by the patient and will probably interfere with growth.

Optimal caloric intake, as mentioned before, is even more important in children than in adults, yet it is often neglected. Some investigators have observed that uremic children who are fed low protein diets, in contrast to healthy individuals fed the same diets, continue to show improvement in nitrogen balance with additional caloric increments above the traditionally accepted "protein sparing" amounts

(Abitbol and Holliday, 1977). Growth failure in uremic children is a common, and often embarrassing, problem for the child. There is evidence indicating that growth failure may in part be related to inadequate energy intake. Growth may improve if energy intake reaches 80 to 100 per cent of the recommended dietary allowance for the individual's height and age (Chantler and Holliday, 1973).

Children with congenital renal anomalies often have problems with sodium wasting, loss of urine-concentrating ability, and inability to acidify the urine. They must, therefore, have these renal functions evaluated, preferably in a hospital under close supervision. Children with sodium wasting are advised not to allow sodium intake to fall below the minimal obligatory amount of sodium excreted in the urine, and to supplement their salt intake when there are additional losses, such as vomiting, diarrhea, or increased sweat losses on hot summer days. Arbitrary sodium restriction in a child with undetected sodium wasting can lead to severe dehydration, shock, and pre-renal failure. Children with excess sodium retention as evidenced by edema, hypertension, or congestive heart failure are urged not to consume salt in excess of the maximal amount they are capable of excreting. Modest dietary sodium restriction (no-added-salt diet and avoidance of foods high in sodium) may be required in these children. More severe restriction is usually poorly tolerated. In such cases, diuretic therapy is probably preferable. Children with defects in concentrating ability should always have free access to fluids and should never be prohibited from having fluids *ad libitum* prior to diagnostic or surgical procedures unless intravenous fluids are running at appropriate rates. Acidosis in these patients can be corrected by administration of sodium bicarbonate. This must be titrated to the patient's need. Usual doses are 2 to 4 mEq/kg of body weight daily, except for cases with proximal renal tubular acidosis where much larger amounts (in the range of 10–15 mEq/kg) are required. Excessive sodium bicarbonate should not be given if full correction of acidosis results in significant volume overload from sodium retention.

Children wih renal osteodystrophy may have impaired growth, rachitic changes, or bone pain, or they may be asymptomatic but have radiologic changes characteristic of osteoporosis and secondary hyperparathyroidism. Serum calcium may be low or normal, serum phosphorus elevated, and, characteristically, both alkaline phosphatase and parathormone may be elevated in parallel. Infants can be started with a daily dose of 10,000 units and this can be increased every 4 to 6 weeks by 5000 to 10,000 unit increments until a fall in alkaline phosphatase and a fall in serum parathormone occur. With time, there will also be evidence of healing of bone lesions. In older children and adolescents, the adult schedule given above can be applied, but these patients must be very carefully monitored to detect the onset of hypercalcemia. Once this occurs, vitamin D should be stopped until serum calcium falls to normal. Marked hypercalcemia may require other therapy including steroids, saline diuresis, and furosemide.

URINARY STONES

The pathogenesis of urolithiasis is complex and incompletely understood. Important influences on stone formation are (1) saturation of urine with respect to precipitating substances, (2) the presence of promoters of crystallization and aggregation, and (3) the presence of inhibitors of crystallization and aggregation. One salt may promote crystallization of another. For example, urate promotes crystallization of calcium oxalate. And both calcium oxalate and monosodium urate promote crystallization of calcium phosphate. A variety of inhibitors, including citrate, pyrophosphate, and magnesium, affect the crystallization of calcium phosphate and calcium oxalate. Rational measures to prevent urolithiasis include prevention of supersaturation, reduction or elimination of promoters of crystallization, and an increase in the concentration of inhibitors of stone formation. Much of current therapy still remains empirical.

Calcium stones, comprising 90 per cent of all renal calculi, may be composed of calcium phosphate, calcium oxalate, or a mixture of both. Less common stones contain struvite or magnesium ammonium phosphate, uric acid, or cystine. Although different therapeutic regimens may be used for different kinds of calculi, high fluid intake to avoid supersaturation is an important feature of all regimens. Patients must be encouraged to drink large quantities of fluids, not only during the day but before retiring at night and during the middle of night if awakening to urinate. Fluid intake must be increased in hot weather and in situations predisposing to dehydration, such as gastroenteritis. Ingested fluids should be checked to avoid excess consumption of calcium (from milk) or oxalates (from tea). Obstruction of the urinary tract and infection must be ruled out as well as excessive dietary intake of alkali, vitamin D, and proprietary drugs with calcium carbonate and sodium carbonate. As mentioned, intake of foods high in calcium, oxalate, or purines may have to be reduced.

Calcium-containing stones may result from distal renal tubular acidosis, urinary tract infection or obstruction, or from diseases associated with hypercalcemia and hypercalciuria (> 300 mg urinary calcium/24-hours in the adult on a normal diet; > 4 mg/kg/24 hours in the child). Diseases associated with hypercalcemia and urolithiasis include primary hyperparathyroidism, immobilization, sarcoidosis, hypervitaminosis D, milk alkali syndrome, Cushing's syndrome, and hyperthyroidism. Whenever possible, prevention of urolithiasis in these conditions should include therapy of the underlying disorder.

Around 80 per cent of cases of urolithiasis are idiopathic. Roughly 50 to 75 per cent of these patients have hypercalciuria, either due to increased gastrointestinal absorption of calcium or due to a renal leak of calcium, sometimes associated with elevated serum parathormone (Coe et al., 1973; Park et al., 1974). The remainder of patients with idiopathic urolithiasis have normal urinary levels of calcium, but may have increased urinary alkalinity, uric acid, or oxalate, or low levels of urinary stone inhibitors.

Treatment of patients with idiopathic hypercalciuria includes decreasing dietary calcium or use of sodium cellulose phosphate, orthophosphate, and thiazide diuretics, or both. Dietary intake of calcium may be reduced by eliminating milk and dairy products as well as vitamin D- and calcium-containing medicines. In addition, diets extremely high in protein, glucose, and salt should be avoided since they have been associated with hypercalciuria.

Because the effect of dietary manipulation in hypercalciuria is variable and may, over an extended period of time, have an ill effect on overall nutrition, other measures are often needed. Sodium cellulose phosphate (5 gm, two to three times daily) specifically inhibits intestinal calcium absorption and may be optimal therapy for absorptive hypercalciuria since it reduces hypercalciuria and urinary supersaturation of calcium phosphate and calcium oxalate, and retards stone formation. Cellulose phosphate also reduces magnesium absorption. Magnesium depletion may occur requiring adjunctive magnesium supplements (Thomas, 1978).

Although the exact mechanism of orthophosphate therapy is unclear, orthophosphate (1500–2000 mg of phosphorus daily) does lower urinary calcium and doubles or triples urinary pyrophosphate, a potent inhibitor of stone formation. The alkaline mixture of dibasic sodium and potassium phosphates, given three times daily in an isotonic dilution, appears to work best, and has the added advantage of increasing urinary citrate, another inhibitor of stone formation. Orthophosphate is not recommended in patients with renal insufficiency, because it may cause hyperphosphatemia and carries a substantial sodium load (Thomas, 1978).

Thiazides (hydrochlorothiazide 25 mg, b. i. d.) have proved remarkably useful in preventing urolithiasis in patients with or without hypercalciuria. They appear to act by inducing volume depletion and increasing tubular resorption of calcium. Although urinary calcium usually falls, there does not appear to be a clear relationship between the extent of decline and the prevention of calculus formation. Thiazides also decrease urinary oxalate and increase urinary magnesium and zinc, both inhibitors of stone formation (Yendt and Cohanian, 1978).

Some cases of urolithiasis are associated with elevated urinary levels of oxalate and urate. Increased urinary oxalate may be due to excessive ingestion of oxalate (spinach, beetroots, Swiss chard, rhubarb, tea, cocoa) or oxalate precursors (ethylene glycol, vitamin C). Primary hyperoxaluria is due to increased endogenous production of oxalate, whereas secondary and enteric hyperoxaluria is due to increased oxalate absorption. Patients with hyperoxaluria from excessive oxalate ingestion should curtail intake of foods high in oxalate. In patients with small bowel disease and acquired or secondary hyperoxaluria, oxalate calculi appear because of increased gastrointestinal absorption of oxalate and episodes of dehydration resulting in very acidic, concentrated urine. Therapy in these patients should include reduction in dietary oxalate and avoidance of dehydration. A diet high in calcium or a substitution of dietary fat by medium chain triglycerides may decrease intestinal absorption of oxalate and decrease urinary oxalate (Williams, 1978). Therapy of primary hyperoxaluria has been disappointing. Magnesium oxide and orthophosphate may be of some benefit (Prien and Gershoff, 1974).

Coe has described patients with calcium urolithiasis associated with hyperuricosuria (> 800 mg urinary uric acid/24 hours in the adult) (Coe and Kavalach, 1974). This may result from excessive intake of purine-rich foods (poultry, fish, meat) or overpopulation of uric acid. Uricosuria may also result from excessive ascorbic acid therapy (Stein et al., 1976). Reduction in dietary purines or use of allopurinol, or both, significantly reduces the incidence of new stone formation.

Struvite or magnesium ammonium phosphate stones are usually seen with very alkaline urine and the presence of high urinary ammonium due to infection with urea-splitting organisms such as Proteus. Therapy is directed toward eradication or containment of infection, relief of obstruction and acidification of the urine with methionine (8–12 grams daily) or ascorbic acid (500 mg every 4–6 hours). A promising new area, but still in the experimental stage, is the use of such urease inhibitors as acetohydroxaminic acid.

Uric acid stones form 5 to 10 per cent of all renal calculi and are seen in conditions leading to concentrated, very acid urine with elevated urinary uric acid. Therapy consists of a low purine intake, allopurinol, high fluid intake and alkali, since urate solubility increases markedly as urinary pH rises to 7.60.

REFERENCES

Abel, R. M., Beck, C. H., Jr., Abbott, W. M., Ryan, J. A., Jr., Barnett, G. O., and Fischer, J. E.: Improved survival from acute renal failure after treatment with intravenous essential L-amino acids and glucose: Results of a prospective, double blind study. New England J. Med. 288:695, 1973.

Abitbol, C. L., and Holliday, M. A.: Total parenteral nutrition in anuric children. Clin. Nephrol. 5:153, 1976.

Adelman, R. D., Abern, S. B., et al.: Hypercalciuria with nephrolithiasis: A complication of total parenteral nutrition. *Pediatrics* 59:473, 1977.

Anderson, C. F., Nelson, R. A., Margie, J. D., Johnson, W. J., and Hunt, J. C.: Nutritional therapy for adults with renal disease. *J.A.M.A.* 223:68, 1973.

Berlyne, G. M., Shaw, A. B., and Nilwarangkur, S.: Dietary treatment of chronic renal failure: experiences with a modified Giovannetti diet. *Nephron* 2:129, 1965.

Black, D. A. K.: *Essentials of Fluid Balance.* Oxford, Blackwell Scientific Publications, 1967.

Brickman, A. S., Coburn, J. W., and Norman, A. W.: Action of 1,25-dihydroxychole-calciferol, a potent, kidney-produced metabolite of vitamin D_3 in uremic man. *New England J. Med.* 287:891, 1972.

Chalmers, T. M., Davie, M. W., Hunter, J. O., Szaz, K. F., Pele, B., and Kodicek, E.: 1-alpha-hydroxycholecalciferol as a substitute for the kidney hormone, 1,25-dihydroxycholecalciferol, in chronic renal failure. *Lancet* 2:696, 1973.

Chantler, C., and Holliday, M. A.: Growth in children with renal disease with particular reference to the effects of caloric malnutrition: A review. *Clin. Nephrol.* 1:230, 1973.

Coe, F. L., Canterbury, J. M., Firpo, J. J., and Reiss, E.: Evidence for secondary hyperparathyroidism in idiopathic hypercalciuria. *J. Clin. Invest.* 52:134, 1973.

Coe, F. L., and Kavalach, A. G.: Hypercalciuria and hyperuricosuria in patients with calcium nephrolithiasis. *New England J. Med.* 291:1344, 1974.

Cohen, B. D.: Abnormal carbohydrate metabolism in renal disease. Blood glucose unresponsiveness to hypoglycemia, epinephrine, and glucagon. *Ann. Intern. Med.* 57:204, 1962.

DeLucca, H. F.: Vitamin D endocrinology. *Ann. Intern. Med.* 85:367, 1976.

Featherston, W. R., Rogers, Q. R., and Freedland, R. A.: Relative importance of kidney and liver in synthesis of arginine by the rat. *Amer. J. Physiol.* 224:127, 1973.

Gallina, D. L., and Dominguez, J. M.: Human utilization of urea nitrogen in low calorie diets. *J. Nutrition* 101:1029, 1971.

Giordano, C.: Use of exogenous and endogenous urea for protein synthesis in normal and uremic subjects. *J. Lab. Clin. Med.* 62:231, 1963.

Giovannetti, S., and Maggiore, Q.: A low nitrogen diet with proteins of high biological value for severe chronic uremia. *Lancet* 1:1000, 1964.

Gulyassy, P. F., Aviram, A., and Peters, J. H.: Evaluation of amino acid and protein requirements in chronic uremia. *Arch. Intern. Med.* 126:855, 1970.

Gulyassy, P. F., and de Torrente, A.: Tryptophan metabolism in uremia. *Kidney International* 7:S311, 1975.

Gutman, R. A., Uy, A., Shalhoub, R. J., Wade, A. D., O'Connell, J. M. B., and Recant, L.: Hypertriglyceridemia in chronic non-nephrotic renal failure. *Amer. J. Clin. Nutr.* 26:165, 1973.

Heidland, A., and Kult, J.: Long term effects of essential amino acids supplementation in patients on regular dialysis treatment. *Clin. Nephrol.* 3:234, 1975.

Hyne, B. E. B., Fowell, E., and Lee, H. A.: The effect of caloric intake on nitrogen balance in chronic renal failure. *Clin. Sci.* 43:679, 1972.

Johnson, W. J., Hagge, W. W., Wagoner, R. D., Dinapoli, R. P., and Rosevear, J. W.: Effects of urea loading in patients with far-advanced renal failure. *Mayo Clinic Proc.* 47:21, 1972.

Josephson, B., Berstrom, J., Furst, P., Hultman, E., Noree, L. O., and Vinnars, E.: Intravenous amino acid treatment in uremia. In *Proceedings of the 4th International Congress of Nephrology, Stockholm, 1969, Volume 2,* N. Alwall, F. Bergland, and B. Josephson (eds.). Basel, Karger, 1970, pp. 203–211.

Kark, R. M.: Nutritional management of chronic renal failure before dialysis or transplantation. *Modern Med.* p. 101, February 21, 1972.

Klahr, S., and Alleyne, G. A. O.: Effects of chronic protein-calorie malnutrition on the kidney. *Kidney International* 3:129, 1973.

Kopple, J. D., Sorensen, M. K., Coburn, J. W., Gordon, S., and Rubini, M. E.: Controlled comparison of 20 g and 40 g protein diets in the treatment of chronic uremia. *Amer. J. Clin. Nutr.* 21:553, 1968.

Kopple, J. D., and Swendseid, M. E.: Evidence that histidine is an essential amino acid in normal and chronically uremic man. *J. Clin. Invest.* 55:881, 1975.

Kopple, J. D., and Swendseid, M. E.: Amino acid and keto acid diets for therapy in renal failure. *Nephron* 18:1, 1977.
Macpherson, C. R., and Pearse, A. G. E.: Histochemical changes in the potassium-depleted kidney. *Brit. Med. J.* 13:19, 1957.
Milne, M. D., Muehrcke, R. C., and Heard, B. E.: Potassium deficiency and the kidney. *Brit. Med. J.* 13:15, 1957.
Norée, L. O., and Bergström, J.: Treatment of chronic uremic patients with protein poor diet and oral supply of essential amino acids. II. Clinical results of long term treatment. *Clin. Nephrol.* 3:195, 1975.
Park, C. Y. C., Ohata, M., Laurence, E. C., and Snyder, W.: The hypercalciurias: Causes, parathyroid functions, and diagnostic criteria. *J. Clin. Invest.* 54:387, 1974.
Pennisi, A. J., Wang M., and Kopple, J. D.: Effects of low nitrogen diets in uremic and control rats. *Proc. Fed. Amer. Soc. Exper. Biol.* 35:257, 1976.
Prien, E. L., Sr., and Gershoff, S. F.: Magnesium oxide-pyridoxine therapy for recurrent calcium oxalate calculi. *J. Urology* 112:509, 1974.
Recommended Dietary Allowances. Eighth revised edition. Washington, D.C., Food and Nutrition Board, National Research Council — National Academy of Sciences, 1974.
Richards, P.: Nitrogen-recycling in uremia: A reappraisal. *Clin. Nephrol.* 3:166, 1975.
Rose, W. C.: Discussion and correspondence: Does the amount of food consumed influence the growth of an animal? *Science* 67:488, 1928.
Siddiqui, J., and Kerr, D. N. S.: Complications of renal failure and their response to dialysis. *Brit. Med. Bull.* 27:153, 1971.
Smith, H. W.: *The Kidney: Structure and Function in Health and Disease.* New York, Oxford University Press, 1951.
Stein, H. B., Hasan, A., and Fox, I. H.: Ascorbic acid-induced uricosuria. A consequence of megavitamin therapy. *Ann. Intern. Med.* 84:385, 1976.
Thomas, W. C., Jr.: Use of phosphates in patients with calcarious renal calculi. *Kidney International* 13:390, 1978.
Toback, F. G.: Amino acid enhancement of renal regeneration after acute tubular necrosis. *Kidney International* 12:193, 1977.
Varcoe, R., Halliday, D., Carson, E. R., Richards, P., and Tavill, A. S.: Efficiency of utilization of urea nitrogen for albumin synthesis by chronically uraemic and normal men. *Clin. Sci. Mol. Med.* 48:379, 1975.
Walser, M., Coulter, A. W., Dighe, S., and Crantz, F. R.: The effect of keto-analogues of essential amino acids in severe chronic uremia. *J. Clin. Invest.* 52:678, 1973.
Williams, H. E.: Oxalic acid and its hyperoxaluric syndromes. *Kidney International* 13:410, 1978.
Yamauchi, H., and Hopper, J., Jr.: Hypovolemic shock and hypotension as a complication in the nephrotic syndrome. *Ann. Intern. Med.* 60:242, 1964.
Yendt, E. R.: Disorders of calcium, phosphorus and magnesium metabolism. In *Clinical Disorders of Fluid and Electrolyte Metabolism*, M. H. Maxwell, and C. R. Kleeman (eds.). New York, McGraw-Hill Book Company, 1972.
Yendt, E. R., and Cohanim, M.: Prevention of calcium stones with thiazides. *Kidney International* 13:397, 1978.
Young, G. A., and Parsons, F. M.: Plasma amino acid imbalance in patients with chronic renal failure on intermittent dialysis. *Clinica Chim. Acta* 27:491, 1971.

11

NUTRITION AND THE RESPIRATORY SYSTEM

Robert E. Hodges, M.D.

At first thought there does not seem to be a logical connection between the food we eat and the functioning of our lungs. Yet, on closer inspection, the relationship assumes surprising importance. Not only are nutrients necessary to optimal functioning of the respiratory organs, but certain common methods of feeding patients carry a high rate of morbidity and mortality; namely, gavage feeding, or worse, semistarvation. As interest in nutrition grows, the number of practical applications also grows to encompass virtually every aspect of medical practice, for nutrients are the pharmaceutical agents of life.

SPECIFIC FUNCTIONS OF THE RESPIRATORY SYSTEM

The most obvious and urgent function of the respiratory system is to ventilate the lungs at just the right rate and depth to meet the metabolic demands of the body at any given moment. This results in gaseous exchanges of oxygen and carbon dioxide and thus maintains body fluids and tissues in an optimal state of oxygenation and at an optimal pH, and, to a minor degree, the rate and depth of respiration aid in regulation of the body temperature. A seldom-recognized fact is the important role of nutrition in these basic functions. As shown by Keys (1950) semistarvation of otherwise healthy young men for twenty-four weeks resulted in significant decreases in their vital capacity (5.17 *versus* 4.78 L), in their minute volume (4.82 *versus* 3.35 L/min), and in their respiratory efficiency (47.93 *versus* 42.65). Their respiratory rate was slowed (11.45 *versus* 9.86), and their tidal volume was reduced (421 *versus* 340 cc/respiration).

Saltman and Salzano (1971) demonstrated, in healthy adults, remarkable increases in minute ventilation, tidal volume, blood lactate production, and oxygen consumption following ingestion of 900 kcal of carbohydrate. $\dot{V}e$ increased from 6.91 to 9.57, $\dot{V}t$ from 628 to 783, and RQ from 0.84 to 1.05. At the same time $\dot{V}CO_2$ rose from 628 to 783 and $\dot{V}O_2$ from 234 to 265.

Wilmore and others (1971) observed similar changes in the respiratory function of a group of burned patients given either 600, 3000, or 6000 kcal of energy daily. They reported significant increases in oxygen consumption and carbon dioxide production, accompanied by a moderate increase in minute ventilation.

An ample supply of glucose is also essential for another aspect of pulmonary function: the synthesis of phosphatidylcholine, or lecithin, which acts as a surfactant at the alveolar air-water interface. Fasting for four days results in a significant decrease in the enzymes of fatty acid and phospholipid synthesis in the lungs of rats (Gross, 1977).

Overnutrition can also impair ventilation and gaseous exchange. Extreme obesity, not surprisingly, limits the ability of the intercostal muscles and the diaphragm to ventilate the lungs. The result is chronic hypoxia and accumulation of carbon dioxide. This condition was described sixty years ago by William Osler, who wrote, ". . . a remarkable phenomenon associated with excessive fat in young persons is an uncontrollable tendency to sleep — like the fat boy in Pickwick." According to Vaisrub (1978), the "Dickensian connection" was missed or ignored by Auchincloss and colleagues (1955), but in the following year it was immortalized by Burwell and others (1956).

These episodes are by no means amusing, for they may result in death: indeed, that was the fate of the patient shown in Figure 11–1, who signed out of the hospital against medical advice and died the next day, apparently of hypoxia and carbon dioxide narcosis. The exact mechnism of death in this syndrome is uncertain; perhaps cardiac arrhythmias explain some deaths.

It is of interest to review the description of the serving boy, Joe (1836–37, by Charles Dickens), who apparently had the syndrome described by Osler and later by Burwell.

> "Damn that boy," said the old gentleman, "he's gone to sleep again."
> "How very odd!" said Mr. Pickwick.
> "Oh! odd indeed," returned the old gentleman; "I'm proud of that boy —
> wouldn't part with him on any account — he's a natural curiosity! Here,
> Joe — Joe — take these things away and open another bottle — d'ye hear?"

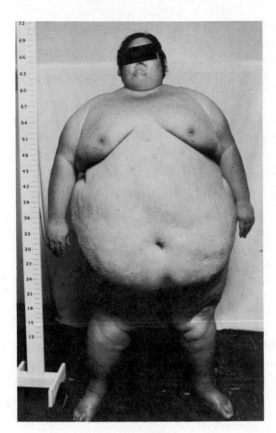

Figure 11-1 This patient, a 27-year-old man, weighed approximately 780 lbs. and was six feet, two inches tall. He had been falling asleep while sitting at the dinner table for several months. Also, he had stopped sleeping in a bed because of severe dyspnea while lying supine. Instead, he slept in an armchair.

On the day after this picture was taken, he signed himself out of the hospital against medical advice. His wife found him dead in bed the following morning.

The fat boy rose, opened his eyes, swallowed the huge piece of pie he had been in the act [of] masticating when he last fell asleep, and slowly obeyed his master's orders. . . .

Few physicians regard the lung as an endocrine organ but Mathé and others (1977) described non-respiratory functions of the lung that respond to catecholamines, steroids, and autacoids (represented by the prostaglandins). Indeed, the lung both synthesizes and destroys prostaglandins. Of the eight known families of prostaglandins — A, B, C, D, E, Fα, Fβ, G, and H — the E and F series are most active in regard to pulmonary vessels and smooth muscle. The most abundant precursor of prostaglandins is arachidonic acid (5,8,11,14 eicosatetraenoic acid), which can be synthesized from linoleic acid in the diet. The actions of the prostaglandins on the pulmonary system are too complex to permit casual understanding, but a general rule is that the PGEs are dilators and the PGFs are constrictors. There are, however, exceptions to this rule, and there are other constrictors and dilators in several other series of prostaglandins.

The question of what, if any, physiologic derangements occur when there is a deficiency of the essential fatty acids has not been answered. Deficiency syndromes occur rarely and then there is little opportunity to study pathophysiology. Presumably, the prostaglandins play a role in regulating both the flow of blood through the lungs and the amount of airway resistance. Another important function of the lung is to inactivate prostaglandins formed elsewhere in the body.

Dietary fatty acids may have another function that could protect the lungs. The polyunsaturated fatty acids have been shown to reduce platelet adhesiveness, and thereby to reduce the likelihood of thrombus formation. Dalen and others (1977) studied pulmonary emboli and found that pulmonary hemorrhage and infarction were more common at the periphery of the lung. It would be of great interest to observe the incidence and type of embolic disease in the lungs of patients who are consuming a diet that supplies ample amounts of polyunsaturated fats, compared with that in a group of patients consuming the usual American diet. At present, there is no evidence that unsaturated fats have any effect, beneficial or otherwise, with regard to pulmonary emboli but neither is there any evidence that vitamin E is useful, as we shall report in the chapter on megavitamins.

PROTECTION AGAINST INFECTION

The pulmonary system has a remarkable array of defense mechanisms that protect the body from infections and toxic inhalants. The first echelon is the epithelial surface which provides a mechanical barrier against microorganisms, particulate foreign matter, and to some extent, noxious gases. Coupled with this epithelial barrier is the ciliated surface of the stratified columnar epithelium that literally sweeps out debris and inhaled particles. Equally important is the layer of mucus secreted by goblet cells and covering most of the epithelial surfaces of the tracheobronchial tree. Reid (1977) demonstrated two types of secretory cells: one mucous, and the other serous. The mechanisms that regulate the mixture of secretions seem to be under control of the autonomic nervous system. Deficiency of either vitamin A or vitamin C results in suppression of seromucous secretions by the salivary, lacrimal, and other epithelial tissues. This is known as Sjögren's syndrome, and may result from such other disorders as rheumatoid arthritis or disseminated lupus erythematosus, regardless of diet.

Similarly, there are both nutritional and non-nutritional factors that impair or stop ciliary action. Heavy cigarette smoking is probably the commonest cause. Deficiency of vitamin A results in loss of cilia and replacement of stratified columnar epithelium with stratified squamous epithelium. Recently, a rare congenital condition known as the immotile cilia syndrome was described by Eliasson and colleagues (1977). In this condition, lack of ciliary action results in recurrent respiratory tract infections, followed by bronchiectasis and sinusitis.

In normal persons, most inhaled microorganisms that escape the mucociliary "escalator" are rapidly engulfed by alveolar macrophages and are carried through lymphatic channels to regional lymph nodes. Little wonder that so few healthy people acquire significant infections when they inhale a few tubercle bacilli or pneumococci.

But what about debilitated or alcoholic patients? Their increased susceptibility to serious respiratory tract infections has been accepted almost as an article of faith. Green and others (1964) studied factors that influence the clearance of bacteria by the lung, and observed that this protective mechanism is inhibited by ethanol intoxication, by adrenocortical steroids, and by hypoxia. Of even greater importance is the observation that clearance of bacteria is impaired by semistarvation, the degree of inhibition being proportional to the amount of weight lost.

Surface fluids contain not only mucilaginous glycoproteins but also immunoglobulins that aid in destruction of many microorganisms. Studies by the author demonstrated impairment of antibody production as a result of specific nutritional deficiencies (Hodges et al., 1962). Little wonder, then, that debilitated hospitalized patients have impaired defense mechanisms of their respiratory membranes (Green et al., 1977).

ATMOSPHERIC POLLUTANTS

Urban living has resulted in pollution of the air with a wide variety of particulate and gaseous material derived from industrial activity and from automobiles. Black smoke, which is the most obvious because of its absorption of light, is the least noxious because the larger carbon particles are deposited chiefly in the nasopharynx and the upper portions of the trachea and bronchi. Smaller particles present in "white smoke" are deposited mostly in the smaller bronchi and in the alveoli.

Noxious gases also are distributed in a characteristic fashion along the airways. The most reactive substances quickly dissolve in or combine with surface fluids. Thus sulfur dioxide concentrates in the nasopharynx where it sets up an intense irritation and causes sneezing and coughing. Nitrogen dioxide and other oxides of nitrogen deposit chiefly in the bronchi where they cause coughing and increased secretion of surface fluids. But the more damaging ozone reaches the alveoli where its presence causes little immediate discomfort. Of course, this regional segregation of gases is not complete and all types of toxic gases can be found in each location.

The effects of air pollutants have been studied extensively and corrective measures have been proposed. Each time a major "smog inversion" covers a city, morbidity and mortality figures show that individuals with pre-existing cardiac or pulmonary disease suffer the most. Efforts at identification of mechanisms involved are beginning to show results.

Ibrahim and others (1976) studied the effects of ozone on the respiratory epithelium and alveolar macrophages of mice exposed to ozone. He found that as little as 0.8 ppm of ozone, inhaled for eleven days, significantly reduced the amount of interferon produced by epithelial cells (in vitro), but has no effect on alveolar macrophages.

Witschi (1977) observed that ozone and nitrogen dioxide are the two main ingredients of photochemical smog, and that these substances, when inhaled by experimental animals, result in peroxidation of unsaturated fatty acids, formation of free radicals, and decreased mitochondrial respiration. Repair of tissue damage may be inhibited by the oxidant gases, and even oxygen can interfere with DNA synthesis in the growing lung of the newborn.

For a number of years, Tappel and his group have studied the effects of antioxidants, especially the tocopherols, on the type of damage produced by the oxidant gases. Fletcher and Tappel (1973) demonstrated a protective effect of dietary α-tocopherol in rats exposed to toxic levels of ozone and nitrogen dioxide. Within the range of 0 to 45 mg/kg of α-tocopherol per day, there was significant evidence of protection against weight loss and death. Pulmonary edema and hemorrhage were the apparent causes of death. Not only α-tocopherol but also other antioxidants — ascorbic acid, methionine, and butylated hydroxytoluene (BHT) — were shown to have protective effects against the noxious effects of oxidant gases.

Apparently, no one has performed the definitive study: administration of appropriate doses of α-tocopherol or administration of a suitable placebo to large numbers of people who live and work in a polluted atmosphere. Obviously, the difficulties inherent in such a study would be great and the cost almost prohibitive. But as yet we do not know whether ingestion of large amounts of α-tocopherol or other antioxidants should be advised for city dwellers, especially those with cardiopulmonary diseases.

The lung, like any other organ, is subject to neoplastic changes when exposed to carcinogenic substances for many years. Undoubtedly, cigarette smoking is the proximate cause of most cases of bronchogenic carcinoma. Perhaps atmospheric pollutants contribute, but this is less certain. Recently, the Federal government announced that, based on extensive studies in experimental animals, it was initiating a cancer-prevention program wherein subjects who presumably have a greater-than-average risk of developing cancer would be given an analog of vitamin A — 13 cis retinoic acid. At present, there is no evidence that this substance can prevent cancer in humans, but it is being given to persons (such as heavy cigarette smokers) with a high level of risk, and only time will tell whether this program is successful.

Various forms of nutritional therapy, dietary or others, have been found to damage or interfere with the functions of the respiratory tract. The most obvious is the taking of mineral oil as a laxative. Not only can this form of self-medication result in loss of essential fatty acids and fat-soluble vitamins, but more importantly, it often results in seepage of the oil down the trachea where it immobilizes the cilia and migrates to the alveoli where it can cause a form of pneumonitis. A good rule is to discourage oral use of mineral oil for any purpose.

Another form of lipid damage to the lung was described by Greene (1974), who reported that a commercial fat emulsion (10 per cent), when given intravenously to normal adult volunteers, resulted in a significant reduction in the pulmonary membrane diffusion in half of the subjects. Infusion of fat emulsion into rabbits resulted in retention of fat in the lung tissues during the early phases of lipid infusion. This cleared within an hour after the infusion was stopped. Greene then repeated studies in human volunteers, but this time the subjects were exercised. As expected, under control conditions pulmonary diffusion capacity increased normally with exercise. After infusion of 500 ml of 10 per cent fat emulsion, the subjects were again exercised. This time six of the ten subjects showed significant impairment of pulmonary diffusion capacity. In separate studies, it has been shown that ingestion of a fatty meal can also impair pulmonary diffusion capacity for a brief period. Administration of heparin can reverse these abnormalities quickly. Presumably, the use of fat emulsions in patients with severe pulmonary disease should be undertaken with caution, if at all.

In the chapter on "Feeding Patients" the problems associated with total parenteral nutrition are described. One of these, hypophosphatemia, has been reported to cause acute respiratory failure in a patient (Newman et al., 1977). The characteristics and methods for avoiding the hypophosphatemic syndrome are described in that chapter.

A disease of childhood, cystic fibrosis, displays a panorama of nutritional problems. Occasionally, these patients survive long enough to become adults; hence internists as well as pediatricians should be familiar with their problems. Their greatest difficulties arise from their inability to secrete adequate amounts of digestive enzymes in their pancreatic juices; hence they have a severe and lifelong malabsorption syndrome. Cramping abdominal distress, flatulence, and diarrhea are common. Retarded growth and development contribute to their self-consciousness. Deficiencies of essential nutrients are very common, but lack of the fat-soluble vitamins and the essential fatty acids are especially troublesome. Although the lung is known to be involved in this multisystems disease, it is probable that nutritional deficiencies contribute substantially to the recurrent infections that often result in bronchiectasis. A humoral factor may account for loss of ciliary motility in the air passages, and lack of essential fatty acids and vitamin A may further reduce resistance to infections by reducing the defensive barriers.

Management of these patients consists of constant attention to their nutritional status and continual awareness of their propensity to develop infections, especially of the respiratory tract. Administration of pancreatic enzymes orally with each meal and provision of generous amounts of the fat-soluble vitamins (including essential fatty acids) will do much to maintain nutritional health. Their tolerance to acute digestive disturbances that cause nausea, vomiting, and diarrhea is far below average because of the salt-losing abnormality of their sweat glands. It is often necessary to hospitalize these patients long enough to replenish their fluids and electrolytes parenterally. Elliott (1976) suggested that deficiency of linoleic acid results in an abnormal accumulation of oleates in the intracellular structures of these patients. He reported observations in seven children with cystic fibrosis who were given infusions of 10 per cent fat emulsions, 20 ml/kg once every three weeks for three years. He feels that restoration of a normal fatty acid pattern allows cellular binding of more oxygen and decreases the common complications of this disorder.

THE HAZARDS OF GAVAGE FEEDING

Although semistarvation is to be deplored in the management of almost any patient, the alternatives are sometimes almost as frightening.

Physicians in general regard nasogastric gavage feeding as an innocuous procedure, but recent evidence suggests another interpretation. A great many patients who need some form of nutritional support other than regular oral feedings are, to some extent, debilitated or mentally obtunded. Nagler and Spiro (1963) demonstrated that prolonged gastric intubation resulted in persistent gastric reflux and a sensation of "heartburn" in three normal subjects when they lay supine. Atkinson (1970) also called attention to the need for elevation of the head of the bed and turning an unconscious patient from side-to-side to reduce the risk of gastric reflux and aspiration of secretions into the trachea.

Olivares and colleagues (1974) reviewed the autopsy records of 720 neurological patients and found that risk of gastric aspiration was six times as great in those who were tube-fed. Of course, one could reason that only the weakest and most debilitated were tube-fed. Hinkle and colleagues (1971) devised a method for measuring the reactivity of the glottis and found that postanesthetic patients were significantly less reactive; hence greater care must be used in giving them fluids by either the gavage or oral route.

Older patients also lose their protective reflexes, according to Pontoppidian and Beecher (1960). Aspiration pneumonitis is increasingly common as the age of patients increases and their glottal reflexes become slower, and administration of depressant drugs further impairs these reflexes. They emphasized that silent tracheal aspiration is very common and may remain unrecognized until autopsy. Even then it is difficult to distinguish between hypostatic pneumonia and aspiration pneumonitis, especially if several days have elapsed before death. Arms and others (1974) reviewed 88 cases of aspiration pneumonia and observed that it most commonly occurred in the right lower lung. Contributing factors included debilitation, impaired consciousness, esophageal and neurologic disorders, cardiac resuscitation, presence of a nasogastric tube, and presence of a tracheostomy tube. The fate of 50 patients who aspirated gastric contents was reviewed by Bynum and Pierce (1976). Twelve per cent died promptly, 62 per cent improved rapidly and remained improved and 26 per cent improved for a time, then worsened. Sixty per cent of these (16 per cent of the total) died. Thus, the overall mortality was 28 per cent of the 50 patients.

Experiments in animals sometimes give surprising answers. The author, like most physicians, regarded aspiration of isotonic glucose as a benign event. But Olson (1970) showed that, in rabbits, introduction of 5 per cent dextrose in water was as damaging as milk, whereas instillation of tap water was less harmful. Greenfield (1969) instilled graded amounts of 0.1 N hydrochloric acid into the tracheas of anesthetized dogs and observed an increasing mortality as the volume increased. Cameron and others (1972) confirmed these observations and attempted to resuscitate dogs by giving positive pressure ventilation. This did decrease intrapulmonary shunting but did not alter mortality.

These reports confirm the frequency and the alarming mortality of aspiration pneumonitis. The only effective form of treatment is prevention. With this in mind, Burgess (1975) studied obstetrical patients in whom aspiration of gastric contents accounts for 2 per cent of maternal deaths. He found that giving 30 ml doses of magnesium trisilicate resulted in a rise in gastric pH to greater than 2.50. This should lessen the severity of pneumonitis if aspiration occurs.

Another relationship between food and the pulmonary system is the "café coronary" syndrome. This usually occurs when a bolus of meat becomes lodged in the pharynx (Haugen, 1963). Many suggestions have been made for dealing with this event, but it is difficult to provide clear and effective instructions that can be followed by a frightened lay-person who attempts to aid a stricken person. Perhaps the most logical is the Heimlich maneuver, in which the person giving aid stands behind the victim, places both arms around his or her chest just below the rib cage and hugs tightly in an effort to "pop the cork out of the bottle." Other methods include a plastic forceps available at all times, which, for the uninitiated, could be more harmful than the first technique described.

Many patients with bronchial asthma or other allergic disorders believe that they have a "food allergy". Often this belief is fortified by skin tests performed by their physician who observes some degree of reaction to a number of substances. Food antigens often give an irritative response, and, in a person who has some degree of dermatographia, the wheal may be quite convincing. A careful history often helps to differentiate real from imaginary allergic reactions. When a food allergy occurs, it usually becomes manifest within a very few minutes. There may be excessive salivation and burning or itching of the lips, tongue, and oropharynx. Laryngeal edema may alter the voice or cause stridor. In this event, immediate treatment is mandatory. A tracheostomy may be necessary. Injections of epinephrine, Benadryl, or hydrocortisone (or prednisone) may be helpful, especially if asthmatic wheezes, anxiety, and cyanosis develop. The most commonly allergenic foods include shellfish and nuts. After recovery from an episode such as that described above, the patient should be examined and tested by a competent allergist. But most cases of "food allergy" with minimal symptoms and no objective signs are unrelated to diet.

REFERENCES

Arms, R. A., Dines, D. E., and Tinstman, T. C.: Aspiration pneumonia. *Chest* 65:136, 1974.

Atkinson, W. J.: Posture of the unconscious patient. *Lancet* 1:404, 1970.

Auchincloss, J. H., Jr., Cook, E., and Renzetti, A. D.: Clinical and physiological aspects of a case of obesity, polycythemia and alveolar hypoventilation. *J. Clin. Invest.* 34:1537, 1955.

Burgess, G. E., III: Antacids for obstetric patients. *Amer. J. Obstet. Gynecol.* 123:577, 1975.

Burwell, C. S., Robin, E. D., Whaley, R. D., and Bickelman, A. G.: Extreme obesity associated with alveolar hypoventilation — A Pickwickian syndrome. *Amer. J. Med.* 21:811, 1956.

Bynum, L. J., and Pierce, A. K.: Pulmonary aspiration of gastric contents. *Amer. Rev. Resp. Dis.* 114:1129, 1976.

Cameron, J. L., Caldini, P., Toung, J-K., and Zuidema, G. D.: Aspiration pneumonia: Physiologic data following experimental aspiration. *Surgery* 72:238, 1972.

Campbell, I. M., Crozier, D. N., and Caton, R. B.: Abnormal fatty acid composition and impaired oxygen supply in cystic fibrosis patients. *Pediatrics 57*:480, 1976.

Dalen, J. E., Haffajee, C. I., Alpert, J. S., Howe, J. P., III, Ockene, I., and Paraskos, J. A.: Pulmonary embolism, pulmonary hemorrhage, and pulmonary infarction. *New England J. Med. 296*:1431, 1977.

Dickens, C.: *The Posthumous Pickwick Papers.* Patten, Robert L., ed. (English Library Series), New York, 1973, Penguin Books, Inc.

Eliasson, R., Mossberg, B., Camner, P., and Afzelius, B. A.: The immotile-cilia syndrome: A congenital ciliary abnormality as an etiological factor in chronic airway infections and male sterility. *New England J. Med. 297*:1, 1977

Elliott, R. B.: A therapeutic trial of fatty acid supplementation in cystic fibrosis. *Pediatrics 57*:474, 1976.

Fletcher, B. L., and Tappel, A. L.: Protective effects of dietary α-tocopherol in rats exposed to toxic levels of ozone and nitrogen dioxide. *Environ. Res. 6*:165, 1973.

Green, G. M., Jakab, G. J., Low, R. B., and Davis, G. S.: Defense mechanisms of the respiratory membrane. *Amer. Rev. Resp. Dis. 115*:479, 1977.

Green, G. M., and Kass, E. H.: Factors influencing the clearance of bacteria by the lung. *J. Clin. Invest. 43*:769, 1964.

Greene, H. L.: Intralipid and respiratory insufficiency. In *Total Parenteral Nutrition,* Philip L. White, and Margarita E. Nagy (eds.). Acton, Mass., Publishing Sciences Group, Inc., 1974, pp. 221–225.

Greenfield, L. J., Singleton, R. P., McCaffree, D. R., and Coalson, J. J.: Pulmonary effects of experimental graded aspiration of hydrochloric acid. *Ann. Surg. 170*:74, 1969.

Gross, I.: Nutritional and hormonal influences on lung phospholipid metabolism. *Fed. Proc. 36*:2665, 1977.

Haugen, R. K.: The cafe coronary. Sudden deaths in restaurants. *J.A.M.A. 186*:142, 1963.

Hinkle, J. E., and Tantum, K. R.: A technique for measuring reactivity of the glottis. *Anesthesiology 35*:634, 1971.

Hodges, R. E., Bean, W. B., Ohlson, M. A., and Bleiler, R. E.: Factors affecting human antibody response. V. Combined deficiences of pantothenic acid and pyridoxine. *Amer. J. Clin. Nutr. 11*:187, 1962.

Ibrahim, A. L., Zee, Y. C., and Osebold, J. W.: The effects of ozone on the respiratory epithelium and alveolar macrophages of mice. 1. Interferon production. *Proc. Soc. Exper. Biol. Med. 152*:483, 1976.

Keys, A. (Editor): Respiration. In *The Biology of Human Starvation,* Volume 1. Minneapolis, University of Minnesota Press, 1950, p. 601.

Mathé, A. A., Hedqvist, P., Strandberg, K., and Leslie, C. A.: Aspects of prostaglandin function in the lung. Part I. *New England J. Med. 296*:850, 1977. Part II. *New England J. Med. 296*:910, 1977.

Nagler, R., and Spiro, H.: Persistent gastroesophageal reflux induced during prolonged gastric intubation. *New England J. Med. 269*:495, 1963.

Newman, J. H., Neff, T. A., and Ziporin, P.: Acute respiratory failure associated with hypophosphatemia. *New England J. Med. 296*:1101, 1977.

Olivares, L., Segovia, A., and Revuelta, R.: Tube feeding and lethal aspiration in neurological patients: A review of 720 autopsy cases. *Stroke 5*:654, 1974.

Olson, M.: The benign effects on rabbits' lungs of the aspiration of water compared with 5% glucose or milk. *Pediatrics 46*:538, 1970.

Pontoppidan, H., and Beecher, H. K.: Progressive loss of protective reflexes in the airway with the advance of age. *J.A.M.A. 174*:2209, 1960.

Reid, L. M.: Secretory cells. *Fed. Proc. 36*:2703, 1977.

Saltzman, H. A., and Salzano, J. V.: Effects of carbohydrate metabolism upon respiratory gas exchange in normal men. *J. Applied Physiol. 30*:228, 1971.

Vaisrub, S.: Pickwickian syndrome? The Dickens! *J.A.M.A. 239*:645, 1978.

Wilmore, D. W., Curreri, P. W., Spitzer, K. W., Spitzer, M. E., and Pruitt, B. A., Jr.: Supranormal dietary intake in thermally injured hypermetabolic patients. *Surg. Gynecol. Obstet. 132*:881, 1971.

Witschi, H.: Environmental agents altering lung biochemistry. *Fed. Proc. 36*:1631, 1977.

12

NUTRITION AND THE INTEGUMENT, INCLUDING MUCOUS MEMBRANES

Robert E. Hodges, M.D.

The epithelial surfaces available for examination include not only the skin and its appendages, the hair and nails, but also the mucous membranes of the eyes, nose, and mouth. In addition, the mucocutaneous junctions of the anogenital regions may reflect important aspects of nutritional status.

Most medical texts of the past half-century have described a variety of "classical" abnormalities of the skin, hair, nails, and mucous membranes, and have ascribed specific nutritional deficiencies to each. For example, scurvy was characterized by swollen, bleeding gums, and pellagra was identified by an actinic dermatitis with accompanying diarrhea and dementia. These word associations were of little value in either diagnosis or treatment of diseases, for patients often failed to respond to administration of the specific nutrient that was presumed to be missing. Furthermore, one "authority" often contradicted another, adding to the confusion. These observers were not entirely wrong; but they provided another example of the age-old error of ascribing a cause-and-effect relationship to a few anecdotal observations. Only recently has there been a return to sound scientific methods in evaluating nutritional problems.

TISSUE ANATOMY AND TYPES OF RESPONSES TO INJURY

The tissues composing the skin and mucous membranes can respond to illness or injury in only a few ways. Therefore, it is important to review the salient features of the anatomy and physiology of these epithelial tissues and structures.

The skin is divided arbitrarily into three layers, the whole of which constitutes the largest organ-system in the body and contains more than one-fourth of all its protein (Sauer, 1973). The innermost layer or subcutaneous tissue is composed of connective tissue cells, collagen strands, and varying amounts of fat in adipocytes. Many nerves and blood vessels pass through this region. The deeper-penetrating hair follicles and sweat glands also occupy this zone.

The dermis, or corium, is composed of denser connective tissue containing cells and a variety of fibers: collagen, elastic, and reticular. Here, the blood supply is very rich and there are many nerve endings, including such specialized receptors as Vater-Pacinian corpuscles and Wagner-Meissner corpuscles, as well as free nerve endings. Motor nerves supply sweat glands, smooth muscle, and arrectores pilorum muscles. Cellular types include reticulohistiocytes, myeloid cells, and lymphoid cells. All of these are surrounded by an amorphous matrix, the ground substance.

The epidermis or outermost layer of skin is itself subdivided into five layers: an inner basal layer which contains both the keratin-forming and the melanin-forming cells, the prickle layer composed of several layers of polyhedral epidermal cells, the granular layer where the epidermal cells are flatter and contain keratohyalin granules, the lucid layer (present only on palms and soles) where the cells are translucent and flat, and the horny superficial layer composed of dead keratinized cells that are constantly being shed. This layer is hydrophilic and can swell visibly when exposed to moisture for a long time.

The appendages of the skin include not only the keratinized tissues (nails and hair), but also the hair follicles themselves, the sebaceous glands, and the sweat glands. Both the hair follicles and the sebaceous glands are greatly affected by the sex hormones, especially at puberty. In addition, the apocrine sweat glands, which are located chiefly in the pubic and axillary regions, are also influenced by the sex hormones.

As we shall see, the principal role played by nutrition is to permit the various structures of the skin to develop, function, and maintain themselves in a normal fashion. The same is true of the exposed mucous membranes. Any nutritional deficit that interferes with the rate of growth and maintenance of epithelial tissues will inevitably alter both the thickness and appearance of these tissues and eventually their continuity. In addition, nutritional deficits may reduce the rate of formation of the end-stage protein, keratin, which is shed from the surface of the skin as well as in the form of hair and nails (Table 12–1).

TABLE 12–1 PATHOPHYSIOLOGIC CHANGES OF THE INTEGUMENT

CHANGES IN COLOR	
(Vascular)	Vasodilatation (redness)
	Vasoconstriction (pallor)
	Extravasation of erythrocytes
(Pigment)	Increased melanin
	Decreased melanin
CHANGES IN PROTEIN SYNTHESIS (DECREASE)	
	Decreased subcutaneous mass
	Decreased skin thickness
	Alterations in skin appendages
	arrest of nail growth
	loss or discoloration of hair
	brittle or deformed hairs
ALTERATIONS IN SECRETIONS	
Skin:	Decreased secretions of sebaceous glands
	plugging of sebaceous ducts
	Increased secretions of sebaceous glands
	seborrheic dermatitis
Mucous Membranes:	Sjögren's syndrome
	loss of secretions in eyes, mouth, and nose

The skin and mucous membranes can respond to injury, illness, or malnutrition in only a few ways. Accordingly, there are few pathognomonic lesions. Nonetheless, careful attention to the details of epithelial abnormalities will allow identification of several nutritional deficiencies.

Alterations in nutritional status can adversely affect the defense mechanisms that protect against infection, impair the thermoregulatory functions of the skin, and even denervate the skin, rendering it more susceptible to mechanical injury. Also, the nutritional status can alter certain metabolic pathways, thereby changing tissue responses to such environmental factors as exposure to actinic light.

The location of various appendages of the skin and mucous membranes can have an important influence on the clinical characteristics of certain nutritional deficiencies. For example, lack of a nutrient that influences the secretory activity of the sebaceous glands may be most apparent on the face, particularly along the nasolabial folds where sebaceous glands are large and numerous (Montagna et al., 1960, (Figure 12–1). It is also important to know that sebaceous glands are absent from palms, soles, and lower lip, and sparse or absent on the dorsum of hands and feet. Seborrheic secretions (the functions of which are still disputed) are sparse in prepubertal children, overabundant during adolescence, and become sparse again after menopause in women and at a similar age in men (Figure 12–2).

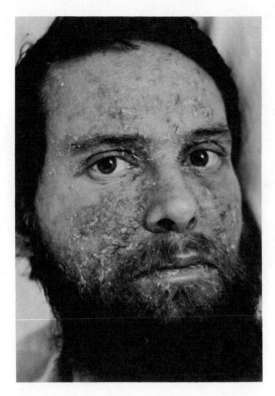

Figure 12–1 Seborrheic dermatitis of essential fatty acid deficiency. This man had received total parenteral nutrition for several months. Since fat emulsions were not then available, he received no linoleic acid. Topical applications of corn oil were without effect.

EFFECTS OF MALNUTRITION ON THE INTEGUMENT AND MUCOUS MEMBRANES

The term "malnutrition" as used in this chapter can indicate a lack of adequate amounts of food energy or lack of protein or deficiency of one or more of the essential nutrients. Other forms of malnutrition which result from excesses of nutrient intake, as in obesity, or from metabolic abnormalities, such as the hyperlipidemic syndromes, are discussed elsewhere in this book.

But the effects of a nutritional deficiency, such as lack of sufficient energy intake, are conditioned by the state of health of the patient prior to the events that resulted in malnutrition as well as the proximate cause of the faulty intake of food. For example, malnutrition resulting from benign pyloric obstruction may differ sharply from that caused by alcoholic cirrhosis of the liver. Furthermore, the rapidity of onset of malnutrition has a profound effect on its clinical manifestations. An acute onset of restricted food intake will result in rapid depletion of those proteins with a short half-life, such as the plasma

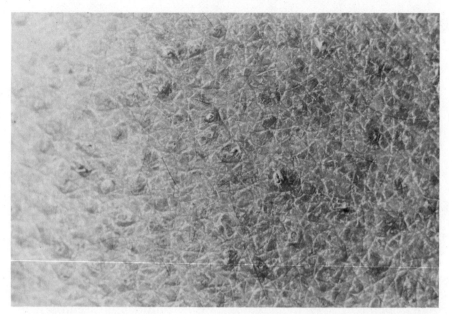

Figure 12–2 Xerosis of skin occurs when seborrheic secretions are scanty or absent. This is especially common in vitamin A deficiency but may occur as a result of general malnutrition.

proteins — transferrin and albumin — while the peripheral tissues — muscle, skin and subcutaneous tissues — may remain intact for some time. By contrast, an illness that results in a gradual and progressive decrease in food intake will result in generalized tissue losses including both the "visceral proteins" of the plasma and the "peripheral proteins" of muscle and supporting tissues.

EXAMPLES OF THE EFFECTS OF NUTRIENT DEFICIENCIES ON INTEGUMENT AND MUCOUS MEMBRANES

One of the commonest deficiencies is lack of sufficient nutrient energy. This may be the result of anorexia nervosa, mental depression, malignant disease, or some prolonged illness. The result is starvation, and the body responds in a characteristic fashion. Energy reserves are utilized and exhausted. Glycogen stores are gone within a day or two, but fat stores may persist for several months. At the same time, the body cannibalizes its own protein tissues: plasma proteins, formed elements of the blood, lymphoid tissue, muscles, skin and subcutaneous tissues, the heart and great vessels, the digestive organs, and even the vital liver and kidneys. Only the central nervous system and peripheral nerves seem to be spared.

Fortunately, the body has developed protective mechanisms that permit survival *despite* advanced starvation. These include a remarkable "shut-down" that greatly reduces all types of metabolic activity. Endocrine functions virtually cease, body temperature falls, the heart rate and respiratory rate are slowed, and most enzyme systems function at a reduced level, if at all. For example, concentrations of blood glucose and of plasma lipids fall to low levels. There is a reduction in both circulating blood volume and red cell mass. Leukocytes are similarly diminished. In this state of malnutrition, the skin appears to be thin and shiny. Subcutaneous tissue loss is evident by the remarkably thin skin-fold thickness as measured by calipers. There may be hair loss, especially the "sexual hair" in the pubic and axillary regions. Bruising and subcutaneous bleeding are common, and muscle atrophy is obvious.

It may seem strange at first, but patients who are severely starved seldom manifest specific deficiency syndromes such as scurvy, beriberi, or pellagra, even though they have had little or no ascorbic acid, thiamin, or niacin in their diets. The reason for this phenomenon is the protective effect of the metabolic, endocrine, and enzymatic function shutdown. As soon as energy and protein are restored to the diet, these deficiencies will become apparent, and may even be fatal.

Lack of sufficient protein is much more common in children than in adults, and it is far more common in the developing countries than in the industrialized nations. It results, of course, in delayed or diminished synthesis of protein and the effects are predictable. Those proteins with the shortest physiologic half-life are depleted first. Thus, the plasma proteins, especially transferrin and albumin, are quickly reduced. One result is hypoalbuminemia with edema. Lack of adequate protein also affects the synthesis of hairs and the production of melanin in the skin and in hair follicles. This explains the common finding, in developing nations, of black children with kwashiorkor who have patches of red or even white skin and red or blond hair. In children who have had a few months of protein deficiency, followed by an improved diet, there may be changes in the scalp hair known as the "flag sign". This consists of normally colored hair in the proximal and distal portions of the hair but depigmentation in the mid-portion which was produced while the diet was deficient in protein.

Other forms of nutritional deficiency can mimic protein deficiency because these nutrients are also essential for protein synthesis. Examples include vitamin A, zinc, and niacin.

Hair follicles also provide a useful indication of metabolic and nutritional status. Normally, the hair follicle produces a smooth cylindrical shaft of keratinized protein that is pigmented according to

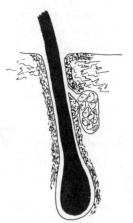

Figure 12-3 A normal hair follicle produces a symmetrical, cylindrical shaft of keratinized protein. A sebaceous gland produces oily secretions that presumably allow easy egress of the hair shaft.

inherited characteristics. The presence of a sebaceous gland that can secrete oily material into the canal may enable the hair shaft to slide easily as it grows (Figure 12-3). Normally, a certain percentage of the hair roots are in the actively growing or anagen stage and others are in the telogen or resting stage (Bradfield and Bailey, 1969; Crounse et al., 1970). The ratio of these two forms of hair roots has been used as an index of protein nutritional status (Figure 12-4).

Thinning of hair and loss of hair occur in a number of nutritional deficiencies but most commonly in patients with lack of sufficient protein intake. This is especially apparent in women but may be indistinguishable from post-menopausal alopecia. In men, who so often develop male baldness, this sign is of little value.

In deficiency of zinc, as in deficiency of essential fatty acids, there is a form of acrodermatitis that appears closely similar. With zinc deficiency, however, the hair of the scalp is easily plucked, whereas the hair remains firmly anchored with essential fatty acid deficiency.

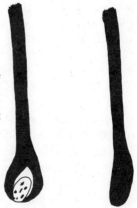

Figure 12-4 In young healthy adults (and in most children) a majority of the hairs in the scalp are in a phase of active growth (anagen stage, left). A few hairs are in the resting phase (telogen stage, right). Some evidence suggests that protein malnutrition increases the number of resting hair follicles.

Although we know little about the relationship between diet and seborrheic secretions, there does seem to be a discernible pattern. Deficiency of either zinc or essential fatty acids can cause a seborrheic type of dermatitis involving those areas where sebaceous glands are most abundant: the scalp, eyebrows, forehead, the nasolabial folds, the upper lip, cheeks, and sometimes the neck and back (Figure 12–1). Similar seborrheic dermatitis may occur in individuals who are deficient in either pyridoxine or riboflavin. In severe cases, there may also be inflammation, itching, and scaling of the anogenital regions where sebaceous glands are relatively abundant.

ABNORMALITIES OF THE BODY HAIRS

In prepubertal boys and girls, the body hairs are fine and inconspicuous. These are referred to as lanugo hairs in infancy, and as vellus hairs in adults. Many of these hairs have an adjoining sebaceous gland that empties into the hair canal. In most adults, but more so in men than in women, many of these body hairs grow in both diameter and length and they may become more deeply pigmented. In men, these hairs become more conspicuous on the face, arms, thighs, calves, anterior thorax, and abdomen. Certain conditions alter their appearance and provide the characteristic lesions that identify important deficiency syndromes; namely vitamin-A deficiency and scurvy. Apparently, these changes result from at least two abnormalities of the hair follicle and its shaft: protein synthesis must be defective and the secretions of the adjoining sebaceous gland must be impaired. But whatever the cause, the result is characteristic: one finds broken hairs, coiled hairs (Plate 5), swan-neck deformities of hairs, and follicular hyperkeratosis (Plate 6). In the latter condition, the structure of the keratinized hair shaft is completely disrupted, and the hair follicle pouts outward as it attempts to extrude an irregular mass of keratin that resembles a piece of broken fingernail. When these lesions are numerous, the skin feels like coarse sandpaper (Figure 12–5).

SPECIFIC NUTRITIONAL DEFICIENCIES

Although mechanisms have been stressed thus far in this chapter, it is useful to consider the major clinical features of the commonest nutritional deficiencies. But it should be emphasized that the classical deficiency syndromes — scurvy, pellagra, beriberi, and rickets — do not occur often in the population of the United States. When these syndromes do occur, it behooves the physician to search for the cause,

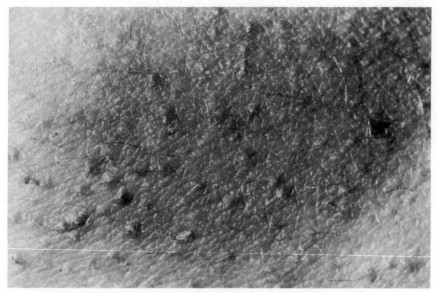

Figure 12–5 Follicular hyperkeratosis in a 17-year-old high school boy. His diet contained few vegetables or fruits and almost no dairy products. These lesions are compatible with but not diagnostic of vitamin A deficiency. The skin feels like coarse sandpaper.

which may be a fad diet, alcohol abuse, or some form of malabsorption.

Thiamin. Deficiency of vitamin B_1, or thiamin, produces a variety of syndromes known collectively as beriberi. There are no characteristic abnormalities of the integument or mucous membranes.

Riboflavin. Lack of riboflavin, or vitamin B_2, is rather uncommon in the United States, largely as a result of the program for enrichment of bread and flour that was initiated in the United States during World War II. The practice is widespread in the United States (Table 12–2) and other affluent countries. Deficiency results in increased vascularity of the conjunctivae, an abnormal redness or magenta discoloration of the tongue, angular lesions at the corners of the mouth, and the aforementioned seborrheic dermatitis of the face and of the anogenital regions (Plate 7).

If deficiency of riboflavin is suspected on the basis of clinical findings, it is desirable to confirm this impression. Specific tests for riboflavin status include: (1) Measurement of urinary excretion of riboflavin in 24 hours (acceptable levels are > 80 μg per g of creatinine); (2) Measurement of erythrocyte content of riboflavin (acceptable levels are > 15 μg per 100 ml of RBCs); and (3) Erythrocyte glu-

TABLE 12–2 STANDARDS FOR ENRICHMENT OF CEREAL PRODUCTS (FIGURES SHOW MINIMUM AND MAXIMUM LEVELS REQUIRED)

PRODUCT	THIAMIN mg/lb	RIBO-FLAVIN mg/lb	NIACIN mg/lb	IRON mg/lb	CALCIUM mg/lb
Bread, rolls, buns (white)	1.1–1.8	0.7–1.6	10–15	8.0–12.5	–
Cornmeal grits	2.0–3.0	1.2–1.8	16–24	13–26	–
Cornmeal, self-rising	2.0–3.0	1.2–1.8	16–24	13–26	–
Farina	2.0–2.5	1.2–1.5	16–20	13–(**)	–
Flour, white	2.0–2.5	1.2–1.5	16–20	13.0–16.5	–
Flour, self-rising	2.0–2.5	1.2–1.5	16–20	12.0–16.5	500–1000
Macaroni } products Noodle	4.0–5.0	1.7–2.2	27–34	13.0–16.5	–
Rice, milled	2.0–4.0	1.2*–2.4*	16–32	13–26	–

*Requirement for riboflavin pending further hearings.
**No maximum level established.

Since World War II, the United States has set standards for enrichment of farinaceous foods. This has been largely responsible for the virtual disappearance of beriberi, pellagra, and riboflavin deficiency. Its impact on iron deficiency anemia has been less apparent.

tathione reductase activity coefficient (acceptable levels are > 1.40) (Sauberlich et al., 1974b).

Unfortunately, few hospitals (even academic institutions) have laboratories that can perform the above tests. The only recourse for the physician is to give a "therapeutic trial" of riboflavin, but once again he or she is thwarted. Pure riboflavin is not readily available as a prescription drug, so the next best thing is to give a multivitamin preparation. Since the average recommended daily allowance for riboflavin for adults is in the range of 1.1 to 1.8 mg daily, it is reasonable to give a patient with suspected deficiency a preparation that contains at least 2.0 mg per unit, three times daily for 7 to 10 days, and a single unit daily thereafter. This should result in clinical improvement within a few days, but the response will be non-specific because of the necessity for giving a multivitamin preparation.

Niacin. Deficiency of niacin or nicotinic acid, as it was once designated, is quite uncommon in the United States for the same reason mentioned in the discussion of riboflavin — most farinaceous foods are enriched with niacin. An occasional patient will be found who has eaten poorly or who has a malabsorption syndrome, but even these are rarely seen.

Deficiency of niacin once occurred chiefly in slaves in the Southern United States. It was seasonal and the cause was elucidated by the brilliant epidemiologic studies of Joseph Goldberger. He demonstrated that blacks eating mostly cornmeal and very little meat had a high incidence of pellagra, whereas people who had better food never developed the syndrome. Later, it was learned that tryptophan (which is not abundant in corn) can be converted in the body to niacin. Now that cornmeal is heavily fortified with niacin, the problem is largely solved.

Pellagra is characterized by inflammation of all of the body orifices, chiefly the mouth and anus, and by a light-sensitive dermatitis. The exposed skin is heavily pigmented and has an inflammatory base with central cracking, crusting, and scaling. Late in the disease, severe diarrhea weakens the patient and may contribute to the onset of mental confusion. Thus, the old adage: "Corn (maize) eaters develop dermatitis, dementia, and diarrhea" is at least partially correct. Foods (such as the millet called *jowar* in India) that are high in lysine content can precipitate the onset of pellagra.

The recommended daily allowance of niacin for adults is in the range of 12 to 20 mg daily, depending upon age and sex. The average American diet contains an abundance of niacin equivalents (60 mg of tryptophan are considered the equivalent of 1 mg of niacin).

If a patient should develop pellagra, it is not necessary to administer the huge quantities of niacin that were once advised (Ruiter and Meyler, 1960). It is sufficient to give approximately 20 mg of niacin three times daily. Once again, it is unlikely that a suitable preparation of pure niacin will be available in desirable doses for either oral or parenteral administration. One could give the "mega doses" that are intended for lowering blood lipids, but a suitable alternative is to give a multivitamin preparation containing the recommended dietary allowances of the water-soluble vitamins. These can be given three times daily, either orally or parenterally, depending upon the patient's condition. If the patient does have pellagra, there will be subjective improvement within hours and noticeable improvement in the oral and cutaneous lesions within a few days. Once the patient has recovered, it is essential that the physician search for the cause of this faulty nutritional status (such as alcohol abuse, fad diets, malabsorption, or some other cause).

Pyridoxine or Vitamin B$_6$. This group of vitamins — pyridoxine, pyridoxal and pyridoxamine — is now known as the "vitamin B$_6$ group." They are responsible for a large number of enzymatic reactions that affect protein and amino acid metabolism. As a result, the requirement for vitamin B$_6$ is increased by a high intake of protein.

As will be shown in another chapter, a number of common drugs affect vitamin B$_6$ metabolism and some may cause frank deficiency. A convenient test for estimating the adequacy of vitamin B$_6$ nutrition is the tryptophan load test. Normally tryptophan is metabolized into a number of end products including serotonin, kynurenine, hydroxykynurenine, anthranilic acid, kynurenic acid, xanthurenic acid, quinolinic acid, and nicotinic acid. When insufficient amounts of vitamin B_6 are present, some of the enzyme systems necessary for normal metabolism of tryptophan are lacking. The result is an accumulation of certain metabolites, especially xanthurenic acid. The test is performed by giving a loading dose of tryptophan, usually 2 g of L-tryptophan or 5 g of DL-tryptophan orally. Urine is collected for 24 hours, and the amounts of tryptophan metabolites are measured, usually kynurenine, hydroxykynurenine, kynurenic acid, and xanthurenic acid. In vitamin B_6 deficiency, all of these metabolites are excreted in increased amounts, but xanthurenic acid is increased the most. The test gives a positive result in normal pregnancy and in persons taking a variety of drugs.

Deficiency of vitamin B_6 is generally considered to be uncommon, but if the tryptophan load test is valid, then some degree of deficiency is widespread. Some experts consider xanthurenuria to be nothing more than a laboratory phenomenon, whereas others regard it as evidence that justifies a higher daily allowance of vitamin B_6 (see chapter on drug-nutrient interactions). The author is inclined to the view that we may have placed undue emphasis on large doses of vitamin C and too little emphasis on ample amounts of vitamin B_6.

At present, the recommended adult allowance for vitamin B_6 is between 1.6 and 2.5 mg daily, depending on age and physiologic status (pregnancy or lactation). High protein diets increase the requirement for vitamin B_6.

Deficiency of this vitamin may result in convulsions, anemia, abdominal distress, vomiting, and weight loss in infants. In adults, it may cause mental depression and confusion, and it may result in abnormal electroencephalographic tracings. A fine, branny scaling of the skin of the forearms and lower legs develops, and in addition, there may be a seborrheic dermatitis involving chiefly the face and the anogenital regions (Vilter et al., 1953).

Folic Acid. Folacin or folic acid (pteroylmonoglutamic acid) has been discussed in the chapter on hematopoiesis. Deficiency of this vitamin is not uncommon in the United States and may account for only a small fraction of all cases of anemia. In pregnancy, its need is exaggerated by the needs of the fetus. Generally, there are few integumentary changes attributable to lack of folic acid (Knowles et al., 1963). Pallor of the skin, nail beds, and mucous membranes may, of course, indicate anemia, and lack of folic acid is a possible cause. But a smooth tongue with filiform papillary atrophy is common in three deficiency syndromes: lack of folic acid, deficiency of iron, and lack of vitamin B_{12} (as in pernicious anemia). It is not known whether the tongue generally is restored to its normal appearance after these deficiencies have been fully treated (Plate 8).

Serum levels of folic acid should be in the range of 6 or more ng/ml, but this, according to Sauberlich and colleagues (1974b), is a poor indicator of folate status. Red blood cell levels of folates are somewhat better, and should be in the range of 160 ng/ml or more. The recommended dietary adult allowance for folic acid is in the range of 400 to 800 μg daily for mixed folates, or one-fourth this amount of the pure forms of folacin. It is of interest to note that acute infectious diseases, such as measles and chicken pox, increase the need for folacin and may precipitate a deficiency (Findlay, 1965). Also, the destruction of erythrocytes by an artificial heart valve results in a need for additional amounts of folic acid.

Vitamin B$_{12}$. Although ancient textbooks of medicine characterized the patient with pernicious anemia as having snow-white hair, lemon-yellow skin, and large ears, it is doubtful that lack of vitamin B$_{12}$ had any effect on pigmentation of the hair or the size of the ears. It seems more likely that many patients were in their seventh and eighth decades of life when white hair and large ears (which keep on growing throughout life) are common. The peculiar skin color results from a severe degree of anemia combined with a mild hemolytic process that raises the plasma level of bilirubin slightly. The smooth, pale tongue has been mentioned before.

Both the neurologic and hematologic aspects of vitamin B$_{12}$ deficiency have been discussed in the chapters on those organ systems.

Pantothenic Acid. Because this important vitamin is present in virtually all unprocessed foods (and in many that have been processed), we know relatively little about its functions. The author (Hodges et al., 1959) observed minor changes in the skin of subjects who volunteered for studies designed to evaluate the functions of this vitamin. There was mild dryness and scaling of their skin, but no inflammatory or pigmentary changes were seen. Spontaneous deficiency of this vitamin is extremely unlikely in a population of free-living individuals. During World War II, pantothenic acid was thought to be the cause of a neurologic disorder, the "burning foot" syndrome, which occurred in American troops imprisoned by the Japanese.

The recommended allowance for pantothenic acid is in the range of 5 to 10 mg daily for adults. The average diet supplies more than this amount.

Biotin. This water-soluble vitamin has been largely ignored by the medical profession, perhaps because deficiency seldom occurs. The vitamin is bound to proteins in foods and is abundant in egg yolk. A peculiar quirk of nature has placed an antivitamin substance in egg whites. This substance, known as avidin, combines with biotin, rendering it useless to the body. The result is that individuals who, for whatever reason, consume large numbers of raw eggs on a daily basis, may develop a deficiency of biotin. The signs and symptoms of this rare deficiency include pallor, a scaling dermatitis, anorexia, nausea, vomiting, and mental depression. (Quite a price to pay for the "pleasure" of eating raw eggs.) Fortunately, avidin is easily destroyed by heat, so most methods of cooking eggs will destroy much of their avidin content.

Presumably, the normal flora of the large bowel produce substantial amounts of biotin. At least, reports (Billings, 1970) indicate that urinary excretion of this vitamin far exceeds dietary intake.

Ascorbic Acid (Vitamin C). Although most physicians look for bleeding gums as the hallmark of scurvy, they should look for skin lesions. One of the earliest changes in adults is acne, which is not in any way different from adolescent acne, except for the fact that most adults have few if any acneiform lesions (Bartley et al., 1953).

The next abnormality to become obvious in a patient with scurvy is the presence of broken hairs (Figure 12–6) and coiled hairs (Figure 12–7). In addition, a number of poorly formed hairs will have "swan-neck" deformity because they are flattened instead of cylindrical (Figure 12–8). But the true hallmark of scurvy is follicular hyperkeratosis (Figure 12–9) with perifollicular hemorrhages (Hodges et al., 1969). These lesions may appear on any part of the body but are most apt to occur on the anterior aspect of the thorax, the forearms, thighs, and legs, and on the anterior abdominal wall (Hodges et al., 1971).

Frank bleeding is a late feature of scurvy, as is the bleeding gingivitis that is usually associated with scurvy. Patients who are edentulous and those whose teeth are clean and in good repair may have little or no evidence of scorbutic gingivitis. But patients with poor dental hygiene and with far-advanced dental caries are apt to have fulminating gingivitis that hastens the loss of already rotten teeth (Figure 12–10).

In far-advanced cases of scurvy, there may be generalized bleeding, not only into the skin, but into any structure that happens to be traumatized (Plate 9).

The amount of vitamin C that should be consumed each day remains a point of controversy. Although the World Health Organization and the United Kingdom consider 30 mg a day as a generous allowance for most adults (excluding pregnancy and lactation), the United States advocates (1974) 45 mg daily and may increase this allowance. Several careful studies have shown that 10 mg daily or slightly less will prevent or cure scurvy. But this vitamin has a mystique that intrigues many people, and so the controversy continues.

THE FAT-SOLUBLE VITAMINS

Of the essential fat-soluble substances, only two, vitamin A and the essential fatty acids, have a major effect on the integument.

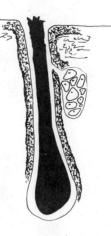

Figure 12–6 Broken hairs. In scurvy, a number of hairs, especially on the legs and thighs, are broken off near the skin surface. Whether this results from defective protein synthesis or from lack of lubrication or from some other cause is uncertain.

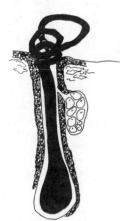

Figure 12–7 Coiled hairs. Scorbutic patients may demonstrate a peculiar lesion: coiled hairs within a hair follicle. This abnormality is seen most commonly on the abdomen and on the forearms. It is highly suggestive of scurvy. It may result from poor lubrication with fracture of the hair shaft, impingement of the broken end against the wall of the hair canal, and continuing growth of the hair itself.

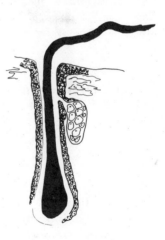

Figure 12–8 Swan-neck deformity of hairs presumably results from faulty synthesis of the hair shaft. Either it is flattened or it is less rigid than normal. This peculiar deformity should bring to mind the possibility of scurvy.

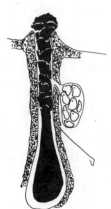

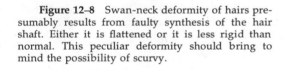

Figure 12–9 Follicular hyperkeratosis. The two commonest nutritional causes of this lesion are deficiency of vitamin C and deficiency of vitamin A. In scurvy there is perifollicular hemorrhage. This lesion is non-specific and may reflect exposure to the elements, contact with detergents that remove skin oils, or other illnesses.

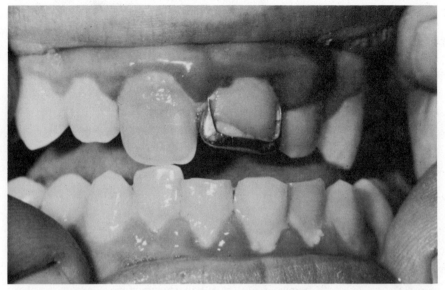

Figure 12–10 Non-specific swelling of interdental papillae. This lesion is particularly common in adolescent boys and girls. There is some evidence that it is more severe in those whose intake of the B-complex vitamins is marginal or low, but the lesion is not diagnostic. Note that the tissue reaction is more severe adjacent to a repaired tooth.

Vitamin A has long been known for its role in maintaining the integrity of the skin and other epithelial membranes (Olson, 1972). The exact mechanism of action is unknown. Indeed, it is not certain which of the forms of vitamin A — retinol, retinal, or retinoic acid — are responsible for maintaining epithelial cells in good health.

Considerable evidence suggests that vitamin A is necessary for protein synthesis. This may explain the development of follicular hyperkeratosis that closely resembles the same lesion in scurvy. But there is one important difference: the hemorrhagic halo that surrounds the hyperkeratotic follicle in scurvy is missing in vitamin A deficiency. But both deficiencies may result in acne and in broken hairs and in coiled hairs; and both deficiency syndromes may result in the sicca syndrome or Sjögren's syndrome. This condition usually is associated with one or another of the collagen-vascular disorders (Kassan and Gardy, 1978) but it probably results more commonly from a nutritional deficiency.

Indeed, suppression of lacrimal and sebaceous secretions probably accounts in large measure for the xerophthalmia, Bitot's spots, and corneal opacification that occur in children of developing countries who are deficient in vitamin A (Figure 12–11).

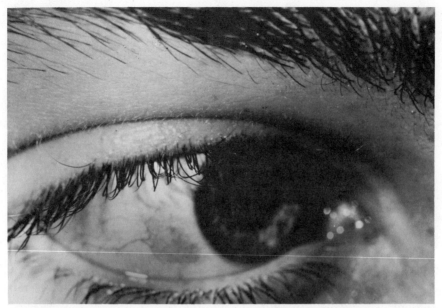

Figure 12–11 Thickening and opacification of the bulbar conjunctiva of a teen-aged girl. This type of lesion is suggestive of vitamin A deficiency, but can occur as a result of exposure to sun and wind or as a result of infection or allergy.

The true requirement for vitamin A has not been established (Sauberlich et al., 1974) but the recommended daily allowance for adults is 800 to 1000 Retinol Equivalents* and slightly higher for lactating women.

Vitamin A has been referred to as the "antikeratinizing" vitamin because lack of this nutrient results in increased keratinization and a surplus (in experimental animals) inhibits keratin synthesis (Logan, 1972).

Therapeutic uses of large doses of vitamin A and β-carotene will be discussed in the chapter on megavitamins.

Vitamin D. The chief relationship between the integument and vitamin D is the long-recognized ability of the skin to synthesize this vitamin when it is exposed to actinic light. This involves conversion of 7-dehydrocholesterol to vitamin D_3, or cholecalciferol. This compound is then hydroxylated in the 25 to 1 positions by the liver and kidney respectively, to form the active substance which is now recognized as a steroid hormone. It, in turn, triggers synthesis of a protein substance

---

*A Retinol Equivalent (RE) is equal to 1.0 μg of retinol or 6.0 μg of β-carotene. For practical purposes, 1 RE $\cong$ 5 IU.

that enhances absorption of calcium by the epithelium of the small bowel.

For many years anthropologists have speculated about the effect of melanin pigments in the skin on the rate of synthesis of vitamin D as a result of a given amount of exposure to actinic light. Supposedly, the black races acquired their heavy pigmentation as a result of genetic survival; excessive formation of vitamin D is presumed to be unfavorable. The evidence in support of this theory is flimsy. Further studies of the ability of black skin to synthesize cholecalciferol are needed. Furthermore, at present it appears that there is a carefully controlled feedback mechanism that limits the rate of hydroxylation of cholecalciferol to 1,25-dihydroxycholecalciferol. In short, the theory that black people cannot synthesize adequate amounts of vitamin D as a result of incidental exposure to sunlight is, in the opinion of the author, unproven.

Vitamin E. Although many claims have been made regarding the supposed beneficial effects of α-tocopherol in preventing wrinkles, fading "age spots", facilitating the healing of burns, and prevention of scar formation, there is no convincing evidence that large amounts of this substance, taken orally or applied to the skin, have any beneficial effects. A few years ago, vitamin E was incorporated in a popular deodorant, but it was removed from the market after a number of people were found to have developed a contact dermatitis. Other alleged effects of vitamin E will be discussed in the chapter on megavitamins.

Vitamin K. This vitamin probably has no effect other than to promote synthesis in the liver of prothrombin and other blood-clotting factors. The only relationship to the skin is the obvious fact that a person who is deficient in vitamin K, and who as a result has low levels of prothrombin activity, is apt to have numerous subcutaneous ecchymoses following minor trauma such as injection of medications, incidental bruises, and venipuncture for collection of blood. This type of bleeding into the skin and subcutaneous tissues is quite different from that seen in scurvy, where the hemorrhages are initially confined to the perifollicular regions of the skin.

The Essential Fatty Acids. Although linoleic, linolenic, and arachidonic acids are all classified as essential, only linoleic acid is needed. The other two compounds can be synthesized from linoleic acid, but the reverse is not true. Hence linoleic acid could be considered to be *the* essential fatty acid, and perhaps should be called a vitamin.

The functions of the essential fatty acids are legion. Many prostaglandins are formed from them. The multiple and complex actions of the prostaglandins cannot be discussed here, but it is sufficient to say that the essential fatty acids appear to be very important nutrients and only a fraction of their role in human nutrition has yet been elucidated.

A deficiency syndrome seemed to be rather unlikely in view of the fact that the average American diet contains at least 4 to 5 per cent of the total energy content as essential fatty acids whereas the requirement is believed to be only 1 to 2 per cent. But the advent of total parenteral nutrition led to continuous infusion of solutions of most nutrients (dextrose, amino acids, vitamins, and minerals) but no fats. As a result, the metabolic activity of these patients was accelerated and at the same time the continuous supply of glucose caused a continuous release of insulin. Since insulin is a "storage" hormone, it is no surprise that this resulted in the body's stores of essential fatty acids becoming imprisoned in the adipose tissues. As a result, there was systemic deficiency of fatty acids with development of a severe acrodermatitis that involved principally the seborrheic areas (Caldwell et al., 1972; Fleming et al., 1976b). Although several reports suggested that topical applications of vegetable oils containing essential fatty acids would cause this dermatitis to subside promptly, we failed to confirm this observation in three consecutive patients who developed this syndrome (Figure 12-1). Fortunately, now that fat emulsions containing essential fatty acids are now available in the United States, it is easy to prevent this deficiency syndrome by infusing 500 ml of the standard 10 per cent emulsion intravenously twice each week.

MINERAL DEFICIENCIES

It is more than a coincidence that total parenteral nutrition, which gave us a clue about the need for the essential fatty acids, also disclosed many features of zinc and copper deficiency. Patients who would have died as a result of disastrous disease or injury to their digestive organs were kept alive and reasonably well-nourished as a result of total parenteral nutrition. In the process, however, it became evident that the nutrient solutions were not complete in that they did not (and still do not) contain *every* essential nutrient (Fleming et al., 1976a). As a result, it became necessary to measure plasma or urinary levels of zinc and copper and to devise methods for giving these trace minerals intravenously. No doubt other trace minerals will also be needed, but our stage of sophistication is still embryonal.

Zinc. Recently, in children, a rare but lethal syndrome was found to result from inability to absorb and utilize zinc. Appropriate supplements of zinc have been reported to result in complete remission of the signs and symptoms of the disease (Moynahan, 1974).

Copper. In addition to the rather unimpressive anemia that seems to develop in patients given total parenteral nutrition without copper supplementation, there has been little evidence of harm. But another genetic defect, known chiefly to pediatricians, called attention to the widespread effects of copper deficiency. In the alliterative style that insures recollection, this disorder has become known as "Menkes's kinky hair" syndrome. Apparently, there is inability to absorb copper, and as a result there may be mental retardation, convulsions, arterial lesions, and bone defects (Danks et al., 1972).

Iron. Although this is generally thought to be involved chiefly in the synthesis of hemoglobin, we know that it plays important roles in a number of enzyme systems. Yet we seldom find that the skin or its appendages provide evidence of iron deficiency. A smooth tongue (Figure 12–12) has been mentioned, but other changes may occur. A peculiar deformity of the finger nails is known as "spoon deformity", or koilonychia. The usually convex surfaces of the finger nails become concave — a striking abnormality (Briggaman and Crounse, 1977).

In addition, several reports have been published indicating that deficiency of iron may cause intense itching of the skin. Correction of the deficiency was reported to result in prompt relief (Lewiecki and Rahman, 1976; Takkunen, 1978).

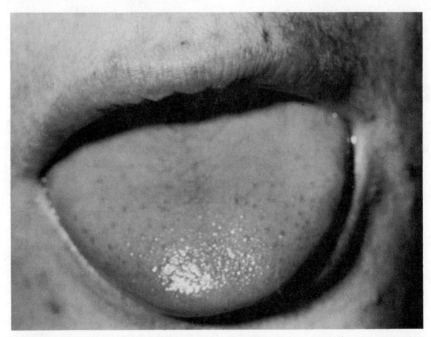

Figure 12–12 A smooth tongue reflects deficiency of iron in an adolescent boy. Many physicians fail to note that the iron requirements of boys between the ages of 11 and 18 years are the same as those of adolescent girls and mature women: 18 mg daily. Many boys and girls fall short of this level of iron intake.

OTHER RELATIONSHIPS BETWEEN
DISEASE, DIET, AND THE SKIN

Tradition supports the concept that adolescent acne vulgaris is adversely affected by diet, and especially by fats, chocolate candy, nuts, and iodized salt. Controlled studies routinely fail to confirm these "old wives' tales" (Fulton et al., 1969). The best advice to the adolescent is to "eat a variety of healthful foods because you enjoy them," and "the acne will disappear as you grow older."

The effects, both real and imagined, of large doses of nutrients on the integument will be reviewed in the chapter on megavitamins.

REFERENCES

Bartley, W., Krebs, H. A., and O'Brien, J. R. P.: *Vitamin C Requirements of Human Adults. A Report by the Vitamin C Subcommittee of the Accessory Food Factors Committee.* London, Medical Research Council, Special Report, Series No. 280, 1953.

Billings, F. L.: *Biotin: An Annotated Bibliography.* Montreal, Vitamin and Chemical Division, Hoffman-La Roche, Limited, 1970, p. 241.

Bradfield, R. B., and Bailey, M. A.: *Hair Root Response to Protein Undernutrition in Hair Growth.* New York, Pergamon Press, 1969.

Briggaman, R. A., and Crounse, R. G.: Skin. In *Nutritional Support of Medical Practice,* Schneider, H. A., Anderson, C. E., and Coursin, D. B. (eds.). Hagerstown, Maryland, Harper & Row, Publishers, 1977, pp. 263–277.

Caldwell, M. D., Josson, H. T., and Otherson, H. B.: Essential fatty acid deficiency in an infant receiving prolonged parenteral alimentation. *J. Pediat. 81:*894, 1972.

Crounse, R. G., Bollet, A. J., and Owens, S.: Quantitative tissue of human malnutrition using scalp hair roots. *Nature 228:*465, 1970.

Danks, D. M., Campbell, P. E., Stevens, B. J., Mayne, V., and Cartwright, E.: Menkes's kinky hair syndrome: an inherited defect in copper absorption with widespread effects. *Pediatrics 50:*188, 1972.

Findlay, G. H.: Pellagra, kwashiorkor, and sun-exposure. *Brit. J. Dermatol. 77:*666, 1965.

Fleming, C. R., Hodges, R. E., and Hurley, L. S.: A prospective study of serum copper and zinc levels in patients receiving total parenteral nutrition. *Amer. J. Clin. Nutr. 29:*70, 1976a.

Fleming, C. R., Smith, L. M., and Hodges, R. E.: Essential fatty acid deficiency in adults receiving total parenteral nutrition. *Amer. J. Clin. Nutr. 29:*976, 1976b.

Fulton, J. E., Plewig, G., and Kligman, A. M.: Effect of chocolate on acne vulgaris. *J.A.M.A. 210:*2071, 1969.

Hodges, R. E., Baker, E. M., Hood, J., Sauberlich, H. E., and March, S. C.: Experimental scurvy in man. *Amer. J. Clin. Nutr. 22:*535, 1969.

Hodges, R. E., Bean, W. B., Ohlson, M. A., and Bleiler, R.: Human pantothenic acid deficiency produced by omega-methyl pantothenic acid. *J. Clin. Invest. 38:*1421, 1959.

Hodges, R. E., Hood, J., Canham, J. E., Sauberlich, H. E., and Baker, E. M.: Clinical manifestations of ascorbic acid deficiency in man. *Amer. J. Clin. Nutr. 24:*432, 1971.

Kassan, S. S., and Gardy, M.: Sjögren's syndrome: an update and overview. *Amer. J. Med. 64:*1037, 1978.

Knowles, J. P., Shuster, S., and Walls, G. C.: Folic-acid deficiency in patients with skin disease. *Lancet 1:*1138, 1963.

Lewiecki, E. M., and Rahman, F.: Pruritus. A manifestation of iron deficiency. *J.A.M.A.* 236:2319, 1976.

Logan, W. S.: Vitamin A and keratinization. *Arch. Dermatol.* 105:748, 1972.

Montagna, W., Ellis, R. A., and Silver, A. F.: *Advances in Biology of Skin, Volume 4: The Sebaceous Glands.* New York, Pergamon Press, The Macmillan Company, 1963.

Moynahan, E. J.: Acrodermatitis enteropathica: A lethal inherited human zinc-deficiency disorder. *Lancet* 2:399, 1974.

Olson, J.: The biological role of vitamin A in maintaining epithelial tissues. *Israel J. Med. Sci.* 8:1170, 1972.

Ruiter, M., and Meyler, L.: Skin changes after therapeutic administration of nicotinic acid in large doses. *Dermatologica* 120:139, 1960.

Sauberlich, H. E., Hodges, R. E., Wallace, D. L., Kolder, H., Canham, J. E., Hood, J., Raica, N., and Lowry, L. K.: Vitamin A metabolism and requirements in the human studied with use of labeled retinol. *Vitamins Hormones* 32:251, 1974a.

Sauberlich, H. E., Skala, J. H., and Dowdy, R. P.: Riboflavin. In *Laboratory Tests for the Assessment of Nutritional Status.* Cleveland, CRC Press, 1974b, pp. 30–37.

Sauer, G. C.: *Manual of Skin Diseases.* Philadelphia, J. B. Lippincott Company, 1973.

Takkunen, H.: Iron deficiency pruritus (Letter to Editor). *J.A.M.A.* 239:1394, 1978.

Vilter, R. W., Mueller, J. F., Glazer, H. S., Jarrold, T., Abraham, J., Thompson, C., and Hankins, V. R.: The effect of vitamin B_6 deficiency induced by desoxypyridoxine in human beings. *J. Lab. Clin. Med.* 42:335, 1953.

Plate 5 This patient with scurvy had neither loose teeth nor swollen gums. He did have follicular hyperkeratosis, perifollicular hemorrhages, broken hairs, and coiled hairs. The diagnosis was made by a medical student who had recently attended a lecture on scurvy.

Plate 6 The classical lesion of scurvy is the hyperkeratotic follicle surrounded by a hemorrhagic halo. In addition there are many hairs showing a "swan-neck" deformity.

Plate 7 Excessive redness of the tongue or magenta (violet-red) color suggests deficiencies of riboflavin, niacin or vitamin B_6. In practice, discoloration of the tongue occurs most often in patients whose general nutritional status is very poor. Usually the color does not change as a result of giving B-complex vitamins but does revert to normal as soon as the patient is restored to a positive caloric and nitrogen balance.

Plate 8 A smooth, shiny tongue suggests the possibility of deficiency of any of three essential nutrients; folic acid, vitamin B_{12}, or iron. If the patient is anemic, the pallor will be even more apparent on a smooth tongue such as this.

Plate 9 Cheilosis or swelling and inflammation of the lips is another non-specific lesion. It is said to occur in riboflavin deficiency (a rare event in this country), and it may occur in patients deficient in vitamin C, niacin, or vitamin B_6. In this photo, there are both swelling and hemorrhage of the lower lip.

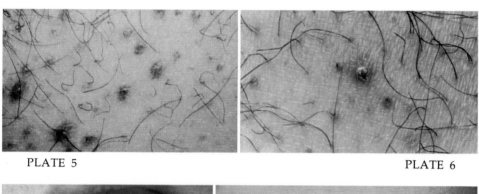

PLATE 5

PLATE 6

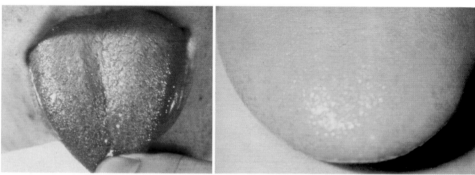

PLATE 7

PLATE 8

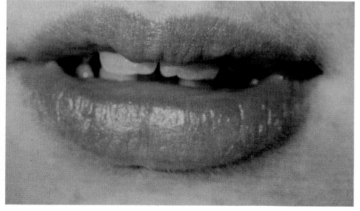

PLATE 9

13

FOOD FADS AND "MEGAVITAMINS"

Robert E. Hodges, M.D.

Humankind seems to be endowed with a strong desire to manipulate its diet in the hope of becoming stronger, more attractive, healthier, and therefore happier. People through the ages have consumed some strange foods in the belief that these would prevent or cure disease. In some instances they were correct: for example, preservation of cabbage with salt resulted in sauerkraut which effectively prevents scurvy; and red chili peppers, which require some training to be enjoyed, are a good source of both vitamin C and vitamin A. Most tribes and races of people developed, through the ages, traditional foods that not only were their favorites but also provided a nutritional advantage by combining plant and animal proteins. Modern-day examples include pizza, goulash, stew, macaroni and cheese, spaghetti and meat sauce, rice and meat (or fish or chicken), and even the hamburger sandwich. The admixture of foods proved to be more nutritious than these same foods consumed at different times. But these advantages were not discovered by scientific experiment; they developed gradually as a result of individual and group preferences or perhaps as a result of the ancient equivalent of our present-day food fads.

Before going further, we should attempt to define the terms "food fad" and "megavitamins". A food fad, as used in this chapter, is any dietary concept that remains unproven scientifically. Thus a food fad may eventually be proven to be either wise or foolish or something in between these extremes.

A "mega" vitamin is a term used originally by non-medical people to refer to very large doses of vitamins. The prefix "mega" means large or great. The metric definition is million. As shown in Table 13–1, nutrients are seldom if ever given in doses one million times the usual or recommended dose. But doses of one hundred times the recommended amount are not uncommon and occasionally doses one thousand times normal are given.

VEGETARIAN DIETS

One of the common food fads is vegetarianism, although some people object to this designation. There is substantial justification for their objections because plant foods can supply all essential nutrients except vitamin B_{12}. Strict vegetarians have less obesity and diabetes mellitus, lower blood levels of cholesterol and triglycerides, and lower prevalence rates for atherosclerotic and certain malignant diseases than the average adult who is omnivorous. Hardinge and Stare (1954) compared the nutritional, physical, and laboratory studies of 112 vegetarian and 88 nonvegetarian adults, adolescents, and pregnant women. These included adult subjects who were lacto-ovo-vegetarians, pure vegetarians, or non-vegetarians. In the adolescent groups and in the pregnant group, lacto-ovo-vegetarians were compared with non-vegetarians.

Their studies indicated that the average intake of nutrients by all groups (with the exception of adolescent pure vegetarians) approximated or exceeded the amounts recommended by the National Research Council. In general, measurements of height, weight, and blood pressure were not significantly different among the three gruops but pure vegetarians on average weighed 20 pounds less. Values for total proteins, albumin, and globulin as well as hematologic findings were not statistically different for all the vegetarian and non-vegetarian groups.

The National Research Council (Committee on Nutritional Misinformation) issued a statement on vegetarian diets (Food and Nutrition Board, 1974). They noted that, "The current trend in the eating habits of certain young adults, away from the familiar Western food patterns toward vegetarianism, has caused concern about the nutritional implications of such changes."

They noted also that, "Vegetarian diets may be based only on plant food sources (total vegetarians), plant foods plus dairy products (lacto-vegetarians), or plant foods plus dairy products and eggs (lacto-ovo-vegetarians)."

After examining the scientific data available, this group of experts summarized their conclusions as follows: "A vegetarian can be well nourished *if* he eats a variety of plant foods and gives attention to the

TABLE 13–1   COMPARATIVE DAILY DOSE-RANGES OF SOME VITAMINS

Vitamin	Minimal Requirement	Recommended Allowance	Therapeutic Dose to Correct Deficiency	Pharmacologic Range	Toxic Range and Abnormalities Induced
Vitamin A	~ 1500 IU	5000 IU	10,000 IU	~ 50,000 IU in malabsorption syndromes	50,000–100,000 IU pseudotumor cerebri
Vitamin D (cholecalciferol)	400 IU	400 IU	800 IU	10,000–50,000 IU in vitamin D–resistant rickets	1000–100,000 IU hypercalcemia renal calcinosis
Ascorbic Acid	~ 10 mg	45 mg	100 mg	1000–2500 mg in attempts to prevent or treat colds	2000–4000 mg teratogenesis, oxaluria interferes with tests for glycosuria
Niacin	~ 10 mg	12–20 mg	60 mg	3000–9000 mg to reduce plasma lipids	1000–10,000 mg flushing of skin rough skin hyperglycemia impaired hepatic function
Folic acid	~ 100 µg* tetrahydrofolate	100–150 µg tetrahydrofolate	300 µg	5000–50,000 µg in malabsorption syndromes	50,000 µg intravenously antagonizes anticonvulsant drugs

*Four times this amount if mixed folates are given.

There are several levels at which most vitamins have been given. The *Minimal Daily Requirement* is that amount necessary to avoid signs and symptoms of deficiency in most persons.
The Recommended Daily Allowance is a generous surplus that should ensure an adequate amount for virtually all healthy persons.
The *Therapeutic Dose* is an arbitrary amount that can be given for a short time to patients who are presumed to be deficient in that nutrient, without undue risk of toxicity.
The *Pharmacologic Range* is a much larger amount intended to produce an effect that is, in most instances, unrelated to the primary vitamin effect.
The Toxic Range is an amount that commonly produces clinical or metabolic abnormalities.

critical nutrients mentioned above [lysine, methionine, calcium, iron, riboflavin, vitamin B_{12}, and for children not exposed to sunlight, vitamin D]. Dairy products and eggs are outstanding sources of the nutrients of greatest concern. Legumes, leafy vegetables, and a source of vitamin B_{12} are important components of the diet containing no foods of animal origin."

Certainly, individuals who limit their food choices to those of plant origin must have a greater-than-average knowledge of nutrient requirements and the nutritional value of food; but a vegetarian diet not only can be healthful and pleasant, it also may prove to be an effective way of postponing such disease processes as atherosclerosis and neoplastic diseases. In this sense, a vegetarian is definitely *not* a food faddist.

FOOD FIBER

The concept of bulk or fiber or undigestible carbohydrates in the diet was discussed in the chapter on Nutrition and the Digestive Tract. Epidemiological studies, buttressed by "armchair logic" seem to indicate that food fiber is a very important part of a healthful diet. But reports of clinical trials are mixed; some investigators believe that food fiber, in the form of bran or other undigestible material, improves their patients who complain of constipation and cramping abdominal pains. But others report no benefit, and some patients complain about embarrassing flatulence. Meanwhile, studies in experimental animals indicate that bran can interfere with absorption of zinc and other divalent cations. The role of fiber in the diet is yet to be established, but the idea is logical and no doubt will be explored by many clinical as well as basic scientists.

MEGAVITAMIN THERAPY

As mentioned above, the term "megavitamin" therapy is non-specific, but implies that a very large amount of a vitamin is to be given. Many patients and a few doctors ask: "If a little is good, why isn't a lot better?" The reason is simple: Herbert (1977) points out that most vitamins (at least the water-soluble ones) function as coenzymes. They are absorbed and carried in the bloodstream to cells whose function depends upon a certain enzyme. Here the vitamin enters the cell and combines with an apoenzyme synthesized by that cell. This results in a holoenzyme that fulfills its purpose within or outside the cell. Since the quantity of apoenzymes is limited, they are generally saturated by modest amounts of their respective coenzymes or vitamins. It is no coincidence that the amounts of vitamins suggested in the Recommended Dietary Allowances (RDAs) (1974) are usually the amounts that will saturate the apoenzymes of cells.

Thus, excessive doses of vitamins serve no additional *nutritional* purpose but may have a pharmacologic or a toxic effect or both. Note in Table 13–1 that large doses of niacin will lower plasma lipids but also may cause toxic side reactions.

Established Uses of Megavitamin Therapy

Although Jukes (1975) and others have cautioned against the irresponsible use of megavitamin therapy in a variety of illnesses, there are a few clinical syndromes that are corrected or alleviated by large doses of specific vitamins. These include two major groups of disorders: the malabsorption syndromes and some of the "inborn errors of metabolism".

Malabsorption Syndromes

Malabsorption of nutrients can result from a variety of disorders including maldigestion, excessively rapid motility, an abnormality of the mucosa of the bowel, and the short bowel syndrome. Of course, this is a gross oversimplification of the many disease syndromes that can impair absorption of nutrients from ingested food, but the end result is nutrient deficiency — sometimes general, sometimes specific.

The most specific deficiency is lack of vitamin B_{12}, which may result from genetic loss of ability to secrete intrinsic factor in the gastric juice or from surgical loss of the terminal portion of the ileum or from a blind-loop syndrome or from infestation with the fish tapeworm, *Diphyllobothrium latum*.

Other forms of malabsorption are less specific; for example, folic acid must be deconjugated before it can be absorbed, and several factors (including ethanol) can limit or interfere with this process.

Any form of steatorrhea, whether it results from pancreatic disease, hepatobiliary disease, or a small bowel disorder, can result in substantial losses of the fat-soluble essential nutrients: vitamin A, vitamin D, vitamin E, vitamin K, and the essential fatty acids, linoleic, linolenic, and arachidonic acid. Most patients with a malabsorption syndrome will benefit from additional amounts of vitamins (Table 13–2 and 13–3). This form of therapy will not cure the primary disorder, but it may improve the patient's general nutritional status, or prevent it from deteriorating further.

Inborn Errors of Metabolism

A large number of inherited abnormalities involve the need for or the metabolism of essential nutrients. Rosenberg (1970) has described the commonest inborn errors that result in vitamin-dependent syndromes. A disproportionate number involve vitamin B_6, perhaps because it plays an important role in a great many enzyme systems. The salient features of a few of the vitamin-dependent syndromes are listed in Table 13–4.

Chopra (1976) reviewed the legitimate uses of megadoses of vitamins one at a time in considerable detail. The fact that some individuals lack the necessary metabolic machinery (apoenzymes, carrier proteins, and so on) to utilize vitamins and essential minerals normally does not imply that normal people should ingest large doses of essential nutrients (Table 13–5). Indeed there is evidence that excessive doses of ascorbic acid (and perhaps of other vitamins) can induce a metabolic change that increases the rate of catabolism of that vitamin and, in effect, makes the individual dependent on large doses. This is discussed later.

Megavitamin Doses of Ascorbic Acid

Perhaps we never will know who first "discovered" the virtues of giving excessive doses of vitamin C to treat infectious diseases and other ailments, but certainly one of the first was Jacques Cartier (quoted in Major, 1945). His fleet was trapped all winter in the ice of the St. Lawrence river outside Montreal, and his sailors were dying of scurvy. Friendly Indians told him how to make an extract of the bark and needles of the arbor vitae tree (a cedar), which he did. Not only were his men saved but, according to his account, "... *and what other disease soever, in such sorte, that there were some bene diseased and troubled with the French Pockes* [syphilis] *foure or five yeres, and with this drink were cleane healed.*"

But we do know that, during the early phases of World War II, German investigators were evaluating vitamin C as a possible means of increasing the resistance of children to infection (Peters, 1939). Peters found little or no evidence of a beneficial effect with regard to colds, but thought that influenza might be a little less common and less severe in children receiving vitamin C. When she combined the data for colds and influenza, she could find no convincing evidence of either prevention or amelioration of respiratory illness.

Since that time, a great many studies have been conducted using a variety of experimental designs. Some of these studies showed absolutely no effect, a few showed an apparent ability of ascorbic acid

TABLE 13–2 APPROPRIATE ORAL DOSES OF VITAMINS*
AND MINERALS FOR PATIENTS WITH ANY TYPE OF
MALABSORPTION SYNDROME

I. WATER-SOLUBLE VITAMINS (IN DIVIDED DOSES)	
Ascorbic acid	150–300 mg daily
Thiamin	5–15 mg daily
Riboflavin	5–15 mg daily
Niacin	30–60 mg daily
Folic Acid	15–30 mg daily
Vitamin B_{12}	100–300 μg daily
Vitamin B_6	5–15 mg daily
II. FAT-SOLUBLE VITAMINS	
Vitamin A (as Retinyl palmitate)	30,000–60,000 IU daily
Vitamin D (as vitamin D_2)	30,000 IU daily
Vitamin E	30 mg daily
Vitamin K	15 mg daily
Essential Fatty Acids (as linoleic)	15 g daily
III. MINERALS	
Calcium (as Ca gluconate)	1.5 g Ca^{++} daily
Magnesium (as Mg sulfate)	600 mg Mg^{++} daily
Iron (as $FeSO_4$)	300 mg daily
Other trace minerals (as indicated by plasma levels or clinical status)	

*Doses for adults. For children give ¼ to ½ depending on age.

Tables 13–2 and 13–3: When a malabsorption syndrome is diagnosed, the physician often will want to give large doses of vitamins in the hope of correcting or preventing deficiencies. But excessive doses can cause undesirable side effects such as nausea, vomiting, or diarrhea. The amounts listed are generally well tolerated, at least for a few weeks. Care should be exercised in the administration of these doses of vitamins A and D for a prolonged period of time.

TABLE 13–3   THE FAT-SOLUBLE VITAMINS

I. VITAMIN D
  a. Hypophosphatemic vitamin D–resistant rickets
     Responds to 25,000 IU cholecalciferol daily
  b. Osteomalacia due to phosphate diabetes
     Vitamin D, 50,000 IU daily
  c. Renal osteodystrophy
     Vitamin D, 50,000–500,000 IU daily
  d. Hepatic rickets
     Vitamin D, 5000–50,000 IU daily
  e. Fanconi syndrome (refractory rickets with multiple and tubular defects)
     Vitamin D, 5000–50,000 IU daily
  f. Cystinosis
     Similar to Fanconi syndrome
  g. Hyperparathyroidism
     Oral phosphates
  h. Hypoparathyroidism
     IV Ca gluconate, then vitamin D, 50,000–100,000 IU daily
  i. Pseudohyperparathyroidism
     Poor response to therapy
  j. Rickets due to anticonvulsant drugs
     Vitamin D, 600 IU daily
  k. Hypercortisolism
     Reduce adrenal steroids

II. VITAMIN A
  a. Pityriasis rubra pilaris (very rare)
     May respond to vitamin A, 150,000–200,000 IU daily
     May be very toxic
  b. Erythropoietic protoporphyria (rare)
     β-carotene, 15–300 mg daily
  c. Acne vulgaris
     Some respond to retinoic acid, 20–50 mg daily
  d. Keratosis follicularis
     Vitamin A, 200,000–300,000 IU daily may produce clearing but is dangerous
  e. Psoriasis
     Retinoic acid (50–200 mg daily)
     170,000–680,000 IU → ? improvement

III. VITAMIN E
  a. Epidermolysis bullosa
     600 IU daily → ? benefit
  b. Tocopherol responsive anemia (premature infants)
     Give Vitamin E, 25 IU daily

TABLE 13-4 SOME VITAMIN-DEPENDENT SYNDROMES

Name	Common Findings	Vitamin Involved	Daily Amount RDA°	Daily Amount Therapeutic Dose
B₆-dependent syndrome	Convulsions	Vitamin B_6	0.5 mg	20 mg
Sideroblastic anemia	Microcytic hypochromic anemia	Vitamin B_6	1–2 mg	10 mg
Xanthurenic aciduria	Mental retardation	Vitamin B_6	1–2 mg	10 mg
Homocystinuria	Mental retardation Vascular occlusions	Vitamin B_6 (or folic acid)	1–2 mg 100 μg	500 mg 20,000 μg
Hartnup's disease	Mental retardation Cerebellar ataxia	Niacin	5–20 mg	200 mg
Methylmalonic aciduria	Mental retardation Ketoacidosis	Vitamin B_{12}	> 0.3 μg	1000 μg
Hypophosphatemic rickets	Bony deformities	Vitamin D	400 IU	50,000 to 200,000 IU

°RDA = Recommended Dietary Allowance.

Some of the more common vitamin-dependent syndromes are listed above. Caution must be exercised in giving large doses of vitamin D for long periods of time.

TABLE 13–5 CONDITIONS SUCCESSFULLY TREATED WITH MEGADOSES OF VITAMINS

I. Pyridoxine Dependency (Presumed to result from enzymatic defects)
Infantile convulsive disorder
Hypochromic (sideroblastic) anemia
Hyperoxaluria (urinary-tract stones)
Homocystinuria
Cystathioninuria
Xanthurenic aciduria (after tryptophan load)

II. Folic Acid
Congenital megaloblastic anemia
Homocystinuria and hypomethioninemia
Formiminotransferase deficiency
Megaloblastic anemia of malabsorption

III. Vitamin B$_{12}$
Juvenile pernicious anemia
Transcobalamin II deficiency
Methylmalonicaciduria
Homocystinuria, hypomethioninemia, and methylmalonicaciduria

IV. The Fat-Soluble Vitamins and the Essential Fatty Acids
Cystic fibrosis
Steatorrhea of any type (such as biliary tract disease, malabsorption)

Some conditions respond to "megadoses" of specific vitamins. These syndromes are quite rare and their responsiveness does not suggest that the average person would benefit from such doses.

to prevent colds, and others seemed to show a therapeutic effect of vitamin C: a shortening of duration of symptoms and fever with a reduction of such complications as sinusitis, streptococcal infections, and rheumatic fever. In all too many studies, the experimental design was unsuitable to permit objective assessment.

For purposes of reference and documentation, representative articles are herewith listed:

Dahlberg and others (1942) studied 2500 Swedish soldiers who spent the winter and spring of 1941–42 in Northern Sweden. Half of the men were given yellow tablets containing 200 mg of vitamin C for 24 days, and 50 mg therafter. The other half were given blue placebo tablets containing citric acid. Although ascorbic acid loading tests indicated a difference in their body loads of this vitamin, there were no differences in either the frequency or the severity of colds.

Glazebrook and Thomson (1942) studied the effects of giving 200 mg of vitamin C daily to 350 boys in a large institution (1500 youths, age 15 to 20 years). The diet of the boys was "rather poor" in vitamin C, and loading tests performed in 77 subjects showed no urinary loss (presumptive evidence of impending scurvy). Vitamin C had no effect on incidence of colds or tonsillitis and there were no differences in duration of colds, but rheumatic fever and pneumonia occurred only in boys who did not receive vitamin C (it is important to recall that the control subjects probably had less than adequate amounts of vitamin C in their diet).

A report that has been widely publicized is that of Cowan and colleagues, (1942), who gave vitamin C or multivitamin preparations to young adults. They concluded that, "This controlled study yields no indication that either large doses of vitamin C alone or large doses of vitamins A, B_1, B_2, C, D, and nicotinic acid have any important effect on the number or severity of infections of the upper respiratory tract when administered to young adults who presumably are on a reasonably adequate diet." Yet this study has been cited as evidence that megadoses of vitamin C can prevent or alleviate colds.

Tarjan-Kassai (1954) observed the effects of giving 300 mg of ascorbic acid daily to factory workers for a total of 18 months. She gave suitable citric acid placebos to a control group. She noted that despite the probability that the Hungarian diet was deficient in vitamin C during winter months, there was no evidence that colds were prevented by ascorbic acid. She did conclude, however, that there was a decrease in anemia and a lessening in the severity of colds.

Franz and others (1956) gave vitamin C with or without bioflavonoids, or a placebo, or bioflavonoids alone to a group of 88 medical students and nurses. There was no reduction in the number of colds, but those receiving vitamin C recovered more quickly. Bioflavonoids had no effect. But Tebrock and others (1956) performed a similar study in 1900 subjects and reported a total lack of effect.

Perhaps the most controversial study of the effects of vitamin C in preventing or treating colds was that of Ritzel (1961). He gave either vitamin C or a placebo to teen-aged boys and girls who were attending either of two ski camps in Switzerland. He reported that there were only 31 days of illness in the group of 139 subjects who took ascorbic acid, but 80 days of illness in the group of 140 persons who took placebo medications. Furthermore, he reported that the average duration of colds was only 1.8 days in the vitamin C group, but 2.6 days in the placebo group.

Walker and others (1967) evaluated the effects of appropriate doses of vitamin C on virus infections in tissue cultures, on mouse influenza, and on human volunteers given five cold viruses by nasal instillation. In none of these three studied did ascorbic acid prevent or modify the infections. In two clinical trials, the group of subjects who were told whether they were receiving ascorbic acid or not, before their colds ended, had appreciably shorter illnesses. In subsequent trials the investigators did not tell the subjects whether they were receiving vitamin C or a placebo and the duration of colds was similar in both groups.

Anderson and colleagues (1972) reviewed the published data on the effects of vitamin C on the common cold and designed a study to determine the facts. They found that giving either ascorbic acid or a placebo resulted in no significant differences in either the number of colds or their duration. But, paradoxically, they found that the number of subjects who remained well was greater in the vitamin C–treated group. [It's marvelous what one can do with statistics—Ed.]

Schwartz and others (1973) evaluated the efficacy of ascorbic acid in preventing induced rhinovirus infections in man. Twenty-one healthy men volunteered for the double-blind study. They received either 3000 mg of ascorbic acid or a placebo each day for two weeks, then they were challenged with rhinovirus 44. The ascorbic acid or placebo therapy was continued for another week. All of the men became ill and the intensity of symptoms was the same except for one day when the placebo group had more severe illness.

A widely publicized study was reported by Coulehan and colleagues (1974), who undertook a double-blind study of 14 weeks' duration in 641 children in a boarding school. The subjects were supposed to receive either 1 g of ascorbic acid daily or 2 g daily or a placebo. There were no differences between the numbers of respiratory episodes in the three groups, but those receiving vitamin C had fewer total days of illness.

Much to his credit, Coulehan, who recognized that there had been irregularities in the conduct of their first (1974) study, organized another group and designed and conducted a second study (1976). This time there were 868 children who received either vitamin C or a placebo in a double-blind fashion. The results were conclusive: There were no differences in the numbers of subjects who became ill or in the total number of respiratory illnesses or in the mean duration of illness. Children receiving vitamin C had fewer positive throat cultures for β-hemolytic streptococci but there were no differences in the complication rates of the two groups. Children with high plasma levels of ascorbic acid had longer-lasting illnesses.

Anderson and others (1974) also decided to repeat their study, but this time they gave graded doses of ascorbic acid: 250, 1000, or 2000 mg daily as prophylaxis and either 4000 or 8000 mg daily on the last day of a cold. They found no differences in the numbers of colds and only a questionably small prophylactic and therapeutic effect. They felt there was some reduction in severity but this was not dose-related. Accordingly, they suggested that the optimal daily dose of vitamin C for preventing colds might be "less than 250 mg."

Anderson and others (1975) then studied the protective effect of 500 mg of ascorbic acid daily versus a placebo. If a cold developed, the individual was given 1500 mg of ascorbic acid the first day followed by 1000 mg daily on the second, third, fourth, and fifth days. Vitamin C was given either in a sustained release or as a regular preparation. A large number of subjects took these medications for an average of 15 weeks. There were no differences between the effects of sustained-release and the regular form of vitamin C. Both groups receiving vitamin C had milder illnesses than those receiving placebo and they spent 25 per cent fewer days indoors. Anderson suggested that smaller doses of vitamin C might be equally effective.

Karlowski and others (1975) conducted a carefully designed study at the clinical center in National Institutes of Health. They summarized their work as follows: "Ascorbic acid had, at best, only a minor influence on the duration and severity of colds. The effects demonstrated might be explained equally well by a break in the double blind."

Chalmers (1975) reviewed 14 published clinical trials and concluded that only eight were creditable. He calculated the difference in the mean number of colds to be only 0.01 ± 0.06 per year, and the difference in duration of colds to be only 0.11 ± 0.24 day. Chalmers remarked that "the minor benefits are not worth the potential risk, however small."

Dykes and Meier (1975) also reviewed the available data regarding the efficacy and the toxicity of ascorbic acid in preventing or treating the common cold. They concluded that: (1) ". . . There is no clear, reproducible pattern of efficacy . . .", (2) "There is currently little adequate evidence on either the presence or the absence of serious adverse reactions to such [large] doses of ascorbic acid . . .", and (3) "The unrestricted use of ascorbic acid for these purposes cannot be advocated on the basis of evidence currently available."

Metabolically, vitamin C plays a number of vital roles, yet it has never been proved to be a coenzyme. Lack of vitamin C causes scurvy, a well-defined and eventually lethal syndrome. Vitamin C, perhaps by virtue of its hydroxylation of proline, plays an important role in the formation of mature collagen, and in the maintenance and repair of connective tissues. It also plays a role in the synthesis of adrenal cortical steroids and of epinephrine. Deficiency of vitamin C in humans and in susceptible experimental animals reduces their resistance to a number of infectious illnesses. Lack of vitamin C also affects the secretory functions of the salivary and lacrimal glands. Impaired secretions may also contribute to dryness of the skin and the follicular hyperkeratosis that accompany scurvy; but the hemorrhagic manifestations of scurvy are still largely unexplained. Generally, the platelet counts are normal and the prothrombin time is within acceptable limits. The bleeding time may be normal, despite widespread hemorrhages into the skin and other tissues. Electron-microscopic studies of cutaneous vessels in skin biopsies from scorbutic patients fail to demonstrate the "loss of intercellular substance" that has been alleged to cause bleeding in scurvy. At present, there is no dependable test that can explain this hemorrhagic tendency.

Pharmacologic Doses of Ascorbic Acid

We know that as little as 10 mg of vitamin C per day will prevent or cure scurvy in adult men. In the United States, the most recent (1974) recommended allowance for ascorbic acid is 45 mg per day.

This was reported by the author and his associates to be sufficient to saturate the body pool of approximately 1500 mg (Hodges et al., 1969; Hodges et al., 1971). Recent evidence suggests that the total body pool of vitamin C may be somewhat larger (Hornig, 1975).

Vitamin C has been given in much larger doses for a variety of reasons. We refer to doses in the range of 100 to 1000 mg daily as pharmacologic because excesses of ascorbic acid cannot perform the same functions as smaller amounts given for the cure of scurvy. Instead, ascorbic acid does a number of things unrelated to its action as a vitamin. For example, excessive amounts are excreted in the urine, which becomes more acidic (Travis et al., 1965). Some physicians use this as a means of preventing or treating urinary tract infections, although better methods are available.

Vitamin C also augments absorption of iron from the digestive tract, a result that could be either useful or harmful (Cook and Monsen, 1977).

Toxic or Undesirable Side Effects of Giving Large Doses of Vitamin C

Protective Mechanisms. When very large (mega) doses of vitamin C are given to (or taken by) patients, there usually are no serious consequences. The body has at least three mechanisms (and the nature of foods provides a fourth) that prevent marked elevations of the level of ascorbic acid in the blood.

The first of these four is the simple fact that few palatable foods contain ascorbic acid in very high concentrations. Scarcely anyone would eat enough parsley to provide 2000 mg of vitamin C daily. Even orange juice becomes tiresome if one is obliged to drink excessive quantities.

The second protective mechanism is the limited capacity of the digestive tract to absorb ascorbic acid (Kübler and Gehler, 1970). These investigators demonstrated that absorption of small doses of vitamin C is very efficient but the efficiency declines with larger and larger doses. Nelson and Cerda (1975) confirmed these observations and showed that only 6 per cent of the largest dose (916 mg per hour) was absorbed. Failure to absorb large doses does not only account for the osmotic diarrhea that results from an excessive intake but also explains why there are so few toxic complications.

A third protective mechanism is the renal threshold for ascorbic acid. When plasma levels are within low or normal ranges, there is very little ascorbic acid excreted in the urine because tubular reabsorption of this vitamin is very effective. But when plasma levels rise above the renal threshold for vitamin C (above 1.7 mg/dl), the rate of ascorbic acid excreted rises abruptly. This has the effect of limiting the concentration of ascorbic acid in the blood (Ahlborg, 1947).

Reference has already been made to the phenomenon of induction of a catabolic mechanism (almost certainly an enzyme) that destroys vitamin C at an unusually rapid rate. This explains the finding of normal or low plasma levels of ascorbic acid in persons who take large amounts of this vitamin. It also explains the occurrence of scurvy in persons who reduce their intake of vitamin C abruptly, even though their new level of intake is adequate for the normal person. Gordonoff (1960) gave large doses of vitamin C to guinea pigs for four weeks, followed by a diet devoid of vitamin C. These animals died in 25 days, while control animals lived 38 days. Schrauzer and Rhead (1973) made similar observations in humans who ingested large amounts of vitamin C for several weeks, then ate a deficient diet. Compared with control subjects, their blood and urinary levels of ascorbic acid fell rapidly to deficient values. Nandi and colleagues (1973) confirmed this finding in guinea pigs, and their work was reconfirmed by Sorensen and others (1974), who observed that the excessive rate of ascorbic acid destruction persisted longer than 68 days.

Reproduction. The idea that vitamin C might be harmful in pregnancy is hotly contested by certain enthusiasts but the facts seem to indicate that this can occur. Neuweiler (1951) reported that large doses of vitamin C given to guinea pigs impaired their fertility and resulted in a high mortality of the embryos. Moriquand and Edel (1953) and Samborskaya and Ferdman (1964) reported that large amounts of ascorbic acid can terminate pregnancy.

Cochrane (1965) observed 42 cases of infantile scurvy in a Halifax hospital, seven of whom were thought to have had an adequate intake of vitamin C. In two cases, the mothers had been giving ascorbic acid in doses of 60 mg daily to their children. But these mothers had been ingesting large amounts of vitamin C during pregnancy and their babies had developed a catabolic mechanism that destroyed much of the vitamin C they received. Cochrane demonstrated this mechanism in pregnant guinea pigs. These observations were confirmed by Norkus and Rosso (1975).

Samborskaya and Ferdman (1966) reported that by giving large doses of vitamin C they interrupted pregnancy in 16 of 20 women who had missed their first menstrual period. They also showed that pregnant rats could be aborted by giving large doses of ascorbic acid. Estrogen excretion in the urine rose during administration of ascorbic acid.

Stitch and others (1976) reported studies of the mutagenic potential of ascorbic acid. Oxidation products of ascorbic acid are mutagenic for both microbial and mammalian cells *in vitro*.

The important message is that, during pregnancy, a woman should eat good food in proper quantities. She should not take large doses of vitamins nor any other medication, unless her physician feels there is a need for her to do so.

Diabetes Mellitus. Ascorbic acid and dehydroascorbic acid, which are in equilibrium with each other, are powerful antioxidants. More than twenty years ago, Levey and Suter (1946) showed that L-ascorbic acid potentiated the diabetogenic effect of alloxan in rats. Patterson (1949) showed that dehydroascorbic acid given to rats would produce diabetes. These studies raised the question of whether large doses of vitamin C, taken in the hope of preventing colds, could either cause or aggravate diabetes. Goldner (1971) reviewed the available evidence and concluded that the greatest problem relates to the interference with tests for glycosuria. Lowering the pH of urine, as a result of large doses of ascorbic acid, will cause false-negative tests for glucose if the popular tape or dipstick method is used. These tests depend upon glucose oxidase which is activated by horseradish peroxidase, which requires an optimal pH.

If the older test for glycosuria is used, in which an effervescent tablet releases a caustic alkali and a copper salt, a positive test results from the reducing action of glucose or other reducing substance. Ascorbic acid will give a false-positive.

Mayson and others (1973) surveyed the results of 47,750 routine urine tests for glucose. Only 170 (0.35 per cent) were false-negatives. The authors found that 41 per cent of these contained a reducing substance, such as ascorbic acid. Thus only 0.14 per cent of these urine tests were abnormal as a result of some reducing substance that may have been vitamin C. Yet it can be a serious problem for those few individuals who are misled by a false test.

Anticoagulants. Among its many biological actions, ascorbic acid can reverse the anticoagulant effects of sodium warfarin (Sigell and Flessa, 1970). It also can reverse the anticoagulant effects of heparin *in vitro* (Owen et al., 1970). Rosenthal (1971) reported a patient who reversed the therapeutic effects of sodium warfarin when she took large amounts of vitamin C, thus verifying the animal studies previously described.

High Altitude Hypoxia. Many young people in our society expose themselves to hypoxic conditions by climbing mountains, sailing in gliders, or even by going to certain ski resorts. Some of these same people may dose themselves with large amounts of vitamin C. Studies initiated in Germany near the beginning of World War II suggest that this practice may be harmful. Pfannensteil (1938) studied the effects of vitamin C on the tolerance of rabbits to simulated high altitudes. Rabbits given no vitamin C had poor tolerance to hypoxia, those given modest supplements had good tolerance, but those given high doses had impaired tolerance. Dörholt (1938) continued these studies and confirmed the deleterious effects of giving vitamin C to rabbits exposed to the "altitude test". After five weeks of vitamin therapy, they manifested a rapid onset of weakness and convulsions when placed in a chamber that was hypoxic.

Schrauzer and others (1975) confirmed these observations in healthy volunteers. The men were placed in separate high altitude chambers adjusted to simulate any altitude between 5000 and 25,000 feet. When men consumed 2000 mg of vitamin C daily for six days there was no measurable change in high altitude performance but after they had consumed 3000 mg daily for six days they were observed to have impairment of functions and the test was terminated at once. Two weeks later they had returned to normal when tested in the chamber.

Urinary Stones. Large doses of vitamin C have been blamed for the development of urinary tract stones. Lamden and Chrystowski (1954) gave increasing doses of ascorbic acid to men and followed their rates of excretion of oxalate in the urine. Doses of less than 4000 mg of vitamin C daily had little effect on the average rate of excretion of oxalates in the urine, but doses in the range of 8000–9000 mg daily increased oxalate excretion significantly. At the highest levels of vitamin C (9000 mg), the men excreted an average of 70 mg more oxalate than normal.

Briggs (1976) reported that some individuals convert more vitamin C into oxalates than others. He found three out of a group of 67 subjects who had this "defect". One apparently healthy young man ingested 4000 mg of ascorbic acid and had a tenfold increase in urinary oxalate. A second young man had an even greater response to 4000 mg of ascorbic acid per day; his urinary oxalate excretion rose from 43 to 738 mg in 24 hours. This patient's father had the same trait.

Roth and Breitenfield (1977) reported a young man with a renal stone, who had been taking 1000 mg of ascorbic acid daily for several months. His urinary excretion of oxalates was found to be 127, 126, and 76 mg per 24 hours on three different days. After he had discontinued taking ascorbic acid his urinary oxalates were 56 and 62 mg per 24 hours on two separate days. The normal for that laboratory was less than 40 mg per 24 hours.

Vitamin C can increase the rate of excretion of uric acid, according to Stein and others (1976). They studied the levels of uric acid in the serum, and in the urine of 14 persons who then ingested 4000 mg of ascorbic acid. Urinary excretion of uric acid doubled, but uricosuria could be inhibited by aspirin. In three persons who took 8000 mg of ascorbic acid daily for three days, the level of uric acid in serum rose 1.2 to 3.1 mg/dl. The authors point out that changes such as these could invalidate studies of gout and might activate latent gout. These changes might also lead to urate stones in the urinary tract.

Large doses of vitamin C given to embryonic chicks can elevate the rate of calcium turnover as measured by radioactive calcium (Ramp and Thornton, 1971). No data are available in humans, but if calcium is mobilized from the skeleton, the rate of urinary loss would likely be increased. More data are needed to evaluate the potential of large doses of ascorbic acid to cause urinary tract stones.

Cholesterol and Fat Metabolism. From time to time various claims have been made to the effect that large doses of vitamin C can aid in regulation of cholesterol metabolism and help prevent athero-sclerotic diseases. Sokoloff and colleagues (1966) studied interactions between dietary cholesterol, ascorbic acid, and plasma levels of lipids. They studied rabbits, rats, and humans. Cholesterol-fed rabbits became very hypercholesterolemic, but much of the rise could be prevented by giving ascorbic acid. In rats, there was a similar but less pronounced effect. In normal humans, the results were conflicting. Doses of 1500 mg of ascorbic acid daily had little or no effect. In patients with elevated levels of cholesterol, doses of 2000 to 3000 mg of ascorbic acid had a "definite" cholesterol-lowering effect in 50 of 60 cases. Along similar lines, Spittle (1971) reported that her own plasma cholesterol level fell markedly when she increased her intake of vitamin C. She gave large doses to a number of persons, and found that while those 25 years old or younger had a fall in cholesterol levels, the response was variable in older persons.

Ginter (1973), who has for years studied the relationships between cholesterol metabolism and vitamin C, believes that cholesterol accumulates in the serum and liver of guinea pigs with chronic deficiency of vitamin C. He claims that vitamin C is necessary for conversion of cholesterol to bile acids.

Tsai and others (1973) studied factors that can inactivate lipase activity and showed that the inactivation requires ATP, Mg^{++}, and ascorbic acid.

Kritchevsky (1974) studied the effects of varying the concentration of ascorbic acid on the rate of 7, α-hydroxylation of cholesterol. He confirmed the observation that scorbutic guinea pigs do not oxidize cholesterol at an optimal rate, but different amounts of ascorbic acid did not change the rate of oxidation of cholesterol *in vitro*. He concluded that the effect of ascorbate on cholesterol metabolism cannot be direct.

The author reported that the cholesterol levels in the plasma of men with mild scurvy were low and increased in proportion to the dose of vitamin C given (Hodges et al., 1971).

Hematologic Values. It would be surprising if large doses of ascorbic acid had no effect on the blood, and several reports seem to indicate that this does occur. We already mentioned that vitamin C enhances absorption of dietary iron. Herbert and Jacob (1974) reported that high doses of ascorbic acid can destroy substantial amounts of vitamin B_{12}. Hines (1975) studied vitamin B_{12} levels in the serum and the microscopic appearance of the blood smears of 90 patients who were ingesting 500 mg or more of ascorbic acid daily. Three subjects who had been taking 1000 mg three times daily, for at least the past three years, had low plasma levels of vitamin B_{12} (65–100 pg/ml). Two of these subjects had hypersegmentation of polymorphonuclear leukocytes and occasional ovalomacrocytes; yet none were anemic. All three had normal Schilling tests for absorption of vitamin B_{12}. Other hematologic effects of vitamin C include an adverse effect on erythrocytes, a decrease in white blood count, and acute hemolysis.

Mengel and Greene (1976) studied the chemical fragility of erythrocytes from 14 healthy white volunteers, using H_2O_2. Daily determinations were done for 3 to 5 days; then the subjects were given 5000 mg of ascorbic acid daily in divided doses for 3 days. Nine subjects, who had been studied before and during ascorbic acid administration, had substantial increases in lysis of red cells by H_2O_2. The clinical significance of this finding is still uncertain.

Robinson and others (1975) observed that the leukocyte counts of subjects who consumed large doses of vitamin C were reduced.

Campbell and others (1975) observed that a patient with genetic glucose-6-phosphate dehydrogenase (G6PD) deficiency had a fatal hemolytic crisis following intravenous infusion of 80 g of vitamin C daily for two days.

Disruption of DNA. As mentioned before, L-ascorbic acid and its metabolic companion, dehydroascorbic acid, are highly reactive substances. Murata and Kitagawa (1973) found that inactivation of double-stranded DNA of bacteriophage Jl could be effected by free radicals formed during auto-oxidation of ascorbic acid.

Wong and colleagues (1974) demonstrated controlled cleavage of RNA of Phage R17 by treatment with ascorbic acid and copper.

Murata and others (1975) studied the mechanism of inactivation of bacteriophage single-stranded DNA by ascorbic acid. They attributed this to a free radical intermediate produced by auto-oxidation of ascorbic acid. Thus, it appears that large amounts of ascorbic acid can have a damaging effect on genetic material.

Other Problems. Jaffe and others (1975) observed that, in persons who consume large doses of ascorbic acid, there is a false negative test for occult blood.

Summary of Vitamin C Effects

The author believes that there is little evidence to support the concept that large doses of vitamin C are worthwhile in prevention or management of colds.

On the other hand, there is substantial evidence that some persons are damaged by the side effects of too much vitamin C. In particular, pregnant women should avoid taking excessive doses of vitamin C, because it may cause abortion, or worse, deformity of the fetus.

Diabetic patients also should avoid taking large doses of vitamin C because of invalidation of the common tests for glycosuria.

Along similar lines, any patient who is receiving anticoagulant therapy should avoid taking large doses of vitamin C.

The same advice applies to persons who may be exposed to hypoxia in high altitudes and to persons with gout or with urinary tract stones or with G6PD deficiency.

In fact, the reasons for *not* taking excessive doses of vitamin C are, in the view of the author, far more compelling than the reasons for taking megadoses of this substance.

In all likelihood, this fad, like so many others, will fade and be replaced by another.

Orthomolecular Psychiatry

Probably the first controlled clinical trials of large doses of vitamins in patients with psychiatric illness were published by Hoffer and Osmond, who had been working in this area since 1952 (Osmond and Smithies, 1952; Hoffer et al., 1957). Despite early encouragement, these investigators soon found that they were regarded by their colleagues as premature in their conclusions that large doses of nicotinic acid and perhaps other vitamins could benefit patients with schizophrenia. Eventually, Dr. Morris Lipton headed a task force that represented the American Psychiatric Association, and was charged with the responsibility of examining the claims of proponents of megavitamin therapy and of reviewing the findings of more than a dozen controlled studies that did not support these claims (Lipton, 1975). Excerpts of their report have been published in a readily available journal (Anonymous, 1974). The original report can be purchased from the American Psychiatric Association, 1700 18th Street, Washington, D.C. The conclusions of this "blue ribbon" committee were not supportive of megavitamin therapy. They summarized their conclusions as follows:

> This review and critique has carefully examined the literature produced by megavitamin proponents and by those who have attempted to replicate their basic and clinical work. It concludes that in this regard the credibility of the megavitamin proponents is low.
>
> Their credibility is further diminished by a consistent refusal over the past decade to perform controlled experiments and to report their new results in a scientifically acceptable fashion.
>
> Under the circumstances, this Task Force considers the massive publicity

which they promulgate via radio, the lay press, and popular books, using catch phrases which are really misnomers like "megavitamin therapy" and "ortho-molecular treatment" to be deplorable.

Vitamin E

Heart Disease

On June 10, 1946 a feature article entitled "The E in Hearts" appeared in *Time Magazine* (Anonymous, 1946). It stated, "Out of Canada last week came news of a startling scientific discovery: a treatment for heart disease (the nation's number one killer) which so far has succeeded against all common forms of the ailment." According to the article, a London, Ontario obstetrician, Dr. Evan Shute, "had a hunch" that vitamin E, "whose natural sources are in whole grain," produced a salutary effect on heart and blood vessels. Shute and a medical student, Floyd Skelton, had worked with vitamin E previously. Another physician, Dr. Vogelsang, had a patient who "was dying of hypertensive heart disease and hemorrhages . . ." This man was given large doses of vitamin E, and "within a week was out of bed . . ."

Since that announcement many investigators have attempted to evaluate the effects of vitamin E in preventing or curing heart disease of many kinds. Some of the most carefully conducted studies are included in Table 13–6. Two points are easily apparent: many clinical investigators have worked diligently on this problem, and the results were largely disappointing. The one encouraging report was by Shute and others (1949). The author reviewed this subject in somewhat greater detail (Hodges, 1974).

Despite overwhelming evidence to the contrary, Wilfred Shute (brother to Evan) published a paperback book, in which he disregarded all negative reports and repeated his belief that vitamin E not only can prevent heart disease, it can cure it.

His logic for believing that vitamin E is *the* critical factor in heart disease is based in part on the fact that between 1900 and 1910 most of the flour mills in North America changed from the old stone method to the new steel drum method of grinding wheat. This results in a flour that is whiter and contains only about one-tenth as much wheat germ (hence vitamin E) as the older stone-ground flour. However, other changes occurred in the diet simultaneously. Vegetable oils from corn, cottonseed, and later, from soybeans, safflower, sunflower, and other plant sources were incorporated into the American diet in the form of cooking oils, salad oils, and margarines. And when "convenience foods" began to become popular, they too were made with vegetable oils.

Since vegetable oils are the richest sources of vitamin E, even after processing and hydrogenation, it is easy to understand why the American diet has, for several decades, contained even more vitamin E than it did prior to 1910.

Wilfrid Shute insists that coronary heart disease was unheard of prior to 1910. Yet the author found, in an 1895 medical text, a detailed discussion of this disease, including a discussion of angina, an anatomical explanation of its cause, and a description of myocardial infarction that follows total occlusion of a coronary artery. Obviously, coronary heart disease occurred before millers learned how to extract most of the wheat germ from flour.

Studies of hospitalized patients with coronary heart disease and of patients of the same age and sex who were hospitalized for some other illnesses have shown that the heart patients have the same amount of tocopherol in their plasma as the other patients (Lemley et al., 1949).

The normal level of tocopherol in human plasma averages 1.05 mg/dl (Harris et al., 1961; Bieri et al., 1964). Harris and Embree (1963) demonstrated that polyunsaturated fatty acids in the diet increase the need for vitamin E. They suggested that the ratio of α-tocopherol in mg to the amount of polyunsaturated fat in grams (E:PUFA) should be about 0.6. Lesser amounts of vitamin E may lead to deficiency, whereas greater amounts are protective. In a study of the effects of prolonged feeding of a diet containing abundant quantities of polyunsaturated fats (PUFA) Dayton and colleagues (1965) found that the subjects consuming PUFA had above-average levels of vitamin E in their plasma. The explanation is that most vegetable oils are rich sources of vitamin E and contain more than enough to compensate for the greater requirement produced by their content of PUFA.

Vitamin E, when given in doses of 400 to 800 IU daily (RDA is 12 to 45 mg), seldom produces significant toxicity. Anecdotal reports of symptoms of fatigue (Cohen, 1973) or of creatinuria and elevated tocopherol levels (Hillman, 1957) have been published. But severe illness must be a rare complication of taking large doses of vitamin E.

Peripheral Vascular Disease

One of the few credible claims relating to beneficial effects of large doses of vitamin E, is that this form of therapy may benefit patients with peripheral arterial occlusion and pain on walking, known as "intermittent claudication". Even this is not entirely convincing but there is some suggestive evidence. Shute and others (1948) claimed that vitamin E may be helpful to patients with varicose ulcers, thrombophlebitis, early gangrene of the legs, and thromboangiitis obliterans; but Pennock (1949) could not confirm this effect. Similarly, Eisen and

TABLE 13-6 CLINICAL TRIALS OF VITAMIN E IN HEART DISEASE

AUTHOR	TYPE OF PATIENTS	VITAMIN E DOSE AND DURATION OF THERAPY	PLACEBO?	NUMBER OF SUBJECTS AND RESPONSE**
Gram and Schmidt, 1948	Chronic atherosclerotic heart disease	200 mg/day 25 days±	No	80 (5+, 12±)
Levy and Boas, 1948	Stable angina (5) Active angina Chronic heart failure	200–800 mg 14–70 days	No	13
Makinson et al., 1948	Stable angina	All subjects given each of 4 therapies/21 days; vitamin E 150 mg/day	Yes Phenobarbital Aminophylline Ca lactate	22 (no value)
Baer et al., 1948	Congestive heart failure Angina pectoris Arteriosclerotic heart disease	300–400 mg 21–210 days	No	22 (6±)
Donegan et al., 1949	7 pts w/hypertensive CVD I* 7 pts w/hypertensive CVD II 7 pts with stable angina	Vitamin E, 150–600 mg/day for 1 month, alternating with 30 days of placebo therapy (5–20 mg)	Yes On alternate months	21 no appreciable benefit
Ravin and Katz, 1949	Angina	250 mg α-tocopherol for 28–118 weeks	No	11 1±

Baum and Stein, 1949	Unselected heart disease, mostly arteriosclerotic or hypertensive or both	200–600 mg/day 9–147 days	No	22 (4+, 8−)
Eisen and Gross, 1940	Arteriosclerotic heart disease (also peripheral vascular disease)	150–800 mg 365 days+	In some pts.	21 no significant changes
Travell et al., 1949	Angina pectoris	200–300 mg/day 70–140 days	Yes	19 + 19 no significant changes
Rush, 1949	Angina pectoris	300 mg/day 90 days+	Yes	54 no benefit
Anderson, 1974	Angina pectoris	400–3200 mg/day	Yes	40 + 15 no significant changes
Ball, 1948	Angina pectoris	300 mg/day 42 days	No	10 (2+, 2±)

*Hypertensive Cardiovascular Disease
  I = Normal heart size by x-ray
  II = Cardiac enlargement

**+ = improved
  ± = equivocal
  − = worse

Some of the clinical trials of vitamin E in heart disease are outlined above. Aside from the reports by the Shutes and their associates, there have been no reports of successful treatment with vitamin E.

Gross (1949) and Hamilton and others (1953) found vitamin E to be worthless in treating peripheral vascular disease. Furthermore, Paul and colleagues (1954) could find no evidence that vitamin E affects blood clotting mechanisms.

Yet Williams and others (1962) reported "encouraging results in 33 patients treated with vitamin E." This was followed by a report by Boyd and Marks (1963) of 13 patients with peripheral vascular disease who improved significantly when treated with vitamin E, and their survival was longer than that of control patients. More recently, Haeger (1968) added support to the concept that vitamin E may benefit patients with peripheral vascular disease. He compared α-tocopherol with vasodilators, anticoagulants, or a multiple vitamin preparation. There was significant improvement in subjective distress, distance the patients could walk, and reduction in the numbers of legs amputated because of gangrene. It is too soon to make a final judgment about the efficacy of vitamin E in treating peripheral vascular disease, but the evidence seems to indicate that it may be beneficial.

Vitamin A

The possible role of vitamin A or its analogs (Sporn et al., 1976) has been discussed previously. The use of large doses of retinol in treating various skin diseases is not recommended because there usually is another drug equally effective, and vitamin A can produce serious, even fatal illness.

WEIGHT-REDUCTION DIETS

Obesity is a serious problem in the United States, yet we do not have a definition that most people can agree with. Some say that 20 pounds above ideal weight represents obesity. Others say more than 15 per cent above ideal weight constitutes obesity. Yet few can agree on what is ideal weight. Estimation of subcutaneous fat by using skin-fold calipers aids in differentiating between overweight resulting from excess fat and that resulting from large skeletal muscles. Numerous formulae based on weight and height have been proposed. The fact is, most of us can agree that one person is fat and another is not. But we can seldom agree on the best way to correct obesity. Dietary and other medical management of obesity will be discussed in the next chapter. Here we want to review the major types of "fad" diets; that is, diets that are based on unproven or incorrect scientific "facts". A very readable little book gives an overview of the diets commonly employed by our population when they want to lose weight (Berland, 1974). Some of these diets are:

1. Low-calorie diets: The patient learns to count calories.

2. The prudent diets: Based on sound nutritional principles, these provide a balanced diet that contains less fat and cholesterol.

3. Low carbohydrate diets: Many different names. This diet causes an initial weight loss of water and salt. Later, ketosis develops and may reduce appetite. This diet often contains too much fat and protein.

4. One-food emphasis diets: Rice, vegetables, yogurt, grapefruit or other fruits, ice cream. The monotony is supposed to suppress hunger. A recent modification of this type of diet is the liquid protein diet, which should be regarded as potentially hazardous.

5. Others: Scores of catchy names such as "miracle diet", "wise woman's diet", the "amazing 'new-you' diet", and so on.

Psychological solutions are becoming popular: TOPS (Take Off Pounds Sensibly), Weight-Watchers, Behavior Therapy Groups, Behavior Modification, and so on.

According to Consumer Union's evaluation, the best diet is the prudent diet or one patterned after it. Low carbohydrate diets are less effective. Group therapy to modify behavior is best. Several "groups" are about equally effective.

OTHER FOOD FADS, CUSTOMS, AND CONCEPTS

Pica

Pica is a peculiar habit of eating non-food substances. Children often engage in pica for a short time, then decide it isn't fun. Adults, particularly pregnant women and obese women, may engage in pica for many years. The commonest form is eating clay. In some of the Southeastern states of the United States, people may travel many miles to dig their favorite clay. Some will sift and moisten the clay, mold it into "cookies" and even sprinkle them with small amounts of sugar and spice. Clay eating may interfere with absorption of some of the essential trace minerals.

Starch eaters consume laundry starch, which is partly digestible. It seems to be harmless aside from providing an excess of calories, and replacing nutritious foods from the diet.

Eating ice seems harmless enough, but some authorities have said that ice eaters are usually deficient in iron. Treatment with medicinal iron is said to end the ice eating (Coltman, 1969). Other forms of pica include eating paper or flakes of paint. Compulsive eating of food may also be considered a form of pica. Usually, this involves some crunchy food such as celery, crackers, or pretzels. Crosby (1976) thinks that all forms of pica may be related to iron deficiency.

Laetrile

Although laetrile is not, strictly speaking, a nutrient, most interested lay persons and many professional authorities turn to nutritionists for answers. They ask: "What is it?" "Is it a vitamin?" "Does it sometimes work as a cancer cure?"

The answers to these questions must be factual rather than emotional. Laetrile is the name applied to a substance found in the seeds of stone-fruit such as apricots, peaches, plums, and to a lesser extent, almonds. This substance is properly named amygdalin but has been incorrectly called vitamin B_{17}. It bears no resemblance to a vitamin and is not an essential nutrient for any known species of animal, including humans.

Amygdalin is a cyanogenetic glycoside that is hydrolyzed by an enzyme, β-glycosidase, to yield mandelonitrile, which decomposes to release benzaldehyde and cyanide. Other plant foods also contain cyanogenetic glycosides; the most familiar example is cassava, which is consumed in Nigeria and other developing countries. Cassava is grated and soaked in water to leach out the toxic cyanides, but people who use it as a staple food may develop a neurologic syndrome known as ataxic neuropathy, which results from chronic exposure to cyanides.

The concept upon which laetrile's anticancer effect is supposed to be based is that malignant cells contain more of the enzyme, β-glycosidase, than do normal cells. Thus, administration of laetrile should, according to theory, result in selective release of cyanide within the malignant cells which would be destroyed in the process.

This optimistic concept was destroyed by two scientific facts: There is very little β-glycosidase in most normal cells but even less in malignant cells; and cyanide, when released by enzymatic action, is rapidly diffused into lymphatic and blood channels, leading to systemic rather than local toxicity.

Unfortunately, laetrile has become a symbol of political freedom and has the support of several powerful legislators. Meanwhile, many who produce and sell laetrile, either legally or otherwise, are reaping huge profits (Jukes, 1976).

Hypoglycemia

Many people feel compelled to diagnose and treat their own ailments, whether real or imaginary. These persons are the favorite targets of certain authors who write popular paper-bound books on health, nutrition, and disease. In recent years, one of the most popular topics has been hypoglycemia, which, according to the popular press, is a widespread and generally unrecognized occurrence in the United States. In an effort to combat misinformation and to provide factual answers, the American Diabetes Association, the Endocrine Society, and the American Medical Association appointed an Ad Hoc Committee on Hypoglycemia to prepare a statement on hypoglycemia (Ad Hoc Committee, 1973). Several portions of this statement are very helpful in explaining hypoglycemia to patients. These are:

1. *Hypoglycemia means low blood sugar.*
2. *Hypoglycemia may be attended by symptoms of sweating, shakiness, trembling, anxiety, fast heart action, headache, hunger, brief feelings of weakness, and occasionally, seizures and coma.*
3. *Most people with these kinds of symptoms do not have hypoglycemia.*
4. *There is no good evidence that hypoglycemia causes depression, chronic fatigue, allergies, nervous breakdowns, alcoholism, juvenile delinquency, childhood behavior problems, drug addiction, or inadequate sexual performance.*
5. *Because there are many causes of hypoglycemia, it is necessary that the diagnosis be accurately established before any form of treatment is given.*

Information that aids in establishing the diagnosis includes:

(a) *Low blood sugar must be documented.*
(b) *Particular symptoms are shown to be related to hypoglycemia.*
(c) *Symptoms are relieved by ingestion of sugar or food.*
(d) *The type of hypoglycemia must be established with regard to:*
    (1) *Reactive hypoglycemia after a meal (most common).*
    (2) *Fasting hypoglycemia (potentially more serious).*

Reactive hypoglycemia occurs for a variety of reasons including postgastrectomy syndromes and mild diabetes mellitus. It also occurs in "a rather large group of individuals who are often nervous, thin women." It is doubtful, however, that their nervousness results from hypoglycemia. Many young or middle-aged men and women have blood sugar levels below normal after ingesting a high-carbohydrate meal, but most do not have symptoms of hypoglycemia. If, however, recurring symptoms can be relieved by food, a diagnosis of reactive hypoglycemia is most likely.

This usually can be controlled by reducing the amount of simple sugars and total carbohydrates in the diet, by increasing the amount of protein moderately, and by feeding frequent small meals throughout the day.

Fasting hypoglycemia is much more likely to result from a serious disorder (Fajans and Floyd, 1976). The major derangements of glucose homeostasis are:

1. Decreased glucose output from the liver.
2. Increased glucose uptake.
3. Increased uptake of amino acids by extrahepatic tissues.

A convenient classification of fasting hypoglycemia is:

1. Organic hypoglycemia (pancreatic disease, liver disease, other endocrine disorders, and others).
2. Enzyme deficiencies (infants and children).
3. Functional hypoglycemia (no recognizable anatomic lesion).
4. Exogenous hypoglycemia (surreptitious use of insulin, alcohol, sulfonylurea drugs, and so on).

The advice given by non-medical persons regarding the management of hypoglycemia is apt to be worthless and potentially harmful. It is important that physicians give their patients a clear and rational explanation of the types, causes, and management of hypoglycemia.

Toxins in Our Food

A surprising number of people in the United States believe that their food and water supply is either poisonous or unwholesome. Part of this attitude arises from the claims of unscientific pundits who write about nutrition and health. Some of the responsibility can be placed at the door of the news media, whose reporters are ever tuned to any topic dealing with food or health. Without question, there have been instances of toxic or spoiled foods being sold in modern retail stores, but the incidence is very small indeed; and there have been reports of toxic or undesirable chemicals in municipal water supplies. Many people feel vaguely anxious about "processed" foods without knowing the exact meanings of the term. It seems, therefore, desirable to include a brief discussion of the nature and magnitude of these problems and the alternatives available.

Naturally Occurring Toxins

Many common foods contain small quantities of potentially toxic substances but few people develop any illness because they eat a variety of foods. Examples of naturally occurring toxins are oxalates in green, leafy plants, solanines in potatoes, and aflatoxins in peanuts.

Food Additives

Most consumers seem to believe that all food additives are sinister and unnecessary chemicals that are added to food by unscrupulous food processing plants for the purpose of earning greater profits.

In fact, food additives are regarded by experts in the field as beneficial substances that allow food manufacturers to produce better quality foods that are safer and more attractive than the unprocessed product.

Food processing has its origin in antiquity. Primitive humans learned to preserve meats by drying and smoking them. Later, salt was found to preserve fish and other protein foods. Still later, honey or sugar was used to preserve fruits and some vegetables. Wine and vinegar are other examples of ancient methods of preserving foods.

These same preservatives are used today, and constitute the bulk of food additives. But many other substances are also added to foods. These include nutrient supplements, preservatives, emulsifiers, stabilizers and thickeners, flavors and flavoring agents, bleaching and maturing agents, colors, and many others.

The public has become alarmed by the large numbers of additives, and some claims have been made that food additives may cause behavior problems in children.

Patients should be advised to read labels and to reject either products that contain an unusual number of additives or those that contain specific substances that they wish to avoid. Actually, no one knows whether one substance or another is potentially toxic if used for many years. This points up a wise policy: eat a wide variety of foods, and change the pattern from time to time. In this way, one will not be as likely to eat the same substances day after day. At present, there is concern among lay people about food colorings, butylated hydroxy toluene (BHT), saccharin, nitrates and nitrites, and substances derived from salicylates. There is little or no evidence that these substances are harmful when consumed in the small amounts present in foods. However, the public has a right to accept or reject foods, and many want to know what they are eating.

Fluoridation

Some individuals and a few non-medical groups condemn the fluoridation of municipal water supplies on the grounds that it constitutes a form of medication of people, willing or not. And a few persons claim that fluorides cause cancer, heart disease, mental illness, and other disorders. Obviously, there is no scientific evidence to support these claims. On the contrary, dentists strongly support fluoridation because it improves dental health substantially. And physicians support it because of the dental benefits and because it reduces the prevalence and severity of osteoporosis in middle-aged and elderly people.

Refined Foods

Our diet is composed of a variety of foods, some of which are highly refined, some only slightly refined, and some not at all. Refining has several purposes: to improve quality, shelf life, appearance, taste, and so on; to eliminate some undesirable component; and to provide greater convenience to the person who prepares meals. There is no question that highly refined foods such as sugar contain no essential nutrients of consequence. White flour loses some of its nutrients in the milling process, but it usually is enriched with thiamin, riboflavin, niacin, and iron. Some refined foods are actually chemical formulas; for example, an artificial fruit drink that contains water, sugar, artificial colors and flavors, citric acid, and a chemical preservative, benzoate of soda.

Most of our foods, however, contain only small amounts of a few additives, and these probably have more effects that are desirable than potentially harmful. The American food market is a miracle of modern agriculture, transportation, processing, preservation, and marketing. There is an abundance of wholesome foods in wide variety. Those who wish to avoid food additives or overly refined foods can take their choice.

REFERENCES

Ad Hoc Committee on Hypoglycemia. Statement on Hypoglycemia. *Arch. Intern. Med.* *131:*591, 1973.

Ahlborg, N. G.: Ascorbic acid excretion by human kidney. *Acta Physiol. Scand.* *12(Suppl. 36)*:1, 1947,

Anderson, T. W.: Vitamin E in angina pectoris. *Canadian Med. Assoc. J. 110:*401, 1974.

Anderson, T. W., Beaton, G. H., Corey, P. N., and Spero, L.: Winter illness and vitamin C: The effect of relatively low doses. *Canadian Med. Assoc. J. 112:*823, 1975.

Anderson, T. W., Reid, D. B. W., and Beaton, G. H.: Vitamin C and the common cold: a double-blind trial. *Canadian Med. Assoc. J. 107:*503, 1972.

Anderson, T. W., Suranyi, G., and Beaton, G. H.: The effect on winter illness of large doses of vitamin C. *Canadian Med. Assoc. J. 111:*31, 1974.

Anonymous: The E in hearts. *Time Magazine,* June 10, 1946, pp. 45–48.

Anonymous: Megavitamin and orthomolecular therapy in psychiatry. Excerpts from a report of the American Psychiatric Association Task Force on Vitamin Therapy in Psychiatry. *Nutr. Reviews (Supplement),* July 1974, pp. 44–47.

Baer, S., Heine, W. I., and Gelfond, D. B.: The use of vitamin E in heart disease. *Amer. J. Med. Sci. 215:*542, 1948.

Ball, K. P.: Vitamin E in angina pectoris. *Lancet 1:*116, 1948.

Baum, G. L., and Stein, W.: Vitamin E therapy in heart disease. *Wisconsin Med. J. 48:*315, 1949.

Berland, T., and editors of *Consumer Guide:* Rating the diets. *Consumer Guide 53:*April 1974.

Bieri, J. G., Teets, L., Belavady, B., and Andrews, E. L.: Serum vitamin-E levels in a normal adult population in the Washington, D.C. area. *Proc. Soc. Exper. Biol. Med. 117:*131, 1964.

Boyd, A. M., and Marks, J.: Treatment of intermittent claudication. A reappraisal of the value of α-tocopherol. *Angiology 14*:198, 1963.
Briggs, M.: Vitamin-C-induced hyperoxaluria (Letter to the Editor) *Lancet 1*:154, 1976.
Campbell, G. D., Jr., Steinberg, M. H., and Bower, J. D.: Ascorbic acid-induced hemolysis in G-6-PD deficiency. *Ann. Intern. Med. 82*:810, 1975.
Chalmers, T. C.: Effects of ascorbic acid on the common cold: an evaluation of the evidence. *Amer. J. Med. 58*:532, 1975.
Chopra, J. G.: *Megadoses of Nutrients in Disease.* Washington, D.C., Bureau of Foods, Food and Drug Administration, Department of Health, Education, and Welfare, 1976.
Cochrane, W. A.: Overnutrition in prenatal and neonatal life: A problem? *Canadian Med. Assoc. J. 93*:893, 1965.
Cohen, H. M.: Fatigue caused by vitamin E? (Letter to the Editor). *Calif. Med. 119*:72, 1973.
Coltman, C. A. J.: Pagophagia and iron lack. *J.A.M.A. 207*:513, 1969.
Cook, J. D., and Monsen, E. R.: Vitamin C, the common cold, and iron absorption. *Amer. J. Clin. Nutr. 30*:235, 1977.
Coulehan, J. L., Eberhard, S., Kapner, L., Taylor, F., Rogers, K., and Garry, P.: Vitamin C and acute illness in Navajo schoolchildren. *New England J. Med. 295*:973, 1976.
Coulehan, J. L., Reisinger, K. S., Rogers, K. D., and Bradley, D. W.: Vitamin C prophylaxis in a boarding school. *New England J. Med. 290*:6, 1974.
Cowan, D. W., Diehl, H. S., and Baker, A. B.: Vitamins for the prevention of colds. *J.A.M.A. 120*:1268, 1942.
Crosby, W. H.: Pica. *J.A.M.A. 235*:2765, 1976.
Dahlberg, G., Engel, A., and Rydin, H.: Om askorbinsyrans värde som profylaktikum mot s.k. Förkylningsinfektioner. [On the value of ascorbic acid as a prophylaxis against so-called colds.] *Nordisk Medicin 14*:1616, 1942.
Dayton, S., Hashimoto, S., Rosenblum, D., and Pearce, M. L.: Vitamin E status of humans during prolonged feeding of unsaturated fats. *J. Lab. Clin. Med. 65*:739, 1965.
Donegan, C. K., Messer, A. L., Orgain, E. S., and Ruffin, J. M.: Negative results of tocopherol therapy in cardiovascular therapy. *Amer. J. Med. Sci. 217*:294, 1949.
Dörholt, G.: Tierexperimentelle Untersuchungen über den Einfluss des Vitamin C auf die Höhenfestigkit. [Experimental research on the influence of vitamin C on the altitude stability.] *Luftfahrtmediz. Abhandl. 2*:240, 1938.
Dykes, M. H. M., and Meier, P.: Ascorbic acid and the common cold. Evaluation of its efficacy and toxicity. *J.A.M.A. 231*:1073, 1975.
Eisen, M. E., and Gross, H.: Vitamin E in arteriosclerotic heart and peripheral vascular disease. *N.Y. State J. Med. 49*:2422, 1949.
Fajans, S. S., and Floyd, J. C.: Fasting hypoglycemia in adults. *New England J. Med. 294*:766, 1976.
Food and Nutrition Board, *Supplementation of Human Diets with Vitamin E*, Division of Biology and Agriculture, National Research Council (Committee on Nutritional Misinformation), National Academy of Sciences, Washington, D.C., June 1973.
Franz, W. L., Sands, G. W., and Heyl, H. L.: Blood ascorbic acid level in bioflavonoid and ascorbic acid therapy of common cold. *J.A.M.A. 162*:1224, 1956.
Ginter, E.: Cholesterol: Vitamin C controls its transformation to bile acids. *Science 179*:702, 1973.
Glazebrook, A. J., and Thomson, S.: The administration of vitamin C in a large institution and its effect on general health and resistance to infection. *J. Hygiene 42*:1, 1942.
Goldner, M. G.: Large doses of vitamin C harmful to diabetics? *Diabetes Outlook 6*:4, 1971.
Gordonoff, T.: Darf man Wasserlösliche Vitamine überdosieren? Versuche mit Vitamin C. [May one overdose water-soluble vitamins to excess? Experiments with vitamin C.] *Schweiz. Med. Wochenschr. 90*:726, 1960.
Gram, N. J., and Schmidt, V.: Ambulant E-Vitamin terapi ved Hjertesygdomme. *Nordisk Medicin 37*:82, 1948.
Haeger, K.: The treatment of peripheral occlusive arterial disease with α-tocopherol as compared with vasodilator agents and antiprothrombin (Dicumarol). *Vasc. Dis. 5*:199, 1968.

Hamilton, M., Wilson, G. M., Armitage, P., and Boyd, J. T.: The treatment of intermittent claudication with vitamin E. *Lancet 1*:367, 1953.

Hardinge, M. G., and Stare, F. J.: Nutritional studies of vegetarians. I. Nutritional, physical, and laboratory studies. *Amer. J. Clin. Nutr. 2*:73, 1954.

Harris, P. L., and Embree, N. D.: Quantitative consideration of the effect of polyunsaturated fatty acid content of the diet upon the requirements for vitamin E. *Amer. J. Clin. Nutr. 13*:385, 1963.

Harris, P. L., Hardenbrook, E. G., Dean, F. P., Cusack, E. R., and Jensen, J. L.: Blood tocopherol values in normal human adults and incidence of vitamin E deficiency. *Proc. Soc. Exper. Biol. Med. 107*:381, 1961.

Herbert, V. D.: Megavitamin therapy. *Contemporary Nutrition 2*:no. 10, October 1977.

Herbert, V., and Jacob, E.: Destruction of vitamin B_{12} by ascorbic acid. *J.A.M.A. 230*:241, 1974.

Hillman, R. W.: Tocopherol excess in man. Creatinuria associated with prolonged ingestion. *Amer. J. Clin. Nutr. 5*:597, 1957.

Hines, J. D.: Ascorbic acid and vitamin B_{12} deficiency (Letter to the Editor). *J.A.M.A. 234*:24, 1975.

Hodges, R. E.: Vitamin E and coronary heart disease. *Cardiac Rehabilitation (Journal of the New York State Heart Assembly) 4*:63, 1973.

Hodges, R. E., Baker, E. M., Hood, J., Sauberlich, H. E., and March, S. C.: Experimental scurvy in man. *Amer. J. Clin. Nutr. 22*:535, 1969.

Hodges, R. E., Hood, J., Canham, J. E., Sauberlich, H. E., Baker, E. M., and Davenport, R. E.: Clinical manifestations of vitamin C deficiency in man. *Amer. J. Clin. Nutr. 24*:432, 1971.

Hoffer, A., Osmond, H., Callbeck, M. J., and Kahan, I.: Treatment of schizophrenia with nicotinic acid and nicotinamide. *J. Clin. Exper. Psychopathol. 18*:131, 1957.

Hornig, D.: Metabolism of ascorbic acid. *World Rev. Nutr. Dietet. 23*:225, 1975.

Jaffe, R. M., Kasten, B., Young, D. S., and MacLowry, J. D.: False-negative stool occult blood tests caused by ingestion of ascorbic acid (vitamin C). *Ann. Intern. Med. 83*:824, 1975.

Jukes, T. H.: Megavitamin therapy (Editorial). *J.A.M.A. 233*:550, 1975.

Jukes, T. H.: Laetrile for cancer. *J.A.M.A. 236*:1284, 1976.

Karlowski, T. R., Chalmers, T. C., Frankel, D. L., Kapikian, A. Z., Lewis, T. L., and Lynch, J. M.: Ascorbic acid for the common cold. A prophylactic and therapeutic trial. *J.A.M.A. 231*:1038, 1975.

Kritchevsky, D.: Vitamin C and cholesterol catabolism (Letter to the Editor). *Nutr. Reviews 32*:96, 1974.

Kübler, W., and Gehler, J.: Zur Kinetic der enteralen Ascorbinsäure Resorption. Eine Beitrag zur Berechnung nicht dosis-proprotionuler Resorptionsvorgänge [Kinetics of enteral ascorbic acid absorption. Computation of non-dose-proportional absorption.] *Internat. Z. Vit. Forschung 40*:442, 1970.

Lamden, M. P., and Chrystowski, G. A.: Urinary oxalate excretion by man following ascorbic acid ingestion. *Proc. Soc. Exper. Biol. Med. 85*:190, 1954.

Lemley, J. M., Gale, R. G., Furman, R. H., Cherrington, M. E., Darby, W. J., and Meneely, G. R.: Plasma tocopherol levels in cardiac patients. *Amer. Heart J. 37*:1029, 1949.

Levey, S., and Suter, B.: Effect of ascorbic acid on diabetogenic action of alloxan. *Proc. Soc. Exper. Biol. Med. 63*:341, 1946.

Levy, H., and Boas, E. P.: Vitamin E in heart disease. *Ann. Intern. Med. 28*:1117, 1948.

Lipton, M. A.: Remarks on the use of megavitamins in the treatment of schizophrenia. In *Nutrition and Mental Functions*, Volume 14, George Serban (ed.). New York, Plenum Press, 1975, pp. 253–258.

Major, R. H. (ed.): Scurvy. In *Classic Descriptions of Disease*, 3rd Edition, Springfield, Illinois, Charles C Thomas, Publisher, 1945, p. 585.

Makinson, D. H., Oleesky, S., and Stone, R. V.: Vitamin E in angina pectoris. *Lancet 1*:102, 1948.

Mayson, J. S., Schumaker, O., and Nakamura, R. M.: False-negative tests for urine glucose. *Lancet 1*:780, 1973.

Mengel, C. H., and Green, H. L., Jr.: Ascorbic acid effects on erythrocytes. *Ann. Intern. Med.* 84:490, 1976.

Mouriquand, G., and Edel, V.: Sur l'hypervitaminose C. *Compt. Rend. Soc. Biol.* 147:1432, 1953.

Murata, A., and Kitagawa, K.: Mechanism of inactivation of Bacteriophage Jl by ascorbic acid. *Agr. Biol. Chem.* 37:1145, 1973.

Murata, A., Oyadomari, R., Ohashi, T., and Kitagawa, K.: Mechanism of inactivation of bacteriophage δ, containing single-stranded DNA by ascorbic acid. *J. Nutr. Sci. Vitaminol.* 21:261, 1975.

Nandi, B. K., Majumder, A. K., Subramanian, N., and Chatterjee, I. B.: Effects of large doses of vitamin C in guinea pigs and rats. *J. Nutrition* 103:1688, 1973.

Nelson, E. W., and Cerda, J. J.: Limitation of intestinal absorption of vitamin C in high doses (abstract). *Clin. Res.* 23:254A, 1975.

Neuweiler, W.: Die Hypervitaminose und ihre Beziehung zur Schwangerschaft. [Effect of hypervitaminosis on outcome of pregnancy.] *Internat. Z. Vit. Forschung* 22:392, 1951.

Norkus, E., and Rosso, P.: Changes in ascorbic acid metabolism in the offspring following high maternal intake of the vitamin in the pregnant guinea pig (abstract). *Fed. Proc.* 34:884, 1975.

Osmond, H., and Smythies, J.: Schizophrenia: A new approach. *J. Mental Sci.* 98:309, 1952.

Owen, C. A., Jr., Tyce, G. M., Flock, E. V., and McCall, J. T.: Heparin-ascorbic acid antagonism. *Mayo Clin. Proc.* 45:140, 1970.

Patterson, J. W.: The diabetogenic effect of dehydroascorbic acid. *Endocrinology* 45:344, 1949.

Paul, R. M., Lewis, J. A., and DeLuca, H. A.: The lack of effect of vitamin E on the blood clotting mechanism. *Canadian J. Biochem. Physiol.* 32:347, 1954.

Pennock, L. L.: Vitamin E (alpha-tocopherol) in treatment of thromboangiitis obliterans and leg ulcers. *Ann. N.Y. Acad. Sci.* 52:413, 1949.

Peters, M.: Zur Frage der resistenzsteigernden wirkung prophylaktischer Dauer-Medikation von Vitamin C. [Question of the resistance-increasing effect of prophylactic medication with vitamin C.] *Z. Kinderheilkd.* 61:179, 1939.

Pfannensteil, W.: Tierversuche über die Vitaminbecinflussarkert der Höhenfestigkeit. [Animal experimentation on the influence of vitamins on altitude stability.] *Luftfahrtmediz. Abhandl.* 2:234, 1938.

Ramp, W. K., and Thornton, P. A.: Ascorbic acid and the calcium metabolism of embryonic chick tibias. *Proc. Soc. Exper. Biol. Med.* 137:273, 1971.

Ravin, I. S., and Katz, K. H.: Vitamin E in the treatment of angina pectoris. *New England J. Med.* 240:331, 1949.

Recommended Dietary Allowances. Eighth Revised Edition, 1974. Food and Nutrition Board, National Research Council, National Academy of Sciences, Washington, D.C., 1974.

Ritzel, G.: Kritische Beurteilung des Vitamins C als Prophylacticum und Therapeuticum der Erkältungskrankheiten. [Critical evaluation of vitamin C as a prophylactic and therapeutic agent against colds.] *Helv. Med. Acta* 28:63, 1961.

Robinson, A. B., Catchpool, J. F., and Pauling, L.: Decreased white blood cell count in people who supplement their diet with L-ascorbic acid (abstract). *ICRS Med. Sci.: Clin. Pharmacol. Therapeutics, Hematol., Immunol. Allergy, Metab. Nutr.* 3:259, 1975.

Rosenberg, L. E.: Vitamin-dependent genetic disease. *Hospital Practice* 5:59, 1970.

Rosenthal, G.: Interaction of ascorbic acid and warfarin (Letter to the Editor). *J.A.M.A.* 215:1671, 1971.

Roth, D. A., and Breitenfield, R. V.: Vitamin C and oxalate stones (Letter to the Editor). *J.A.M.A.* 237:768, 1977.

Rush, H. P.: Experience with vitamin E in coronary disease. *Calif. Med.* 71:391, 1949.

Samborskaya, E. P., and Ferdman, T. D.: [The problem of the mechanism of artificial abortion by use of ascorbic acid]. *Byull. éksp. biol.* 4:105, 1964.

Samborskaya, E. P., and Ferdman, T. D.: The mechanism of termination of pregnancy by ascorbic acid. *Bull. Exper. Biol. Med.* 62:934, 1966.

Schrauzer, G. N., Ishmall, D., and Kiefer, G. W.: Some aspects of current vitamin C usage: Diminished high-altitude resistance following overdose. *Ann. N.Y. Acad. Sci.* 258:377, 1975.

Schrauzer, G. N., and Rhead, W. J.: Ascorbic acid abuse: Effects of long term ingestion of excessive amounts on blood level and urinary excretion. *Internat. J. Vit. Nutr. Res.* 43:201, 1973.

Schwartz, A. R., Togo, Y., Hornick, R. B., Tominaga, S., and Gleckman, R. A.: Evaluation of the efficacy of ascorbic acid in prophylaxis of induced rhinovirus infection in man. *J. Infect. Dis.* 128:500, 1973.

Shute, E. V., Vogelsang, A. B., Skelton, F. R., and Shute, W. E.: The influence of vitamin E on vascular disease. *Surg. Gynecol. Obstet.* 86:1, 1948.

Shute, W. E., Shute, E. V., and Vogelsang, A.: The physiological and biochemical basis for the use of vitamin E in cardiovascular disease. *Ann. Intern. Med.* 30:1004, 1949.

Sigell, L. T., and Flessa, H. C.: Drug interactions with anticoagulants. *J.A.M.A. 214:*2035, 1970.

Sokoloff, B., Hori, M., Saelhof, C. C., Wrzolek, T., and Imai, T.: Aging, atherosclerosis and ascorbic acid metabolism. *J. Amer. Geriatr. Soc.* 14:1239, 1966.

Sorensen, D. I., Devine, M. M., and Rivers, J. M.: Catabolism and tissue levels of ascorbic acid following long-term massive doses in the guinea pig. *J. Nutrition 104:*1041, 1974.

Spittle, C. R.: Atherosclerosis and vitamin C. *Lancet* 2:1280, 1971.

Sporn, M. B., Dunlop, N. M., Newton, D. L., and Smith, J. M.: Prevention of chemical carcinogenesis by vitamin A and its synthetic analogs (retinoids). *Fed. Proc.* 35:1332, 1976.

Stein, H. B., Hasan, A., and Fox, I. H.: Ascorbic acid-induced uricosuria. A consequence of megavitamin therapy. *Ann. Intern. Med.* 84:385, 1976.

Stich, H. F., Karim, J., Koropatnik, J., and Lo, L.: Mutagenic action of ascorbic acid. *Nature* 260:722, 1976.

Tarjan-Kassai, S.: Ascorbinsav tartós adagolásának hatása Üzemi dolgozókon. [Effect of ascorbic acid intake on factory workers]. Különlenyomat az Orvosi Hetilap Számából 21:577, 1954.

Tebrock, H. E., Arminio, J. J., and Johnston, J. H.: Usefulness of bioflavonoids and ascorbic acid in treatment of common cold. *J.A.M.A.* 162:1227, 1956.

Travell, J., Rinzler, S. H., Bakst, H., Benjamin, Z. H., and Bobb, A. L.: Comparison of effects of alpha-tocopherol and a matching placebo on chest pain in patients with heart disease. *Ann. N.Y. Acad. Sci.* 52:345, 1949.

Travis, L. B., Dodge, W. F., Mintz, A. A., and Assemi, M.: Urinary acidification with ascorbic acid. *J. Pediat.* 67:1176, 1965.

Tsai, S-C., Fales, H. M., and Vaughan, M.: Inactivation of hormone-sensitive lipase from adipose tissue with adenosine triphosphate magnesium and ascorbic acid. *J. Biol. Chem.* 248:5278, 1973.

Walker, G. H., Bynoe, M. L., and Tyrrell, D. A. J.: Trial of ascorbic acid in prevention of colds. *Brit. Med. J.* 1:603, 1967.

Williams, H. T. G., Clein, L. J., and Macbeth, R. A.: Alpha-tocopherol in the treatment of intermittent claudication: A preliminary report. *Canadian Med. Assoc. J.* 87:538, 1962.

Wong, K., Morgan, A. R., and Paranchych, W.: Controlled cleavage of phage R17 RNA within the virion by treatment with ascorbate and copper (II). *Canadian J. Biochem.* 52:950, 1974.

14

DRUG-NUTRIENT INTERACTIONS

Robert E. Hodges, M.D.

Until recent years, neither physicians nor pharmacologists gave much thought to any possible relationships between drugs and food or the nutrients food contains. Occasionally, patients were advised to take a prescribed medication with or after meals, especially if it had a propensity to cause nausea or other distress. Indeed the author, while a house-officer in the 1950s, often advised patients to drink a glass of milk with each dose of tetracycline, a practice that we now know will reduce absorption of the antibiotic by more than two-thirds (Visconti, 1977).

Each year we learn of more drug-nutrient interactions. Most of these are either detrimental by virtue of interfering with the normal metabolism of an essential nutrient or because the pharmaceutical agent is inactivated or otherwise rendered useless. Sometimes these reactions are harmless, but rarely are they beneficial.

It is tempting to suggest that physicians who prescribe drugs use a computerized data bank to alert them and their patients to potential drug-nutrient interactions. This suggestion may yet be worth implementing. The problem is, however, that over-the-counter drugs, which constitute the major share of all medications, may also have undesirable interactions with nutrients. Aspirin, which is so widely used by people in the United States, is known to have several important interactions with nutrients.

The problem becomes even more complex when we discover that the distinction between drugs and nutrients is sometimes indistinct and arbitrary. For example, both iron and calcium properly belong in both groups: nutrients and drugs. The same can be said about nicotinic acid, and even glucose.

In the following discussion, the author has chosen to place each substance in one column or the other (nutrient or drug), arbitrarily. This facilitates organization of an otherwise amorphous collection of data that are derived from various sources, some excellent, some anecdotal. The reader should keep in mind that a given type of drug-nutrient interaction may occur rarely, often, or invariably, depending upon a variety of conditions. Any effort at bringing these reports together into a compact and responsible evaluation of the available evidence is tenuous and subject to change as more data (and more accurate information) become available.

In the following pages, the interactions between drug and nutrients will be presented in three ways:

1. Pharmaceutical agents that affect nutrients;
2. Nutrients that may be affected by drugs;
3. Clinical syndromes that may result from drug-nutrient interactions.

MECHANISMS OF ACTION

Much of the information we now have about the interactions between nutrients and pharmaceutical agents has been collected, classified, and interpreted by Daphne Roe, who also has made major contributions through her well-designed investigations. She has offered logical explanations for a number of the seemingly inexplicable observations made by others (Roe, 1976a). Drugs can interfere with endogenous synthesis of nutrients or impair digestion and absorption or affect transport, storage, metabolism, and excretion. Yet the types of abnormalities produced by drugs is limited to manifestations of deficiency of a relatively small number of nutrients. Obviously, those nutrients that are involved in a large number of metabolic activities, such as pyridoxine and folic acid, are most likely to be affected by a variety of drugs.

Some of the obvious mechanisms involved in drug-nutrient interactions include changes in solubility, absorption, transport mechanisms, rate of renal excretion; interference with synthesis of carrier proteins, enzymes and coenzymes; altered rates of degradation; competitive cell binding; and direct competition for enzyme systems.

There are numerous factors that affect the requirement for essential nutrients in situations where drugs have been given. These include the obvious effects of the dose and duration of administration of the drug, and simultaneous administration of other medications that may have a synergistic effect, augmenting the first drug's action on nutrients.

Other factors include characteristics of the person taking a medication. These include genetic differences, malabsorption, individual rates of utilization and other physiologic processes, presence of diseases that alter nutrient needs, rates of cell turnover, and rates of nutrient losses (Roe, 1976b).

Similarly, the incidence and risk of malnutrition resulting from drugs vary from one person to another and from one population to another, depending upon a number of variables. These include dose and duration of drug use, habitual diet, psychological stress, presence of disease, and environmental factors, to name a few (Roe, 1976c). Table 14–1 lists a number of drugs that commonly or occasionally affect essential nutrients. An attempt has been made to list the probable mechanisms whereby these drugs alter nutritional status. No doubt this list will grow longer and more complex as we gain more knowledge about drug-nutrient interactions.

From this table, it is obvious that the diagnosis of drug-induced malnutrition can be very difficult. Roe (1976d) pointed out that awareness of the types of interactions and prior experience are important in making this type of diagnosis. Physicians would be well advised to limit the duration of drug therapy whenever possible and to keep the number of medications to a minimum.

Indeed, physicians unwittingly prescribe drug combinations that are especially prone to limit absorption, hasten excretion, and impair tissue storage of essential nutrients. Examples include antacids, laxatives and cathectics, diuretics, and chelating agents (Roe, 1976a); Mueller, 1976).

In certain diseases or conditions, the intentional use of antivitamins can be advantageous. The most important examples are the anti-folates used in treating neoplastic diseases, malaria, and trypanosomiasis, and the anti–vitamin K drug (sodium warfarin) which retards blood coagulation. Other drugs (isoniazid, penicillamine, and L-dopa) induce deficiency of vitamin B_6 and, in the case of L-dopa, administration of vitamin B_6 antagonizes the desired drug effect (Roe, 1976f); Brin, 1976; Roe, 1976j).

In Table 14–2, some nutrients that are commonly affected by drugs are listed individually, and the drugs affecting them are shown on the right. This list is representative, but not all-inclusive.

The most commonly used (and abused) drug in the world is ethanol. The very remarkable ubiquity of this drug and the wide variety of forms in which it is marketed attest to its widespread popularity. It is a drug of extremely variable effects; many people feel that alcohol, taken in moderation, improves the quality and perhaps the length of life. Everyone knows, however, that excesses of alcohol can destroy both body and mind.

TABLE 14–1 PHARMACEUTICAL AGENTS THAT AFFECT NUTRIENTS*

DRUGS	NUTRIENTS	MECHANISMS
Alcohol; in excess of 20% kcal	Folates Thiamin Vitamin B₆ Zinc and magnesium	↓ absorption and utilization ↑ need, ↓ absorption ↓ conversion to active forms ↓ absorption
Antacids; aluminum hydroxide and others	Phosphates	↓ absorption
Anticoagulants; sodium warfarin	Vitamin K	↓ synthesis of coagulation factors
Anticonvulsants; barbiturates and diphenylhydantoin	Folates Vitamin D Vitamin K	unknown inhibition of 25-hydroxylation ↑ enzymatic destruction of sodium warfarin (Coumadin)
Antibiotics; chloramphenicol	Phenylalanine	competes for binding to tRNA direct antagonism
isoniazid	Vitamin B₆, niacin and tryptophan	
neomycin	Fats and fat-soluble vitamins	sequesters bile acids
tetracyclines	Calcium	chemical combination
Anti-inflammatory agents; salicylates indomethacin phenylbutazone	Ascorbic acid Folates	↑ urinary excretion ↓ absorption
Corticosteroids	Vitamin D and calcium Vitamin B₆ Zinc	↑ metabolism of vitamin D, ↑ calcium absorption ↑ requirement** ↑ urinary excretion
Cholesterol-lowering agents; cholestyramine clofibrate	Fats and fat-soluble vitamins Vitamin K	bile acid sequestration potentiates sodium warfarin (Coumadin) drugs

Diuretics; thiazides	Sodium and potassium	↑ urinary excretion
	Glucose	? impaired glucose utilization
	Uric acid	hyperuricemia, cause ?
Antimetabolites; methotrexate, pyrimethamine, 5-fluorouracil	Folates	direct antagonism
	Protein	↓ absorption and impaired synthesis
Antihypertensives; hydralazine	Vitamin B$_6$	uncertain
Hypoglycemias; metformin, phenformin	Vitamin B$_{12}$	↓ absorption
Oral contraceptive steroids	Vitamin B$_6$	↑ requirement
	Folates	↓ absorption
	Ascorbic acid	↓ WBC concentration
	Riboflavin	↑ requirement
	Vitamin B$_{12}$	↓ levels of B$_{12}$ in plasma
	Iron and copper	↑ serum levels, ↑ hemoglobin
	Calcium	better absorption
	Vitamin A	marked ↑ in plasma levels
Laxatives; mineral oil, high fiber diet, others	Fat-soluble vitamins	GI excretion (disputed)
	Zinc and iron	impaired absorption
	Potassium loss	fecal excretion
Miscellaneous; antihistaminics, tricyclic antidepressants, L-dopa	↓ food intake	dry mouth, ↓ appetite
	↑ food intake	uncertain
	Vitamin B$_6$	competitive antagonism; large dose of B$_6$ reduces effect of L-dopa
colchicine	Vitamin B$_{12}$	↓ absorption

*Weinsier et al., 1977
**Theuer and Vitale, 1977

TABLE 14–2 NUTRIENTS THAT MAY BE AFFECTED
BY DRUGS

NUTRIENTS	DRUGS THAT AFFECT NUTRIENT STATUS
Protein	5-fluorouracil; neomycin
Carbohydrates	metformin; phenformin; corticosteroids ↑ ; chlorothiazide ↑
Fats and fatty acids	neomycin; cholestyramine; clofibrate
Thiamin	antacids; ethanol; carbohydrates
Riboflavin	boric acid; oral contraceptive steroids
Niacin	isoniazid; 6-mercaptopurine; 5-fluorouracil
Vitamin B_6	isoniazid; ethanol; oral contraceptive steroids; penicillamine; hydralazine; cycloserine; L-dopa
Folates	diphenylhydantoin; methotrexate; pyrimethamine; ethanol; oral contraceptive steroids; phenylbutazone
Vitamin B_{12}	para-aminosalicylic acid; barbiturates; colchicine; cholestyramine; phenformin; oral contraceptive steroids
Vitamin C	aminopyrine; cigarettes; diphenylhydantoin; oral contraceptive steroids; paraldehyde; salicylates
Vitamin A	mineral oil (disputed); cholestyramine; oral contraceptive steroids ↑
Vitamin D	phenobarbital; diphenylhydantoin; cholestyramine; mineral oil
Vitamin E	mineral oil; iron; polyunsaturated fatty acids; cholestyramine
Vitamin K	sodium warfarin (Coumadin); barbiturates; ascorbic acid ↑ ; mineral oil
Essential fatty acids	continuous infusions of glucose
Sodium	thiazides; ethacrynic acid; Aldactone
Potassium	thiazides; cathartics
Calcium	oxalates; fatty acids; phytates; phosphates
Phosphorus	aluminum hydroxide; total parenteral nutrition
Magnesium	ethanol; ethacrynic acid
Iron	phytic acid; oxalates; phosphates; ascorbic acid ↑
Zinc	ethanol; penicillamine; oral contraceptive steroids
Copper	ethanol; penicillamine; phytates; corticosteroids

TABLE 14–3 SOME CLINICAL SYNDROMES THAT MAY RESULT FROM DRUG-NUTRIENT INTERACTIONS

SYNDROME	NUTRIENT	MOST LIKELY DRUG
Anemia	folic acid vitamin B_{12} iron	ethanol colchicine phosphates
Steatorrhea	tryglycerides	cholestyramine
Hypophosphatemia	phosphates	aluminum hydroxide
Tetany	calcium magnesium	oxalates and phytates ethanol
Muscular weakness	potassium	thiazides
Impaired taste and smell	vitamin A	cholestyramine
Peripheral neuropathy	vitamin B_6	isoniazid
Hypoprothrombinemia Spontaneous hypoprothrombinemia Resistance to sodium warfarin (Coumadin)	vitamin K vitamin K vitamin K	sodium warfarin (Coumadin) mineral oil ascorbic acid
Mood changes	vitamin B_6	oral contraceptive steroids
Yellow mottling of teeth	calcium	tetracyclines in children
Wernicke-Korsakoff's psychosis	thiamin	ethanol
Night blindness and follicular hyperkeratosis	vitamin A	mineral oil (?)
Weakness, mental confusion, and hypotension	sodium	thiazides
Rickets in children, osteomalacia in adults	vitamin D	phenobarbital and diphenylhydantoin
Seborrheic dermatitis	vitamin B_6	L-dopa
Stomatitis and mucositis	folates	methotrexate

But how much alcohol is too much? The best data available (and these are indeed meager) suggest that habitual ingestion of more than 20 per cent of total calories as ethanol will cause damage over a period of months or years. No doubt there are individual differences based on genetics, state of nutritional and general health, and physical activity.

Alcohol has an adverse effect on a remarkable number of nutrients (see Table 14-2) and affects food intake and nutrient absorption, metabolism, storage, and excretion. In some instances it may increase nutrient requirements (Roe, 1976g; Isselbacher, 1977).

Alcohol can also potentiate or alter the effects of other drugs, including anticoagulants, anticonvulsants, and oral hypoglycemic drugs (Hansten, 1976).

Certain groups or classes of drugs are especially prone to have an adverse effect on nutritional status. Accordingly, it seems appropriate to close with a brief mention of these drugs. The anticonvulsant drugs are especially deleterious to vitamin D and the folates. Administration of large doses of folic acid can counteract the anticonvulsant effect (Roe, 1976h) as well.

Oral contraceptive steroids, which are taken by millions of women in the United States (Roe, 1976i), adversely affect a wide range of nutrients: folates, ascorbic acid, riboflavin, vitamin B_6. Some nutrients are favorably affected (if we can assume that higher blood levels are good). These include vitamin A, iron, and copper. Calcium absorption is also improved.

The antituberculous drugs, which have proved to be highly effective in this debilitating disease, have strong antivitamin effects, especially with regard to vitamin B_6. It is strongly suggested that any patient taking isoniazid or cycloserine should be given pyridoxine in a dose of 50 mg daily; and it is well to remember that paraaminobenzoic acid (PABA) can cause deficiency of vitamin B_{12} (Roe, 1976k).

A number of clinical syndromes that can suggest drug-induced nutrient deficiencies are listed in Table 14-3. This is not a complete list, and many of the drugs that might produce these disorders have, of necessity, been omitted. It may become necessary to resort to a computerized data bank to alert physicians to the many possible side effects of medications.

REFERENCES

Brin, M.: Drug-vitamin interrelationships. *Nutrition and the M.D.,* Volume III, no. 1, pp. 1-2, November, 1976. Los Angeles, PM Inc.

Hansten, P. D.: *Drug Interactions,* 3rd Edition. Philadelphia, Lea and Febiger, 1976.

Isselbacher, K. J.: Metabolic and hepatic effects of alcohol. *New England J. Med.* 296:612, 1977.

Mueller, J. F.: Drug-nutrient interrelationships. *Nutrition and the M.D.*, Volume II, no. 5, pp. 2–3, March, 1976. Los Angeles, PM Inc.

Roe, D. A.: Basic concepts. In *Drug-induced Nutritional Deficiencies*, Daphne A. Roe (ed.). Westport, Connecticut, The AVI Publishing Company, 1976a, pp. 1–69.

Roe, D. A.: Factors affecting nutritional requirements. In *Drug-induced Nutritional Deficiencies*, Daphne A. Roe (ed.). Westport, Connecticut, The AVI Publishing Company, 1976b, pp. 70–91.

Roe, D. A.: Variables determining incidence and risk. In *Drug-induced Nutitional Deficiencies*, Daphne A. Roe (ed.). Westport, Connecticut, The AVI Publishing Company, 1976c, pp. 92–101.

Roe, D. A.: Diagnosis of drug-induced malnutrition. In *Drug-induced Nutritional Deficiencies*, Daphne A. Roe (ed.). Westport, Connecticut, The AVI Publishing Company, 1976d, pp. 102–128.

Roe, D. A.: Iatrogenic hyperexcretion and tissue depletion of minerals and vitamins. In *Drug-induced Nutritional Deficiencies*, Daphne A. Roe (ed.). Westport, Connecticut, The AVI Publishing Company, 1976e, pp. 145–153.

Roe, D. A.: Antivitamins. In *Drug-induced Nutritional Deficiencies*, Daphne A. Roe (ed.). Westport, Connecticut, The AVI Publishing Company, 1976f, pp. 154–186.

Roe, D. A.: Aclohol and alcoholism. In *Drug-induced Nutritional Deficiencies*, Daphne A. Roe (ed.). Westport, Connecticut, The AVI Publishing Company, 1976g, pp. 202–210.

Roe, D. A.: Nutritional effects of anticonvulsants. In *Drug-induced Nutritional Deficiencies*, Daphne A. Roe (ed.). Westport, Connecticut, The AVI Publishing Company, 1976h, pp. 211–221.

Roe, D. A.: Nutritional effects of oral contraceptives. In *Drug-induced Nutritional Deficiencies*, Daphne A. Roe (ed.). Westport, Connecticut, The AVI Publishing Company, 1976i, pp. 222–238.

Roe, D. A.: Nutritional effects of antiparkinson drugs: L-DOPA. In *Drug-induced Nutritional Deficiencies*, Daphne A. Roe (ed.). Westport, Connecticut, The AVI Publishing Company, 1976j, pp. 247–252.

Roe, D. A.: Nutritional effects of antituberculous drugs. In *Drug-induced Nutritional Deficiencies*, Daphne A. Roe (ed.). Westport, Connecticut, The AVI Publishing Company, 1976k, pp. 239–246.

Theuer, R. C., and Vitale, J. J.: Drug and nutrient interactions. In *Nutritional Support of Medical Practice*, Howard A. Schneider, Carl E. Anderson, and David B. Coursin (eds.). Hagerstown, Harper and Row, 1977, pp. 297–305.

Visconti, J. A.: Drug-food interaction. In *Nutrition in Disease*, Robert A. Dell (ed.). Columbus, Ohio, Ross Laboratories, 1977, pp. 2–28.

Weinsier, R. L., Butterworth, C. E., and Sahm, D. N.: Drug-nutrient interactions. In *Handbook of Clinical Nutrition. Physician's Manual for the Diagnosis and Management of Nutrition Problems*, R. L. Weinsier, C. E. Butterworth, and D. N. Sahm (eds.). Birmingham, Department of Nutritional Sciences, University of Alabama, 1977, pp. 89–96.

15

FEEDING PATIENTS

Robert E. Hodges, M.D.

The practical application of all of the studies of the biochemistry of foods, the physiology of nutrients, human requirements, and nutritional assessment is the *feeding of patients*. Here the physician needs both a broad knowledge of nutrition and practical experience in dealing with patients.

In office practice, a physician is most often concerned with weight control, while in hospital practice he or she often deals with seriously ill patients whose recovery hinges in part on their nutritional status.

But another, and equally important, application of nutritional knowledge is in community service, for here the physician advises groups of people regarding the best ways to feed themselves and their children. In this area of preventive medicine, there is a need for expansion of information and for its dissemination.

OBJECTIVES OF NUTRITIONAL PRACTICE

Until recently, relatively few physicians practiced nutrition as a subspecialty of pediatrics or medicine or surgery. More often, they were interested in a narrower aspect of medicine, such as hematology or diabetes mellitus or renal failure, for in these areas nutritional management is clearly a substantial part of their task.

Data Base

No matter what the discipline or specialty, nutrition in the practice of medicine employs the same principles, methods, and philosophy as any other. The first task is to collect a data base, starting with a history and a physical examination. As described in the chapter on nutritional evaluation, special emphasis is placed on food choices and eating habits as they may relate to the patient's problems. Similarly, in conducting the physical examination, emphasis is placed on height, weight, musculature, and the integument.

Modern automated laboratory procedures allow the physician to obtain 18 or 20 biochemical measurements on the blood of his or her patients, in addition to the complete blood count and the urine analysis. This information will be of considerable value in assessing the nutritional status of most patients. Occasionally, it is desirable to request additional tests such as the prothrombin time, the levels of folic acid and vitamin B_{12} in serum, and the concentrations of iron, zinc, and copper in serum.

Assessment

From this information, the physician can make an assessment of the patient's current nutritional status. We have found it convenient to score each patient with regard to energy status and protein status on a scale of I to IV. Class I patients are within normal range, Class II patients have significant abnormalities, Class III patients have serious defects that may interfere with or retard recovery, and Class IV patients have life-threatening defects that must be given immediate and appropriate attention.

It is wise to pay close attention to hematologic values, especially hemoglobin, hematocrit, and total lymphocyte counts. If there is evidence of any specific deficiency syndrome, such as scurvy, beriberi, zinc deficiency, and so on, these must be treated promptly.

Therapeutic Plan

Once the patient's status has been established, a plan for nutritional therapy should be completed. This is based on:

1. *An estimate of normal body weight* (from height-weight tables; see page 4).

2. *An estimate of the target level for energy needs.* At rest, a healthy person will use about 25 kcal/kg of *normal* body weight per day. Physical activity, tissue injury, fever, or metabolic derangements will increase this need. Approximately 90 per cent of all hospitalized patients can be effectively repleted with diets containing 30 to 40 see page 4).

kcal/kg normal body weight per day. Remember, this is only a target level and can be revised as often as necessary.

3. *An estimate of the target level for protein.* A healthy adult may need only 0.5 g protein per kg of normal body weight per day, but the recommended dietary allowance (RDA) in the United States is 0.8 g/kg per day. Even this is far less than the average amount of protein (1.0 to 1.2 g/kg) consumed each day by adults in the United States. Many physicians and most surgeons give very generous amounts of protein to their patients. Not uncommonly, they prescribe 1.2 to 2.4 g/kg per day. The evidence that these large amounts are either helpful or harmful is incomplete and controversial. The author favors a target level of 1.0 g/kg of normal body weight per day unless the patient is losing large amounts of protein (1) from the skin, as in burns; (2) from the digestive tract, as in protein-losing enteropathy; or (3) from the urinary tract, as in the nephrotic syndrome. Even in these conditions, excessive amounts of protein are unnecessary. Fortunately, an effective and inexpensive method is readily available to monitor the amount of protein a patient is utilizing from day to day. This is the ratio of the blood urea nitrogen (BUN) to creatinine (Cr) in the plasma. This ratio normally falls between ten and twenty. When it is below ten, the patient may need larger amounts of protein. When it is above twenty, the patient may be catabolizing more protein than normal. This can indicate an excessive intake of protein, a catabolic process such as infection or burns, or inadequate intake of carbohydrate to protect amino acids from catabolism. It also can result from bleeding into the upper portion of the digestive tract. Whatever the cause, an abrupt rise in the BUN/Cr ratio is a signal that something is wrong and further investigation is needed.

4. *Determination of the best route for feeding patients.* This rests on clinical judgment. By far the best route is the digestive tract, and any patient who *can* eat should be *encouraged* to do so. Sometimes a simple problem such as absence of teeth can be solved by providing a soft diet. Some patients who are hospitalized will eat familiar foods but reject "regular" meals. This is particularly true of ethnic minority groups who may speak little or no English and who are embarrassed to ask for special treatment. For this reason, a visit by the physician at mealtimes may solve many problems.

Any patient who cannot or will not eat foods, even after efforts have been made to make it acceptable, must be given another form of nutrients.

Assuming that the patient has a reasonably normal digestive tract, the next step is to give gavage feedings by tube. The commonest method is the nasogastric tube (Pareira, 1959), which usually is effective despite its objections (discomfort, danger of regurgitation). An alternative that may be preferable in patients who will require long-term gavage feedings is a gastrostomy, which avoids nasopharyngeal discomfort and probably reduces the frequency of regurgitation.

In any patient who is comatose or obtunded, the risks of regurgitation, aspiration, and pneumonia are very substantial. These patients may be fed through a jejunostomy tube or they can be given parenteral feedings.

5. *Initiation of feedings in graduated stages.* Any patient who has been severely undernourished for many days should not be given his or her full target level of nutrients abruptly. Starvation causes a decrease in circulating blood volume and in blood pressure and cardiac output of humans (Brozek et al., 1948). Rapid refeeding can result in cardiovascular overload. It may be necessary to start with about one-fourth of the target level, then after one to three days increase the amount given to one-half of the target level. If this is well tolerated, the amount can be increased again in a few days, then the full amount given a few days later. This is not time wasted because it usually avoids the setbacks engendered by gastrointestinal malfunctioning.

6. *Monitoring a patient's progress.* This is done by assessing the daily progress in terms of vital signs, intake and output of fluids, body weight, general sense of well-being, and a few well-chosen laboratory tests and anthropometric measurements. The first evidence of an anabolic trend may be improvement in the patient's sense of well-being. Cahill (1970) called attention to the consequences of human starvation, which constitute a series of metabolic adaptations to derive energy from fat and conserve protein. The result is exclusion of glucose from most tissues, modification of the Cori cycle so as to conserve glucose, and adaptation of the brain to a state of "balanced, benign ketoacidosis".

Restoration of sufficient amounts of glucose to reverse these adaptations can result in prompt improvement in sense of well-being. But the body must adapt to increased supplies of energy and of protein. And, if the patient is fed enterally, restoration of digestive enzymes will require a few days, at least.

As mentioned before, the quantity of protein that is converted into urea can be estimated by measuring the BUN/Cr ratio. It can also be estimated by measuring the total amount of urea excreted in the urine each 24 hours. This is an effective indicator of nutrient needs, for a rise in urea excretion means that more protein is being wasted, and implies that not enough glucose energy is being provided or that too much protein is being given. This concept was introduced by Cuthbertson (1932), who studied the catabolic effects of fractures.

The clinical syndrome of "protein-calorie-malnutrition," that is, a disparity between energy metabolism and protein metabolism, was first clearly understood in children. At one end of the spectrum is lack of protein in the diet of a child who is receiving adequate or nearly adequate energy from carbohydrates. Anemia, edema, and integumentary changes are characteristic of this syndrome, which is termed "kwashiorkor". At the opposite end of the spectrum is marasmus, in which the intake of *all* foods is grossly inadequate. In short, these children are the victims of chronic starvation or semistarvation.

Several recent investigators have called attention to "hospital malnutrition" (Leevy et al., 1965) and its clinical manifestations (Bollet and Owens, 1973). Law and others (1974) and Munster (1976) and Bistrian and others (1975) demonstrated the deleterious effects of malnutrition on immune mechanisms. Consolazio and colleagues (1972) showed that as few as 10 days of caloric restriction can greatly alter the metabolism of tryptophan and niacin in young men.

Butterworth (1974) and Butterworth (editorial, 1974) called attention to the high prevalence (as high as 50 per cent) of hospital malnutrition. Many patients had deteriorated nutritionally after two weeks of hospitalization. The high level of malnutrition among hospitalized patients speaks in favor of nutritional monitoring of any patient who does not seem to be prospering (Blackburn and Bistrian, 1976; Bistrian et al., 1976).

The use of anthropometric measurements, as described in the chapter on nutritional assessment, applies equally to the monitoring of patients who are receiving nutritional care on a daily basis. This type of measurement can help a physician differentiate between lack of sufficient protein and lack of energy (Martorell et al., 1976).

7. *Final counseling.* After a patient has recovered and is ready to return home, the nutrition-oriented physician will want to give specific advice about food habits and nutritional needs. Often the cause is abuse of alcohol, but sometimes it reflects food fads or indifference or ignorance of foods and nutrition. In some instances, a multivitamin supplement is needed, but more often all the patient needs is sensible and practical advice.

NUTRITION IN PRACTICE

Advice to the Community

In many towns and in some cities it is common practice for municipal governmental officials and officers of the school board or the Parent-Teachers Association or other groups interested in community health to invite physicians to lecture on some topic related to health. This topic might be "Food Vending Machines in Schools",

"Junk Foods", "Fast Foods", "Fluoridation of Water", or the alleged "Relationship between Food Additives and Hyperkinesis in Children".

Favorite topics for service clubs and fraternal organizations include: "Organic" or "Natural Foods", "Processed Foods", "Alcoholism", or "Fats, Cholesterol, and Heart Disease".

The practicing physician may find that non-medical friends and neighbors have their own questions to ask about fad diets, vitamin supplements, diet pills, or orthomolecular psychiatry.

Office Nutrition Counseling

Fats, Cholesterol, and Heart Disease

As described in the chapter on cardiovascular disease, the average physician can offer valuable advice to his or her patients and can identify these who have a greater-than-normal level of risk.

Alcoholism

Few patients will volunteer information regarding excessive use of alcohol, but the telltale signs of flushed faces, paper-money skin, and intention tremor of the hands may suggest the diagnosis.

Diabetes Mellitus

At least 80 per cent of diabetic patients are obese at the time the diagnosis is made and most remain obese. A physician can induce many to control their eating, but it requires constant reinforcement.

Obesity

Few medical problems are as common and none so difficult to treat as obesity. The very fact that there are so many forms of treatment attests to the futility of our efforts. Nonetheless, the situation is far from hopeless and, when put into perspective, is much easier to deal with.

In the opinion of the author, most methods of classifying obesity are artificial and unrealistic. The vast number of obese patients who come into a physician's office fall into one or the other of two categories: childhood-onset obesity, and middle-aged obesity. Rarely is there an endocrine disorder, and even less often can obesity be attributed to a metabolic error.

Childhood-onset Obesity. Childhood-onset obesity (or familial obesity) probably is more common in women than in men—at least in our clinic women outnumber men by a ratio of about five-to-one. The history is usually one of a child who was normal at birth but who soon outgrew her peer group. In preschool years she was taller and larger than other children her age. The same pattern prevailed in the grade-school years (ages 6 to 12) but often the "large" child had an early menarche at age 9, 10, or 11 years. Within two years, her epiphyses had closed so by the time she entered junior high school she was shorter than many of her classmates and much fatter. From this time on she had one discouraging event after another. Many of these girls married early and became teen-aged mothers. Each pregnancy seemed to increase the degree of obesity. Often these individuals reach a weight level that is two hundred to three hundred per cent of normal for their height. Diets and a variety of reducing schemes are largely ineffective. These patients are angry and discouraged. They feel they have been abandoned by their families, their friends, their physicians, and by society itself.

Middle-aged Spread. By contrast, this group of patients was normal in weight through childhood, adolescence, and early adult life. There was no need to diet — their appetite regulated their food intake with uncanny precision. But by the time they reached their late 20s or early 30s they began to gain slightly. At first the gain was only about 2 pounds per year for men and 3 pounds per year for women. Sometimes they dieted for a few weeks and found it rather easy to take off 5 to 10 pounds but they usually regained this weight in a few months. These people, who represent the vast majority of adults in the United States, continue to gain weight slowly until about age 55 for men and about 65 for women, then their weight plateaus or declines slightly thereafter.

The idea that the first group of patients has a "weak will" and "doesn't care," while the second group is "too proud to let themselves get fat" is sheer nonsense. The author is conviced that the first group of patients was born with a defective feeding center in the hypothalamus or elsewhere.

Of course, obesity does not always fall into one or the other pattern; there are some in between. But it is convenient and helpful to keep these two stereotypes in mind because the treatment of the two is vastly different.

One of the first objectives in dealing with obese patients is to convince them that you are not going to criticize them. They have had more than their share of this.

The next point to make is that fad diets, including low-carbohydrate diets, are not effective in the long run (Anonymous, 1964; Krehl et al., 1967; Council on Foods and Nutrition, 1973).

There is evidence that starvation *in utero* during the last half of pregnancy prevents obesity in adult life (Ravelli et al., 1976). And other evidence suggests that starvation and refeeding of animals, if done repeatedly, can lead to hypertension and cardiovascular disease (Smith et al., 1964).

For mildly obese persons of the adult-onset type, diets are reasonably effective. The author favors an allowance of 25 kcal/kg of *normal* body weight. Surprisingly, this usually gives the patient about 1000 kcal less than he or she had been eating.

Kempner and colleagues (1975) reported successful treatment of massive obesity with a rice diet, similar to that used in treating malignant hypertension three decades ago. It is true that obesity is rare in countries where rice is the dietary staple (and animal foods are scarce) but most Americans will not accept a vegetarian diet, much less a rice diet.

But diets for most patients with familial or childhood-onset obesity are almost useless. What, then, are the choices for them? Drugs are dangerous and, after a few weeks, ineffective. Exercise alone was reported by Gwinup (1975) to be effective in causing weight loss in 11 women, but most patients did not persist in this activity. Exercise, for many of these people, is almost out of the question; they either can't or won't continue with an exercise program. Surgical procedures have received much notoriety in treating these massively obese patients. These can be divided into three major classes: Wiring the teeth together is a cruel and temporary way to reduce the amount of food eaten by obese patients. After the wires are removed, most patients regain all of the weight they lost (Malt and Guggenheim, 1976). The gastric bypass operation has been reported to cause substantial weight loss but without serious metabolic derangements. But the most popular (and most dangerous) operation is the jejunoileal bypass, which produces a severe malabsorption syndrome (Bray and Drenick, 1972; Anonymous, 1978). These patients often lose 100 pounds or more in the first year but the persistent diarrhea, their change in eating habits, and serious metabolic complications make this a hazardous procedure. The last and probably most effective and safe approach is behavior modification. This is based on the theory that many obese people eat excessively not because they are hungry but for a host of others reasons: habit, frustration, loneliness, sadness, anger, anxiety, depression, and so on. If they can identify the factors that trigger their eating behavior, and if they can substitute a more appropriate response, then they should be able to curtail their excessive eating (Penick et al., 1971; Howard, 1975).

This, of course, is a gross oversimplification of a very complex form of therapy, but the success rate is better than that of most other conservative approaches and there are no undesirable side effects. Until medical science can regulate the feeding centers of the brain, this seems to be the choice method for managing obesity of the childhood-onset variety.

Hospital Nutrition

In the hospital, a physician finds the greatest need for nutritional competence and knowledge. After he or she has made an assessment of a patient who obviously needs nutritional therapy, the physician will estimate the degree and type of nutritional deficit and set target levels for kilocalories and for protein.

Next, this physician will decide upon oral feedings, gavage feedings, or parenteral infusions. If oral feedings are selected, the type of diet must be designated.

Few people realize that, of the thousands of diets that have been prescribed over the years, all can be classified into just four categories, for there are only four ways in which dietary changes can be made. These are:

1. Quantitative changes. More or less of a given nutrient, such as sodium or protein or fat.

2. Frequency of meals. Patients are usually fed three times daily (unless diagnostic procedures interfere) but meals can be given as often as once every hour or, with gavage feedings, continuously.

3. Texture. The diet may be of normal texture or soft or liquid or high in fiber or low in residue.

4. Qualitative changes (seldom used). Removal of some offensive substance from a diet is termed a "qualitative" change. Examples are removal of gluten from the diet of a patient with celiac sprue, or prescription of a copper-free diet for a patient with hepatolenticular degeneration.

Formula Feedings by Tube

As indicated above, formula feedings can be very effective if a few simple precautions are taken. There are commercial formulas marketed in the United States but many are closely similar. The two basic types are: (1) those made with whole proteins, complex carbohydrates, and triglyceride fats; and (2) an "elemental" diet which contains either crystalline amino acids or protein hydrolysate, simple sugars, and small amounts of essential fatty acids. The elemental diets have certain advantages and disadvantages. Since they are "predigested" they do not require pancreatic enzyme action before absorption. Also, the very low fat content reduces the need for micelle formation, hence for bile salts; and total absence of fiber is thought to "place the bowel at rest," a theoretically desirable effect in patients with inflammatory bowel disease.

The disadvantages of the elemental diets are substantial: their cost is high and the taste of free amino acids is well-nigh impossible to mask. Few patients will drink enough of these formulas to meet their nutritional needs. In addition, the high osmolality of these formulas causes nausea, abdominal distress, and diarrhea in some patients. The very low fat content may not favor absorption of the fat-soluble vitamins, especially vitamin A; and the total lack of fiber may not be as "restful" for the bowel as we once thought. In some patients, the only alternative to administration of an elemental diet by tube is the use of parenteral feedings.

The commonest reasons for dissatisfaction with gavage feedings are regurgitation or diarrhea or both. These may be attributed to common mistakes on the part of physicians and nurses. They are: (1) excessive amounts of formula at the start. It is wise to begin with one-fourth of the target level and increase by stages; (2) excessively concentrated formula with an osmolality of 500 or greater. Even though regular meals may have much higher potential osmolality than this, the hypertonic formula can cause vomiting or hypermotility of the bowel; (3) presence of lactose in formula. Many formula diets, especially the older ones, are based on milk as the principal source of protein. Milk also contains lactose, which may cause gastrointestinal distress in persons who lack sufficient lactase in their bowel mucosa to hydrolyze milk sugar. This pertains not only to those with a racial predisposition to lactase deficiency (Blacks, Orientals, American Indians, Eskimos, Jews, and those whose ancestors inhabited the Mediterranean shores) but also to many patients who have developed some degree of malabsorption as a result of illness or poor dietary habits; and (4) bacterial contamination of the formula. Great care is taken in the diet kitchen to maintain sterility and cleanliness in areas where food is prepared. Once a formula reaches the patient area, however, a number of things may happen to contaminate it. One is the practice of pouring a large amount of formula (perhaps enough for 12 hours) into a hanging bottle to which the feeding tube is attached. As the formula runs out, air enters the bottle and introduces bacteria which grow abundantly in the culture medium of the formula, which is no longer refrigerated. The result may be iatrogenic food poisoning with the usual symptoms of diarrhea and abdominal pain, nausea, vomiting, and dehydration.

The obvious solution to these problems is to start gavage feedings slowly, avoid lactose, avoid hyperosmolality, and be certain that only small quantities (enough for 3 hours) of formula are hung at one time and that a *clean, sterile* container is used with each new portion of formula. If, because of injury or illness, any patient is unable to tolerate food in the digestive tract, there is still an opportunity to provide ample amounts of nutrients.

Parenteral Feedings

Introduction and Indications. Although many physicians still are hesitant to use parenteral nutrition in the management of their patients, it represents a great advance in medical and surgical therapy. If one accepts the concept that *every* patient has a right to adequate nutrition (as well as adequate medical care), then it becomes axiomatic that certain patients who cannot use their digestive tract adequately, if at all, must be given some form of parenteral nutrition or they will die (Johnston, 1978).

Every physician who attends patients recognizes that patients who are hopelessly ill or injured have a "right to die". But parenteral nutrition will not maintain life indefinitely in such patients and certainly should be withheld from these patients who are denied other life-support systems such as a respirator or a cardiac pacemaker. There is no need to list specific indications for parenteral feeding, but some of the most dramatic successes have been reported in treatment of infantile diarrhea and congenital defects of the digestive tract of newborn infants; management of adults or children with massive injuries including burns (Wilmore, 1976), gunshot wounds, and automobile accidents; and supportive care of patients with inflammatory bowel disease, renal failure, and even hepatic failure.

Contraindications. As experience is gained in the use of parenteral nutrition there are fewer and fewer absolute contraindications. Even cancer patients who have received immunosuppressive therapy or patients with septicemia sometimes benefit from parenteral feedings (Copeland and Dudrick, 1978). Some patients with fluid overload syndromes can be effectively managed by restricting the fluid volume while administering needed nutrients.

Three conditions that were at one time considered to be contraindications to parenteral feeding are acute renal failure (Abel, 1976; Meng et al., 1976; Chini et al., 1976; Briggs et al., 1976; Sofio and Nicora, 1976), hepatic coma (Aguirre et al., 1976), and cerebral edema. Experience now indicates that parenteral feeding may be highly advantageous even in such patients as these. The important point to remember is that *each case should be judged individually* and potential benefits are weighed against risks.

Methods and Procedures. As described above, the first step is to take a history and perform a physical examination. Special attention should be paid to evidence for or against the ability of the digestive tract to perform, even at a reduced level. Also, such factors as fever, blood loss, and intestinal fistula have an important influence on the patient's needs for energy and for protein (James, 1978). Another important and often neglected piece of information is the patient's *normal body weight,* for this is the basis upon which nutritional needs are calculated. (Some experts prefer to use nomograms for estimating body surface area and metabolic activity but these are based on height and weight.) (Blackburn and others, 1974).

Once the target levels for energy and for protein have been established on the basis of normal body weight, present metabolic needs, and present protein needs, it is convenient to select the therapeutic level closest to your estimates. We have found it convenient and economical to have our pharmacy formulate solutions of parenteral nutrients according to the following standards:

Most experts suggest that the desirable level of non-protein energy to nitrogen (kcal/N) is in the range of 150 to 250. (Remember that commercial preparations of dextrose use *hydrated* dextrose which provides 3.4 kcal/g. Also remember that protein ÷ 6.25 = nitrogen in grams.) This is easily calculated as:

$$\frac{\text{grams dextrose} \times 3.4}{\text{grams protein} \div 6.25}$$

If one uses 40 grams of protein equivalent (amino acids) and 400 grams of dextrose, this ratio becomes 212:1, which is in the middle of the range as established by others.

We have found it convenient to have several stages of parenteral nutrition solutions as follows:

Protein	Dextrose	Non-protein kcal
40 g	400 g	1360
60 g	600 g	2040
80 g	800 g	2720
100 g	1000 g	3400

These amounts of nutrients are dissolved in the appropriate volume of water, usually 3 liters per day.

Most patients are given one liter of the "40/400" formulation the first day (that is, 13.3 g protein and 133 g dextrose), then 2 liters (27 g protein and 267 g dextrose) the second day, and 3 liters daily thereafter.

The concentration of the infusion fluid is increased as tolerated, usually every 2 to 3 days to "60/600", then "80/800", and sometimes to "100/1000".

Choice of Products. There are several brands of parenteral nutrition products available in the United States. These are made either from hydrolyzed protein such as casein, or from crystalline amino acids. There is some evidence that the crystalline products are more desirable because they cause less hyperchloremic acidosis and less hyperammonemia, but the differences are small. Among the crystalline products the differences seem to be relatively unimportant, although excesses of glutamic and aspartic acids may be undesirable and additional amounts of arginine may be beneficial under certain circumstances. Of greater importance, however, is avoidance of either a deficiency or a surplus of any single amino acid. Munro (1978) called attention to the biological factors that are altered when amino acids are infused rather than absorbed from the digestive tract. The full implications of these factors are yet to be determined but it seems prudent to avoid radical departures from established regimens that have been found both safe and effective. Nonetheless, studies of various amino acid formulations are of great interest and may have important therapeutic implications (Ghadimi, 1975; Ghadimi and Tejani, 1975). In a related area, Walser and others (1976) reported the use of the alpha-keto analogues of essential amino acids in patients with renal failure.

Recently, the concept of "protein sparing" by infusing amino acids into a peripheral vein along with minimal amounts of dextrose has received considerable attention (Greenberg et al., 1976; Blackburn and Bistrian, 1977b; Tweedle et al., 1977).

Vitamins and Minerals. Patients who are fed parenterally are presumed to have about the same nutrient requirements as they would if they were fed orally. This does not, however, take into account the biochemical transformations that occur in the mucosa of the bowel nor the many functions of the liver in metabolizing nutrients that are concentrated in the portal blood stream. It is doubtful that such nutrients as vitamin A are as effectively transported if they are not attached to their respective carrier proteins. We have, nonetheless, for the past decade relied upon vitamin preparations that allow little flexibility in prescribing for patients who are to receive all of their nutrients intravenously. The same can be said for the trace minerals (Greene, 1975). It is common practice to give iron, iodine, zinc, copper, cobalt, magnesium, chromium, and fluoride, although not all of these elements are available from commercial sources. In addition, we believe that a number of other nutrients are essential for the human economy, but the evidence of deficiency syndromes is meager or totally lacking. For practical purposes, calcium, phosphorus, and magnesium are added by pharmacists along with sodium, potassium, and chloride. Cobalt is contained in the vitamin B_{12} routinely given, and iodine, which is present in the antiseptic used at the catheter site, is absorbed through the skin. Fluoride is usually present in the water used to formulate these solutions. Manganese, copper, and zinc can be added by the pharmacist in appropriate amounts as suggested by Fell and Burns (1977):

Manganese	2–3 mg daily
Zinc	15 mg daily
Copper	2 mg daily

We have not added iron to the infusion fluid because it reacts with tocopherol, ascorbic acid, and several amino acids. Iron is given as needed on a basis of hematologic values, serum levels of this element, and per cent saturation of transferrin.

It is possible to provide enough protein as amino acids to meet the usual daily requirements, but only about 20 per cent of the energy needs can be given as dextrose into a peripheral vein. This procedure, referred to as peripheral parenteral nutrition (PPN) in contradistinction to total parenteral nutrition (TPN), has been shown to reduce the net loss of nitrogen by about half. Accordingly, it may have utility in providing some nutritional support for those patients who are in reasonably good nutritional health (Class I) and who should be able to eat adequately within three or four days. But for the patient who may be unable to eat for a week or who is less well nourished initially, it is better to give total parenteral nutrition from the start.

Energy Sources. Much has been written about the use of various alternatives to dextrose as the major energy source in TPN solutions (Long et al., 1977). This is a very complex issue, but it appears to the author that dextrose is as good as any other product and better than most (Bessman, 1975). Hyperglycemia does occur in a few patients, but clinicians have learned how to deal with this problem effectively.

Fat emulsions have been used as a supplemental energy source for many years in Europe and for a shorter period of time in the United States. Fats have several advantages: they contain linoleic acid which meets requirements for essential fatty acids, they do not increase the osmotic activity of the infusion fluid, and they do not require insulin for oxidative metabolism (Meng, 1976; Greene, 1976; Jeejeebhoy et al., 1976).

Therapeutic Successes. In pediatric practice, TPN has been especially useful in those cases where growth and development are retarded by illness and undernutrition (Harries, 1978). In both children and adults with inflammatory bowel disease, many experts report favorable responses, especially with Crohn's disease (McFadyen and Dudrick, 1976; Layden et al., 1976; Reilly et al., 1976; Goode et al., 1976; Feliciano and Telander, 1976).

Perhaps the most spectacular results of TPN therapy are seen in patients with fistulas of the bowel. Most of these will close without surgical intervention and the remainder usually can be closed by a combination of an operation plus TPN (Aguirre and Fischer, 1976).

Complications of TPN and How to Avoid Them. When parenteral nutrition was first introduced into general use, it was widely acclaimed as a great boon to medicine, but then the negative reports began to appear. These included mechanical hazards, infection, metabolic and deficiency syndromes. Some said that TPN was too dangerous to use in clinical practice and many viewed it as a last resort.

Fortunately Dudrick and many others devised routines that drastically reduced the mechanical hazards, the risks of infection, and the prevalence of metabolic derangements; and recent developments have largely eliminated the deficiency syndromes.

The complications and their management are listed and discussed briefly:

1. Mechanical problems including hemorrhage, pneumothorax, thrombosis, or injury to some intrathoracic structure usually can be avoided by a skilled operator. Problems arise when physicians view parenteral nutrition as "just another I.V." and delegate the placement of a central line to the least experienced member of the team. The presence of a skilled TPN nurse, who anticipates errors and thus avoids them, helps immeasurably.

2. Infections occur either because bacteria or fungi are introduced with the catheter or because the TPN solution is infected or because the central catheter is a foreign body that becomes coated with fibrin on which organisms can become implanted. Infections introduced with or through the catheter are termed "catheter related" and those that occur following a bacteremia that arose from some other source are called "secondary". We feel that most catheter-related infections can and should be avoided, whereas secondary infections cannot. In either event, when the catheter becomes infected it should be removed within 24 hours and replaced, preferably on the opposite side (Maki, 1976; Sanders and Sheldon, 1976; Allen, 1978). The incidence of catheter-related infections should be in the range of 2 to 5 per cent, whereas the incidence of secondary infections varies with the type of patient. Most burned patients and many cancer patients will have daily episodes of bacteremia. Under these circumstances, infection of the catheter usually recurs about twice each week and is anticipated in hospitals where these patients are cared for. Indeed, changes of the central catheter are made a part of the routine in cancer hospitals and in burn units.

3. Metabolic problems: One of the most serious and yet easily avoided syndromes is that of hypophosphatemia (Silvis and Paragas, 1971; Silvis and Paragas, 1972). This syndrome is most apt to develop when a semistarved patient is given a large load of dextrose too abruptly. The normal need for phosphates to phosphorylate glucose and its metabolic derivatives is overwhelmed by an abrupt increase in the amount of glucose substrate. Furthermore, constant infusion of glucose results in a constant release of insulin, which in turn favors the storage of organic phosphates in the liver. The result is a fall in the concentration of inorganic phosphorus in the plasma and a secondary fall in the concentrations of ATP and of 2,3-diphosphoglycerate in erythrocytes. This causes a shift-to-the-left in the hemoglobin-oxygen dissociation curve, and results in tissue hypoxia. The clinical results are complex: There is loss of elasticity of erythrocytes and decreased phagocytosis by polymorphonuclear leukocytes. Most important of all, however, is cerebral hypoxia, which causes confusion, coma, convulsions, and death. Treatment is effective if initiated promptly: the infusion of glucose must be slowed, phosphates given intravenously (40 mEq in 24 hours), and oxygen and other supportive measures instituted. Prevention of this syndrome can be achieved by: (1) introducing TPN at a low level, with increases by stages over a period of time; (2) inclusion of phosphates in the infusion fluid (40 mEq daily); (3) avoidance of aluminum hydroxide antacids that trap phosphorus; and (4) careful monitoring of blood chemistries, including phosphorus levels, at appropriate intervals.

Hypertonic, hyperglycemic, non-ketotic coma can develop in patients who are receiving TPN, especially in middle-age or older patients who are obese, physically inactive, and mildly diabetic. Their blood sugar levels may rise slowly to the 200 to 300 mg/dl range without causing alarm in the minds of the medical team; then abruptly the glucose level may rise above 500 mg/dl and the patient may become obtunded. The hyperglycemia causes an osmotic diuresis that may result in hyponatremia, hypotension, and decreased perfusion of the brain. Once the syndrome begins to develop, it is important to recognize the need for salt and water. Administration of insulin alone is ineffective (Ryan, 1976).

Other metabolic abnormalities include metabolic acidosis, cholestatic jaundice, and hyperammonemia (Ausman and Hardy, 1978). Each of these can be anticipated and dealt with effectively by experienced physicians.

4. Deficiency syndromes: One of the most unexpected events was the appearance of an essential fatty-acid deficiency syndrome in patients receiving TPN therapy. Despite an abundance of linoleic acid in their fat stores, they develop very low plasma levels and a rise in the concentration of an abnormal fatty acid, 5,8,11(9W)-eicosatrienoic acid. This syndrome results in a scaling dermatitis of the face and other areas, and may interfere with wound healing, among other things (Caldwell, 1976; Fleming et al., 1976b).

Deficiencies of zinc and copper, which rarely occur in healthy people in the United States, may develop in patients receiving TPN for a prolonged period of time, unless these elements are added to the infusion fluid (Fleming et al., 1976a).

The Team Approach. Despite some opinions to the contrary, the author strongly opposes the use of parenteral nutrition by unskilled and untrained physicians and paramedical personnel. This valuable form of therapy fully justifies the formation of a "TPN Team" which should include a specially trained nurse, one or more physicians, a pharmacist, and a dietitian (Phillips, 1976). Standard protocols should be prepared and closely followed. Accurate records permit self-appraisal (Fischer, 1976). Even "home TPN" is feasible for a few selected patients (Shils, 1975).

SUMMARY

Optimal nutritional support of patients, in or outside the hospital, has become more than a reality — it has become a right. No longer can we justify the development and worsening of malnutrition without making a conscientious effort to correct it. There are failures, to be sure, but the existing knowledge and skills we have are successful in changing the outlook of several specific disorders; and nutritional support of both surgical and medical patients has improved their response to therapy in terms of decreased infections, increased wound healing, and better sense of well-being.

REFERENCES

Abel, R. M.: Total parenteral alimentation in the treatment of renal failure. In *Total Parenteral Alimentation*, C. Manni, S. I. Magalini, and E. Scrascia (eds.). Amsterdam-Oxford, Exerpta Medica; New York, American Elsevier Publishing Company, 1976, pp. 125–137.
Aguirre, A., and Fischer, J. E.: Intestinal fistulas. In *Total Parenteral Nutrition*, Josef E. Fisher (ed.). Boston, Little, Brown and Company, 1976, pp. 203–218.
Aguirre, A., Funovics, J., Wesdorp, R. I. C., and Fischer, J. E.: Parenteral nutrition in hepatic failure. In *Total Parenteral Nutrition*, Josef E. Fischer (ed.). Boston, Little, Brown and Company, 1976, pp. 219–230.
Allen, J. R.: The incidence of nosocomial infection in patients receiving total parenteral nutrition. In *Advances in Parenteral Nutrition*. Proceedings of an International Symposium, Bermuda, 16–19 May, 1977, I. D. A. Johnston (ed.). Baltimore, University Park Press, 1978, pp. 339–377.
Anonymous: The role of carbohydrates in the diet. *Nutr. Reviews* 22:102, 1964.
Anonymous: What's new in weight control. *Dairy Council Digest* 49:2, 1978.
Ausman, R. K., and Hardy, G.: Metabolic complications of parenteral nutrition. Proceedings of an International Symposium, Bermuda, 16–19 May, 1977, I. D. A. Johnston (ed.). Baltimore, University Park Press, 1978, pp. 403–410.

Bessman, S. P.: Glucose metabolism (the glycolytic cycle). In *Total Parenteral Nutrition. Premises and Promises*, H. Ghadimi (ed.). New York, John Wiley and Sons, 1975, pp. 57–63.

Bistrian, B. R., Blackburn, G. L., Hallowell, E., and Heddle, R.: Protein status of general surgical patients. *J.A.M.A. 230*:858, 1974.

Bistrian, B. R., Blackburn, G. L., Scrimshaw, N. S., and Flatt, J. P.: Cellular immunity in semistarved states in hospitalized adults. *Amer. J. Clin. Nutr. 28*:1148, 1975.

Bistrian, B. R., Blackburn, G. L., Vitale, J., Cochran, D., and Naylor, J.: Prevalence of malnutrition in general medical patients. *J.A.M.A. 235*:1567, 1976.

Blackburn, G. L., and Bistrian, B. R.: Careers in nutrition from the clinical viewpoint. *Nutr. Reviews 34*:97, 1976.

Blackburn, G. L., and Bistrian, B. R.: Curative nutrition: Protein-calorie management. In *Nutritional Support of Medical Practice*, Howard A. Schneider, Carl E. Anderson, and David B. Coursin (eds.). Hagerstown, Harper and Row, 1977, pp. 80–100.

Blackburn, G. L., and Bistrian, B. R.: Nutritional support resources in hospital practice. In *Nutritional Support of Medical Practice*, Howard A. Schneider, Carl E. Anderson, and David B. Coursin (eds.). Hagerstown, Harper and Row, 1977, pp. 139–151.

Bollet, A. J., and Owens, S. O.: Evaluation of nutritional status of selected hospitalized patients. *Amer. J. Clin. Nutr. 26*:931, 1973.

Bray, G. A., and Drenick, E. J.: Obesity: A serious symptom. *Ann. Intern. Med. 77*:779, 1972.

Briggs, W. A., Kaminski, M. V., Kyle, R. W., Light, J. A., and Yeager, H. C.: Hyperalimentation in anephrics. *Acta Chir. Scandinavica, Supplementum 466*:100, 1976.

Brozek, J., Chapman, C. B., and Keys, A.: Drastic food restriction. Effect on cardiovascular dynamics in normotensive and hypertensive conditions. *J.A.M.A. 137*:1569, 1948.

Butterworth, C. E., Jr.: The skeleton in the hospital closet. *Nutr. Today 9*:4, 1974.

Butterworth, C. E., Jr.: Malnutrition in the hospital (Editorial). *J.A.M.A. 230*:879, 1974.

Cahill, G. F., Jr.: Starvation in man. *New England J. Med. 282*:668, 1970.

Caldwell, M. D.: Human essential fatty acid deficiency: A review. In *Fat Emulsions in Parenteral Nutrition*, H C. Meng, and D. W. Wilmore (eds.). Chicago, American Medical Association, 1976, pp. 24–28.

Chini, G., Santino, F. F., Rosa, E. R., Imbassahy, F. E., Villela, R. A., Silva, J. C., Dutra, S. L., Cerosimo, E., Gomes, E. P. R., and Gomes, S.: Parenteral nutrition in the management of acute renal failure. *Acta Chir. Scandinavica, Supplementum 466*:96, 1976.

Consolazio, C. F., Johnson, H. L., Krzywicki, H. J., and Witt, N. F.: Tryptophan-niacin interrelationships during acute fasting and caloric restriction in humans. *Amer. J. Clin. Nutr. 25*:572, 1972.

Copeland, E. M. III, and Dudrick, S. J.: The importance of parenteral nutrition as an adjunct to cancer treatment. In *Advances in Parenteral Nutrition*. Proceedings of an International Symposium, Bermuda, 16–19 May, 1977, I. D. A. Johnston (ed.). Baltimore, University Park Press, 1978, pp. 473–495.

Council on Foods and Nutrition: A critique of low-carbohydrate ketogenic weight reduction regimens. A review of Dr. Atkin's Diet Revolution. *J.A.M.A. 224*:1415, 1973.

Cuthbertson, D. P.: The distribution of nitrogen and sulphur in the urine during conditions of increased catabolism. *Biochem. J. 25*:236, 1932.

Feliciano, D. V., and Telander, R. L.: Total parenteral nutrition in infants and children. *Mayo Clin. Proc. 51*:647, 1976.

Fell, G. S., and Burns, R. R.: Zinc and other trace elements. In *Advances in Parenteral Nutrition*. Proceedings of an International Symposium, Bermuda, 16–19 May, 1977, I. D. A. Johnston (ed.). Baltimore, University Park Press, 1978, pp. 241–261.

Fischer, J. R.: The organization of a Parenteral Nutrition Unit. In *Total Parenteral Nutrition*, Josef E. Fischer (ed.). Boston, Little, Brown and Company, 1976, pp. 127–131.

Fleming, C. R., Hodges, R. E., and Hurley, L. S.: A prospective study of serum copper and zinc levels in patients receiving total parenteral nutrition. *Amer. J. Clin. Nutr.* 29:70, 1976a.

Fleming, C. R., Smith, L. M., and Hodges, R. E.: Essential fatty acid deficiency in adults receiving total parenteral nutrition. *Amer. J. Clin. Nutr.* 29:976, 1976b.

Ghadimi, H.: Newly devised amino acid solutions for intravenous administration. In *Total Parenteral Nutrition. Premises and Promises,* H. Ghadimi (ed.). New York, John Wiley and Sons, 1975, pp. 393–442.

Ghadimi, H., and Tejani, A.: Protein and amino acid requirements. In *Total Parenteral Nutrition. Premises and Promises,* H. Ghadimi (ed.). New York, John Wiley and Sons, 1975, pp. 213–230.

Goode, A., Hawkins, T., Feggetter, J. G. W., and Johnston, I. D. A.: Use of an elemental diet for long-term nutritional support in Crohn's disease. *Lancet* 1:122, 1976.

Greenberg, G. R., Marliss, E. B., Anderson, G. H., Langer, B., Spence, W., Tovee, E. B., and Jeejeebhoy, K. N.: Protein-sparing therapy in post-operative patients. *New England J. Med.* 294:1411, 1976.

Greene, H. L.: Vitamins and trace elements. In *Total Parenteral Nutrition. Premises and Promises,* H. Ghadimi (ed.). New York, John Wiley and Sons, 1975, pp. 351–371.

Greene, H. L.: Effect of Intralipid on pulmonary function. In *Fat Emulsions in Parenteral Nutrition,* H. C. Meng, and D. W. Wilmore (eds.). Chicago, American Medical Association, 1976, pp. 95–98.

Gwinup, G.: Effect of exercise alone on the weight of obese women. *Arch. Intern. Med.* 135:676, 1975.

Harries, J. T.: Aspects of intravenous feeding in childhood. In *Advances in Parenteral Nutrition.* Proceedings of an International Symposium, Bermuda, 16–19 May, 1977, I. D. A. Johnston (ed.). Baltimore, University Park Press, 1978, pp. 267–280.

Howard, A. N.: Dietary treatment of obesity. In *Obesity: Its Pathogenesis and Management,* T. Silverstone (ed.). Lancaster, England, Medical and Technical Publishing Company, Ltd., 1975, pp. 123–153.

James, W. P. T.: Research in malnutrition and its application to parenteral feeding. In *Advances in Parenteral Nutrition.* Proceedings of an International Symposium, Bermuda, 16–19 May, 1977, I. D. A. Johnston (ed.). Baltimore, University Park Press, 1978, pp. 521–531.

Jeejeebhoy, K. N., Marliss, E. B., Anderson, G. H., Greenberg, G. R., Kuksis, A., and Breckenridge, C.: Lipid in parenteral nutrition: Studies of clinical and metabolic features. In *Fat Emulsions in Parenteral Nutrition,* H. C. Meng, and D. W. Wilmore (eds.). Chicago, American Medical Association, 1976, pp. 45–54.

Johnston, I. D. A.: Metabolic foundations of intravenous nutrition. In *Advances in Parenteral Nutrition.* Proceedings of an International Symposium, Bermuda, 16–19 May, 1977, I. D. A. Johnston (ed.). Baltimore, University Park Press, 1978, pp. 3–20.

Kempner, W., Newborg, B. C., Peschel, R. L., and Skyler, J. S.: Treatment of massive obesity with rice/reduction diet program. *Arch. Intern. Med.* 135:1575, 1975.

Krehl, W. A., Lopez-S, A., Good, E. I., and Hodges, R. E.: Some metabolic changes induced by low carbohydrate diets. *Amer. J. Clin. Nutr.* 20:139, 1967.

Law, D. K., Dudrick, S. J., and Abdou, N. I.: The effects of protein calorie malnutrition on immune competence of the surgical patient. *Surg. Gynecol. Obstet.* 139:257, 1974.

Layden, T., Rosenberg, J., Nemchausky, B., Elson, C., and Rosenberg, I.: Reversal of growth arrest in adolescents with Crohn's disease after parenteral administration. *Gastroenterology* 70:1017, 1976.

Leevy, C. M., Cardi, L., Frank, O., Gellene, R., and Baker, H.: Incidence and significance of hypovitaminemia in a randomly selected municipal hospital population. *Amer. J. Clin. Nutr.* 17:259, 1965.

Long, J. M. III, Wilmore, D. W., Mason, A. D., Jr., and Pruitt, B. A., Jr.: Effect of carbohydrate and fat intake on nitrogen excretion during total intravenous feeding. *Ann. Surg.* 185:417, 1977.

Maki, D. G.: Preventing infection in intravenous therapy. *Hospital Practice* 11:95, 1976.

Malt, R. A., and Guggenheim, F. G.: Surgery for obesity (Editorial). *New England J. Med.* 295:43, 1976.

Martorell, R., Yarbrough, C., Lechtig, A., Degaldo, H., and Klein, R. E.: Upper arm anthropometric indicators of nutritional status. *Amer. J. Clin. Nutr.* 29:46, 1976.

McFadyen, B. V., Jr., and Dudrick, S. J.: Inflammatory bowel disease — A new method of treatment. *Acta Chir. Scandinavica, Supplementum 466*:90, 1976.

Meng, H. C.: Fat emulsions in parenteral nutrition. In *Total Parental Nutrition,* Josef E. Fischer (ed.). Boston, Little, Brown and Company, 1976, pp. 305–334.

Meng, H. C., Sandstead, H. H., Walker, P. J., Ackerman, J. R., and Johnson, K. H.: The use of essential amino acids for parenteral nutrition in patients with chronic and acute renal failure. *Acta Chir. Scandinavica, Supplementum 466*:94, 1976.

Munro, H. N.: Biological limiting factors to parenteral amino acid feeding in man. In *Advances in Parenteral Nutrition.* Proceedings of an International Symposium, Bermuda, 16–19 May, 1977, I. D. A. Johnston (ed.). Baltimore, University Park Press, 1978, pp. 107–118.

Munster, A. M.: Post-traumatic immunosuppression is due to activation of suppressor T cells. *Lancet* 1:1329, 1976.

Pareira, M. D.: *Therapeutic Nutrition with Tube Feeding.* Springfield, Ohio, C C Thomas, 1959.

Penick, S. B., Filion, R., Fox, S., and Stunkard, A. J.: Behavior modification in the treatment of obesity. *Psychosom. Med.* 33:49, 1971.

Phillips, K. J.: Nursing care in parenteral nutrition. In *Total Parenteral Nutrition,* Josef E. Fischer (ed.). Boston, Little, Brown and Company, 1976, pp. 101–110.

Ravelli, G-P., Stein, Z. A., and Susser, M. W.: Obesity in young men after famine exposure in utero and early infancy. *New England J. Med.* 295:349, 1976.

Reilly, J., Ryan, J. A., Strole, W., and Fischer, J. E.: Hyperalimentation in inflammatory bowel disease. *Amer. J. Surg.* 131:192, 1976.

Ryan, J. A., Jr.: Complications of total parenteral nutrition. In *Total Parenteral Nutrition,* Josef E. Fischer (ed.). Boston, Little, Brown and Company, 1976, pp. 55–100.

Sanders, R. A., and Sheldon, G. F.: Septic complications of total parenteral nutrition. *Amer. J. Surg.* 132:214, 1976.

Shils, M. E.: A program for total parenteral nutrition at home. *Amer. J. Clin. Nutr.* 28:1429, 1975.

Silvis, S. E., and Paragas, P. V., Jr.: Fatal hyperalimentation syndrome. Animal studies. *J. Lab. Clin. Med.* 78:918, 1971.

Silvis, S. E., and Paragas, P. D., Jr.: Paresthesias, weakness, seizures, and hypophosphatemia in patients receiving hyperalimentation. *Gastroenterology* 62:513, 1972.

Smith, G. S., Smith, J. L., Mameesh, M. S., Simon, J., and Johnson, B. C.: Hypertension and cardiovascular abnormalities in starved–re-fed swine. *J. Nutrition* 82:173, 1964.

Sofio, C., and Nicora, R.: High calorie essential amino acid parenteral therapy in acute renal failure. *Acta Chir. Scandinavica, Supplementum 466*:98, 1976.

Tweedle, D. E. F., Fitzpatrick, G. F., Brennan, M. F., Culebras, J. M., Wolfe, B. M., Ball, M. R., and Moore, F. D.: Intravenous amino acids as the sole nutritional substrate. Utilization and metabolism in fasting normal human subjects. *Ann. Surg.* 186:60, 1977.

Walser, M., Sapir, D. G., and Maddrey, W. C.: The use of alpha-keto analogues of essential amino-acids. In *Total Parenteral Nutrition,* Josef E. Fischer (ed.). Boston, Little, Brown and Company, 1976, pp. 413–430.

Wilmore, D. W., and Pruitt, B. A., Jr.: Parenteral nutrition in burn patients. In *Total Parenteral Nutrition,* Josef E. Fischer (ed.). Boston, Little, Brown and Company, 1976, pp. 231–252.

INDEX

Page numbers in italic type refer to illustrations; those followed by t refer to tables.

Appendix

TABLE 1 FOOD AND NUTRITION BOARD, NATIONAL ACADEMY OF SCIENCES-NATIONAL RESEARCH COUNCIL RECOMMENDED DAILY DIETARY ALLOWANCES,[a] Revised 1979

Designed for the maintenance of good nutrition of practically all healthy people in the U.S.A.

	Age (years)	Weight (kg)	Weight (lbs)	Height (cm)	Height (in)	Protein (g)	Vitamin A (μg R.E.)[b]	Vitamin D (μg)[c]	Vitamin E (mg α T.E.)[d]
Infants	0.0–0.5	6	13	60	24	kg × 2.2	420	10	3
	0.5–1.0	9	20	71	28	kg × 2.0	400	10	4
Children	1–3	13	29	90	35	23	400	10	5
	4–6	20	44	112	44	30	500	10	6
	7–10	28	62	132	52	34	700	10	7
Males	11–14	45	99	157	62	45	1000	10	8
	15–18	66	145	176	69	56	1000	10	10
	19–22	70	154	177	70	56	1000	7.5	10
	23–50	70	154	178	70	56	1000	5	10
	51+	70	154	178	70	56	1000	5	10
Females	11–14	46	101	157	62	46	800	10	8
	15–18	55	120	163	64	46	800	10	8
	19–22	55	120	163	64	44	800	7.5	8
	23–50	55	120	163	64	44	800	5	8
	51+	55	120	163	64	44	800	5	8
Pregnant						+30	+200	+5	+2
Lactating						+20	+400	+5	+3

[a] The allowances are intended to provide for individual variations among most normal persons as they live in the United States under usual environmental stresses. Diets should be based on a variety of common foods in order to provide other nutrients for which human requirements have been less well defined. See text for detailed discussion of allowances and of nutrients not tabulated. See Tables (pp. 5–12) for weights and heights by individual year of age.

[b] Retinol equivalents. 1 Retinol equivalent = 1 μg retinol or 6 μg β carotene. See text for calculation of vitamin A activity of diets as retinol equivalents.

[c] As cholecalciferol, 10 μg cholecalciferol = 400 I.U. vitamin D.

[d] α tocopherol equivalents. 1 mg d-α-tocopherol = 1 α T.E. See text for variation in allowances and calculation of vitamin E activity of the diet as α tocopherol equivalents.

[e] 1 NE (niacin equivalent) is equal to 1 mg of niacin or 60 mg of dietary tryptophan.

Appendix

TABLE 1 FOOD AND NUTRITION BOARD, NATIONAL ACADEMY OF SCIENCES-NATIONAL RESEARCH COUNCIL RECOMMENDED DAILY DIETARY ALLOWANCES,[a] Revised 1979

Designed for the maintenance of good nutrition of practically all healthy people in the U.S.A. (*Continued*)

	WATER-SOLUBLE VITAMINS						MINERALS					
Vitamin C (mg)	Thiamin (mg)	Riboflavin (mg)	Niacin (mg N.E.)[e]	Vitamin B_6 (mg)	Folacin[f] (µg)	Vitamin B_{12} (µg)	Calcium (mg)	Phosphorus (mg)	Magnesium (mg)	Iron (mg)	Zinc (mg)	Iodine (µg)
35	0.3	0.4	6	0.3	30	0.5[g]	360	240	50	10	3	40
35	0.5	0.6	8	0.6	45	1.5	540	360	70	15	5	50
45	0.7	0.8	9	0.9	100	2.0	800	800	150	15	10	70
45	0.9	1.0	11	1.3	200	2.5	800	800	200	10	10	90
45	1.2	1.4	16	1.6	300	3.0	800	800	250	10	10	120
50	1.4	1.6	18	1.8	400	3.0	1200	1200	350	18	15	150
60	1.4	1.7	18	2.0	400	3.0	1200	1200	400	18	15	150
60	1.5	1.7	19	2.2	400	3.0	800	800	350	10	15	150
60	1.4	1.6	18	2.2	400	3.0	800	800	350	10	15	150
60	1.2	1.4	16	2.2	400	3.0	800	800	350	10	15	150
50	1.1	1.3	15	1.8	400	3.0	1200	1200	300	18	15	150
60	1.1	1.3	14	2.0	400	3.0	1200	1200	300	18	15	150
60	1.1	1.3	14	2.0	400	3.0	800	800	300	18	15	150
60	1.0	1.2	13	2.0	400	3.0	800	800	300	18	15	150
60	1.0	1.2	13	2.0	400	3.0	800	800	300	10	15	150
+20	+0.4	+0.3	+2	+0.6	+400	+1.0	+400	+400	+150	[h]	+ 5	+25
+40	+0.5	+0.5	+5	+0.5	+100	+1.0	+400	+400	+150	[h]	+10	+50

[f] The folacin allowances refer to dietary sources as determined by *Lactobacillus casei* assay after treatment with enzymes ("conjugases") to make polyglutaryl forms of the vitamin available to the test organism.

[g] The RDA for vitamin B_{12} in infants is based on average concentration of the vitamin in human milk. The allowances after weaning are based on energy intake (as recommended by the American Academy of Pediatrics) and consideration of other factors such as intestinal absorption; see text.

[h] The increased requirement during pregnancy cannot be met by the iron content of habitual American diets nor by the existing iron stores of many women; therefore the use of 30–60 mg of supplemental iron is recommended. Iron needs during lactation are not substantially different from those of nonpregnant women, but continued supplementation of the mother for 2–3 months after parturition is advisable in order to replenish stores depleted by pregnancy.

Appendix

TABLE 2 ESTIMATED SAFE AND ADEQUATE DAILY DIETARY INTAKES OF ADDITIONAL SELECTED VITAMINS AND MINERALS[a]

	Age (years)	Vitamins			Trace Elements[b]						Electrolytes		
		Vitamin K (µg)	Biotin (µg)	Pantothenic Acid (mg)	Copper (mg)	Manganese (mg)	Fluoride (mg)	Chromium (mg)	Selenium (mg)	Molybdenum (mg)	Sodium (mg)	Potassium (mg)	Chloride (mg)
Infants	0–0.5	12	35	2	0.5–0.7	0.5–0.7	0.1–0.5	0.01–0.04	0.01–0.04	0.03–0.06	115–350	350–925	275–700
	0.5–1	10–20	50	3	0.7–1.0	0.7–1.0	0.2–1.0	0.02–0.06	0.02–0.06	0.04–0.08	250–750	425–1275	400–1200
Children and Adolescents	1–3	15–30	65	3	1.0–1.5	1.0–1.5	0.5–1.5	0.02–0.08	0.02–0.08	0.05–0.1	325–975	550–1650	500–1500
	4–6	20–40	85	3–4	1.5–2.0	1.5–2.0	1.0–2.5	0.03–0.12	0.03–0.12	0.06–0.15	450–1350	775–2325	700–2100
	7–10	30–60	120	4–5	2.0–2.5	2.0–3.0	1.5–2.5	0.05–0.2	0.05–0.2	0.1–0.3	600–1800	1000–3000	925–2775
	11+	50–100	100–200	4–7	2.0–3.0	2.5–5.0	1.5–2.5	0.05–0.2	0.05–0.2	0.15–0.5	900–2700	1525–4575	1400–4200
Adults		70–140	100–200	4–7	2.0–3.0	2.5–5.0	1.5–4.0	0.05–0.2	0.05–0.2	0.15–0.5	1100–3300	1875–5625	1700–5100

[a] Because there is less information on which to base allowances, these figures are not given in the main table of the RDA and are provided here in the form of ranges of recommended intakes.

[b] Since the toxic levels for many trace elements may be only several times usual intakes, the upper levels for the trace elements given in this table should not be habitually exceeded.

From: Recommended Dietary Allowances, Revised 1979. Food and Nutrition Board National Academy of Sciences-National Research Council, Washington, D.C.